P. G. Lankisch P. A. Banks **Pancreatitis**

Springer

Berlin
Heidelberg
New York
Barcelona
Budapest
Hong Kong
London
Milan
Paris
Santa Clara
Singapore
Tokyo

P. G. Lankisch   P. A. Banks

Pancreatitis

With 99 Figures and 61 Tables

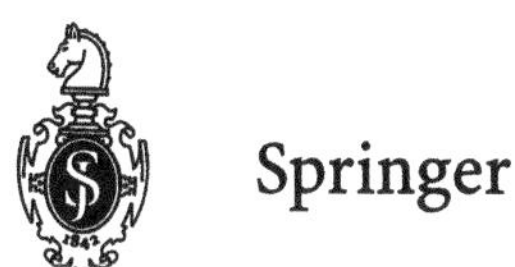

Springer

Prof. Dr. P. G. Lankisch
Städtisches Krankenhaus
Medizinische Klinik
Bögelstraße 1, D-21339 Lüneburg, Germany

Peter A. Banks, M.D.
Associate Professor of Medicine, Harvard Medical School
Director, Clinical Gastroenterology Service
Gastroenterology Division
Brigham and Women's Hospital
75 Francis Street, Boston MA 02115, USA

ISBN-13:978-3-642-80322-2   e-ISBN-13:978-3-642-80320-8
DOI: 10.1007/978-3-642-80320-8

Library of Congress Cataloging-in-Publication Data applied for

Die Deutsche Bibliothek – CIP-Einheitsaufnahme
Lankisch, Paul Georg:
Pancreatitis / P. G. Lankisch ; P. A. Banks. – Berlin ; Heidelberg ; New York ; Barcelona ; Budapest ;
Hong Kong ; London ; Milan ; Paris ; Santa Clara ; Singapore ; Tokyo : Springer, 1998
  ISBN-13:978-3-642-80322-2

Production: PRO EDIT GmbH, D-69126 Heidelberg
Cover design: Design & Production, D-69121 Heidelberg
Typesetting: Zechnersche Buchdruckerei, D-67330 Speyer

SPIN: 10507818   23/3134-5 4 3 2 1 0   Printed on acid-free paper

Preface

As we began to plan this book about 10 years ago, we wanted to write a practical book for medical students, doctors in training, internists, gastroenterologists, and surgeons faced with everyday clinical problems in the care of patients with acute and chronic pancreatitis. Now, 10 years later, our book has become much more than what we had originally intended, with so many new findings that have expanded our knowledge of pancreatic diseases, not to mention new imaging procedures and controlled studies on the effectiveness of various therapies. Consequently, we decided to include:

- The state-of-the-art on diagnosis and therapy in inflammatory pancreatic diseases
- Recommendations for diagnosis and therapy based on the published results from experienced clinicians. In the many areas still untested we have relied on the decades of experience of the two authors on both sides of the Atlantic
- A discussion of unanswered questions for future research by physicians interested in pancreatitis who can draw upon our bibliography of almost 1900 references complete through 1996.

We also wanted to demonstrate with this work that two authors from two continents can come to common conclusions that can help physicians and students in their everyday clinical work and their clinical research.

It is with deep gratitude that we acknowledge the assistance of Mrs. Gisela Ropte for years of patient cooperation, great precision, and initiative, as well as that of Dr. Dr. Chris Jones for fine-tuned editing and translations on the German side of the Atlantic.

We would also like to thank Ms. Margie Orifice on the American side of the Atlantic for her dedicated assistance in the preparation of the manuscript.

Last, but certainly not least, we are most grateful to our families for their steady encouragement and loving support.

Summer 1997

Paul G. Lankisch
Peter A. Banks

Table of Contents

1 General Considerations: Embryology

1.1
Normal Development

The pancreas is formed by two separate anlagen, a large dorsal and a smaller ventral endodermal bud. The development of the gland starts at about the 4th week of gestation when the organ first appears as two diverticula arising from the primitive foregut just distal to the stomach [46]. The dorsal bud eventually forms the tail, body and part of the head of the pancreas, the ventral anlage contributes most to the head of the pancreas. The ventral anlage is initially a paired structure. The left part atrophies, the right component is gradually pulled posteriorly as the duodenum rotates (Fig. 1.1) [64]. At about the end of the 6th week of gestation, the ventral primordium fuses with the dorsal part to form the remainder of the head of the pancreas and the uncinate process.

Each anlage possesses its own duct system. The duct of the ventral part arises from the common bile duct and maintains its association with the biliary system by opening into a common duodenal papilla, the ampulla of Vater. During fusion of both anlagen, the ventral and the dorsal duct form the main pancreatic duct, the duct of Wirsung. The duct of the dorsal bud arises from the duodenal wall, undergoes varying degrees of atrophy to remain as the accessory duct of Santorini (Fig. 1.1) [64].

1.2
Congenital Abnormalities

Congenital abnormalities of the pancreas are related to the two critical events during embryological development: rotation and fusion. Congenital abnormalities are uncommon, mostly asymptomatic, and discovered incidentally during surgery, or endoscopy, or at autopsy. Occasionally they produce symptoms and require therapy [34].

Table 1.1. Congenital abnormalities of the pancreas

- Aplasia
- Hypoplasia
- Dysplasia
- Pancreas divisum
- Heterotopic pancreas
- Annular pancreas
- Congenital cyst(s)

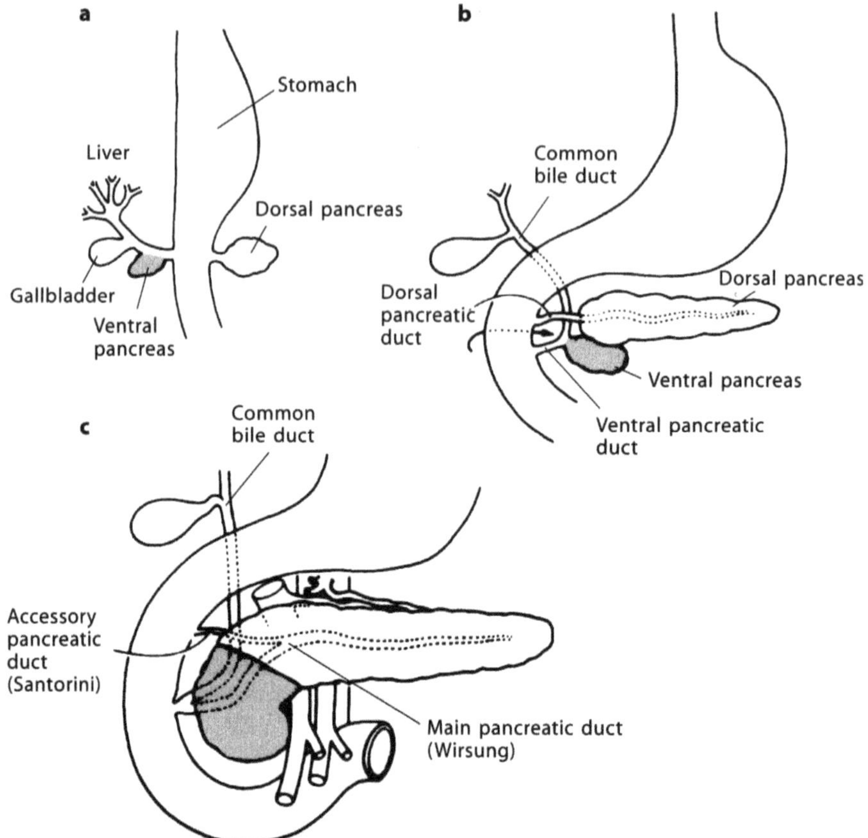

Fig. 1.1 a–c. Embryonic development of the pancreas. **a** Formation of dorsal and ventral pancreatic primordia. **b** Rotation of the ventral pancreas. **c** Fusion of the primordia to form adult pancreas. (From [64] with permission)

Those which are associated with acute and chronic pancreatitis or exocrine pancreatic insufficiency, or which are suspected to be associated with certain symptoms, are reported briefly in this chapter (Table 1.1).

1.2.1
Aplasia, Hypoplasia, and Dysplasia

1.2.1.1
Definition

Complete and partial agenesis of the pancreas results from a primary defect in early organic embryogenesis. Complete agenesis is probably incompatible with life. There is only one case of long-term survival which has been described as *functional pancreatic agenesis*, because of the lack of postmortem confirmation of the anatomic defect [36].

In partial agenesis, the pancreas is histologically normal, but defective in size and shape owing to failure of development of structures of the pancreatic primordia, usually involving the dorsal bud.

In hypo- and dysplasia of the pancreas, the organ is of normal size and shape, but defective in cellular differentiation. Hypoplasia is characterized by replacement of the normal epithelial structures with fatty tissue and reduction of the number of ducts and their terminal differentiation. In dysplasia, the parenchyma is disorganized, with dilated ducts surrounded by a fibromuscular layer.

There are only a few reports on these congenital abnormalities [7], probably due to the fact that these patients have enough exocrine and endocrine tissue left for a normal life.

Combinations with other congenital defects are possible [80].

1.2.1.2
Clinical Presentation

A recent report summarizes 11 cases of complete agenesis of the dorsal pancreas in adults, most of them having presented with symptoms of diabetes mellitus and some with abdominal pain [60]. The latter had been attributed to diabetic neuropathy, but pain relief after sphincteroplasty in one case suggests that the sphincter of Oddi is involved in this symptom [73].

Familial occurrence of agenesis of the dorsal pancreas has been reported suggesting that hereditary mechanisms may play a role [78].

1.2.1.3
Diagnosis

The diagnosis is made by endoscopic retrograde cholangiopancreatography (ERCP) and computed tomography (CT). In agenesis of the dorsal pancreas, the minor papilla is absent, and the pancreatogram shows a short ventral duct with complete absence of the accessory and dorsal ducts.

In contrast, the dorsal pancreatic duct can be demonstrated by cannulation of the minor papilla in pancreas divisum, while abrupt obstruction, tapering, or stenosis of the pancreatic duct can be found in tumor.

An association between partial agenesis and recurrent or chronic pancreatitis has been discussed [9, 25].

1.2.1.4
Treatment

In all abnormalities described, exocrine pancreatic insufficiency requires intensive treatment to ensure satisfactory growth [34].

1.2.2
Pancreas Divisum

1.2.2.1
Definition

Pancreas divisum results from incomplete fusion of the dorsal and ventral ductal systems (Fig. 1.2). It is the most common congenital abnormality of the pancreas and has been reported in 3.4%–12.9% of patients undergoing ERCP [5, 10, 12, 17, 29, 51, 56, 59]. As these patients represent a selective group, the true incidence in the population not undergoing any upper abdominal investigation is unknown.

1.2.2.2
Pathogenetic Implications

Whether pancreas divisum is a cause of acute and/or chronic pancreatitis, is controversial [5, 10, 12, 13, 17, 18, 29, 31, 32, 51, 59, 71]. Those in favor of an association have put forward the hypothesis that the accessory papilla and Santorini's duct are too small to accept total pancreatic secretion, resulting eventually in obstructive pain and pancreatitis (Fig. 1.2). Some reports have also shown a significantly higher incidence of pancreas divisum in patients with documented pancreatitis as compared to those with biliary tract disease [54], and very high incidence rates of this duct abnormality in patients with acute idiopathic pancreatitis: Cotton [12] 25.6%, Bernard [5] 50%.

An association with chronic pancreatitis appears in Fig. 1.3 [6].

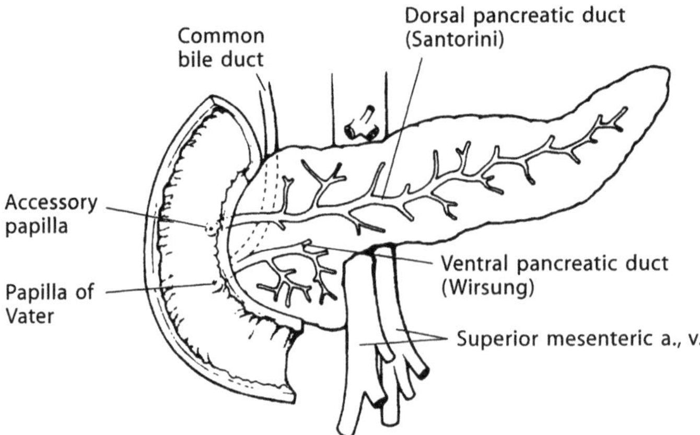

Fig. 1.2. Pancreas divisum with nonunion of the dorsal and ventral pancreatic ducts. The ventral duct (Wirsung's duct) drains the smaller part of the gland with the common bile duct at the papilla of Vater, i.e., via the bigger papilla. The dorsal duct (Santorini's duct) drains at the smaller minor papilla approximately 2 cm anterosuperior to the papilla of Vater. (From [6] with permission)

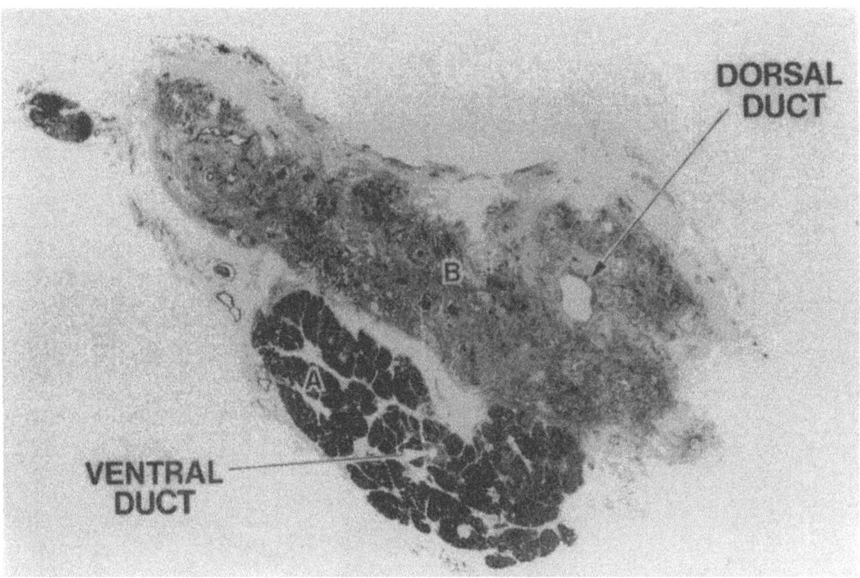

Fig. 1.3. Cross section of the head of the pancreas obtained after pancreaticoduodenectomy. The ventral pancreas has normal parenchyma with a normal-sized duct, the dorsal gland demonstrates chronic pancreatitis with atrophy, fibrosis, and a grossly dilated duct. (From [6] with permission)

1.2.2.3
Clinical Presentation

Those in favor of an association with pancreatitis report on patients with pancreas divisum admitted with typical abdominal pain and raised serum amylase levels. When compared with patients with pancreatitis and normal duct development, patients with pancreatitis associated with pancreas divisum tended to be younger and to have a clinical pattern of recurrent acute attacks of pancreatitis [54].

1.2.2.4
Diagnosis

The diagnosis is best made by ERCP. After intubation of the major duodenal papilla, injection of the contrast medium fills only a small portion of the pancreatic duct in the head of the pancreas. Careful inspection of the ductal morphology is required to distinguish pancreas divisum from duct obstruction due to benign or malignant obstruction of the main duct [43, 74]. Figure 1.4 represents a female patient, in whom this differentiation was difficult.

With pancreas divisum, a short, small-caliber duct is opacified, smaller than would be expected for the normal pancreatic duct in the head of the pancreas. The termination of the column of contrast medium is by arborization rather than obstruction. It is then necessary to independently cannulate the minor duodenal papilla to opacify the remaining larger portion of the pancreatic duct system.

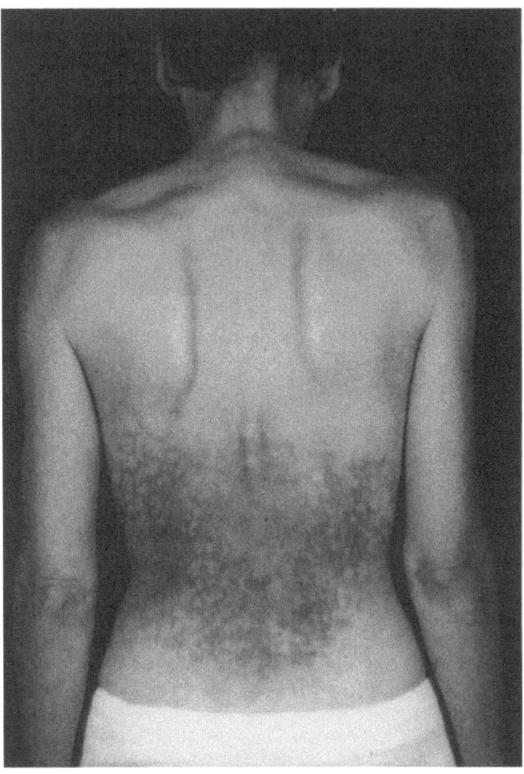

Fig. 1.4. 39-year-old patient with abdominal pain radiating into the back. An ERCP showed a short duct wrongly interpreted as the ventral part of a pancreas divisum. Only when an erythema ab igne occurred, due to the use of hot waterbottles to overcome severe pain, was the patient re-evaluated. The ERCP finding then correctly attributed to an inoperable pancreatic carcinoma. (From [43] with permission)

Further diagnostic procedures include manometric measurement of intraductal pressure via the minor papilla and measurement of the diameter of the dorsal duct following secretin stimulation under ultrasound or CT control.

Intraductal pressure was largely increased versus controls in a small series of patients with pancreas divisum and abdominal pain [66]. Functional obstruction of the dorsal pancreatic duct was diagnosed by ultrasound demonstration of ductal dilatation during secretin provocation [76]. Reliability and significance, however, remain controversial [47]. When secretin provocation had been performed under CT control, dilatation of the dorsal duct in patients with unexplained upper abdominal pain had revealed the presence of pancreas divisum without morphologic evidence of pancreatitis [45].

1.2.2.5
Treatment

The management of patients with pancreas divisum and symptoms of recurrent pancreatitis is controversial. Patients with mild to moderate symptoms should be medically treated. For those with severe recurrent pain, a number of procedures including balloon dilatation, papillotomy, and stenting, as well as surgical procedures such as ductal drainage or distal pancreatic resection, with or without distal drainage, have been attempted with varying success [40, 54, 57, 58, 63, 77]. Surgical treatment has been recommended once chronic pancreatitis is established [75].

In symptomatic patients with pancreas divisum, we recommend a check for gallstones and alcohol abuse and, in their presence, suggest cholecystectomy and alcohol abstinence, but otherwise to maintain medical treatment as long as possible. We have tried pancreatic enzymes for pain relief (see Sect. 19.1) but have been disappointed with results. Experience with endoscopically placed pancreatic stents and/or dilatation of the minor papilla has suggested some benefit, but there is a paucity of randomized prospective well-controlled studies. Accordingly, the role of endoscopic stenting remains unproven. In severe cases, we recommend surgical treatment as the last result, either a sphincteroplasty of the accessory papilla or ductal drainage in patients with a dilated dorsal duct.

1.2.3
Heterotopic Pancreas

1.2.3.1
Definition

Heterotopic, ectopic, aberrant, or accessory pancreas is defined as the presence of pancreatic tissue that lacks anatomic and vascular continuity with the main body of the pancreas.

Pathogenetic theories include in situ errors of pluripotent endodermal stem cell differentiation, multiple ventral pancreatic buds that fail to atrophy, adhesion of embryonic pancreatic cells to neighboring structures during migration of the ventral anlage, and budding of pancreatic tissue from the embryonic anlagen or pancreatic ducts with separation and attachment to the gut wall during elongation of the intestinal tract [34].

1.2.3.2
Clinical Presentation

In most cases patients with heterotopic pancreas are asymptomatic [42]. Location in almost 70% of the cases is within the gastrointestinal tract [16, 42, 55], and in the remaining 30% elsewhere in the abdomen (liver, gallbladder), or even extraabdominally, including the lung and the umbilicus [34].

Ectopic tissue may cause a number of secondary complications such as biliary obstruction, cholecystitis, pyloric obstruction, intussusception, intestinal obstruction and even jejunal atresia [34].

Acute pancreatitis in ectopic pancreas has been described [4, 28], and even calcification of ectopic pancreas similar to that in chronic pancreatitis has been reported [24]. Furthermore, malignant degeneration of ectopic pancreas has been found [30, 39, 53].

1.2.3.3
Diagnosis

A definitive diagnosis requires histological confirmation, but most cases seen by upper gastrointestinal endoscopy do not require surgery. Usually, a well-defined dome-shaped structure with central umbilication is found, usually <1 cm in diameter on the greater curve of the antrum or in a prepyloric position. The nodule may resemble an adenomatous polyp, leiomyoma, lymphoma, carcinoma, or peptic ulcer, all of which require histological evaluation in order to be ruled out. Endoscopic biopsy of the nodule often yields normal gastric mucosa because the pancreatic tissue is submucosal or subserosal in location.

1.2.3.4
Treatment

Management of heterotopic pancreas is controversial. Local excision may be very helpful in symptomatic patients [15], but it may be very difficult to define whether abdominal symptoms are due to heterotopic pancreas [19]. In an effort to refine indications for surgery, it has been suggested that clinically significant lesions tend to be greater than 1.5 cm in diameter and are adjacent to, or directly involve, the mucosa [2].

Incidental lesions should be left alone.

1.2.4
Annular Pancreas

1.2.4.1
Definition

An annular pancreas is a thin, flat band of normal pancreatic tissue surrounding the second part of the duodenum and continuing into the head of the pancreas on either side (Fig. 1.5). The band may be wholly or partially free from the duodenum, or the pancreatic tissue may penetrate the duodenal muscularis. The ring of pancreatic tissue contains a large duct that usually enters the duodenum independently. Duodenal stenosis at the level of the pancreatic ring is usual [64].

Currently, three main theories for its development are as follows:
- Hypertrophy of both anlagen resulting in complete constriction around the duodenum
- Persistence and enlargement of the left bud of the paired ventral primordium
- Fixation of the tip of the ventral bud prior to rotation resulting in persistence of the ventral bud completely around the duodenum. This theory would account for the most common variants of annular pancreas [34]

Annular pancreas is an uncommon congenital disease, which, however, has been more frequently reported during the last decades. A Mayo Clinic review revealed 15 cases seen over a 20-year period [41].

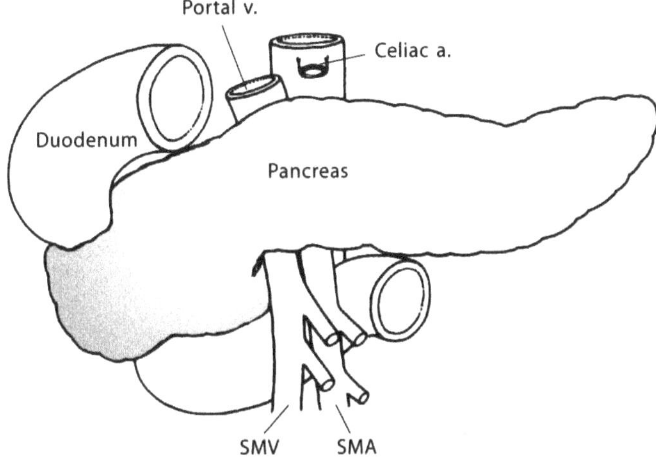

Fig. 1.5. Annular pancreas. *SMV* = superior mesenteric v., *SMA* = superior mesenteric a. (From [64] with permission)

The coexistence of annular pancreas and pancreas divisum (annular pancreas divisum) has been described in 5 cases [21], and of annular pancreas and ectopic pancreas in another case [52].

1.2.4.2
Clinical Presentation

Onset of symptoms may occur at any stage from birth to adulthood. In a review of 281 cases, 50% presented in the pediatric age group, and of these, 86% in the neonatal period [41].

In the newborn period, annular pancreas may be associated with polyhydramnios and typically presents with failure to tolerate feedings, persistent bile-stained vomiting, and upper abdominal distension. A number of other abnormalities may be associated, such as intestinal malrotation, cardiac defects, Meckel's diverticulum, imperforate anus, duodenal bands, spinal defects, and cryptorchidism. A high incidence of Down's syndrome has been reported [41].

In adults, symptoms include upper abdominal or epigastric pain, nausea and vomiting, postprandial fullness and bloating, weight loss and upper gastrointestinal hemorrhage. Peptic ulcer may occur in about half of the patients. Astonishingly, annular pancreas becomes first manifest in the aged in almost half of the patients (Fig. 1.6 a, b) [3, 8, 14, 20, 23, 26, 27, 37, 41, 44, 61, 67, 70, 72].

Both acute [1] and chronic pancreatitis [20, 26, 37], and also an association with pancreatic carcinoma [79], have been reported. Annular pancreas may cause symptoms of gastric outlet obstruction and recurrent pancreatitis [21].

Several reports of annular pancreas in families have suggested an autosomal-dominant transmission of this congenital abnormality [11, 33, 38, 48].

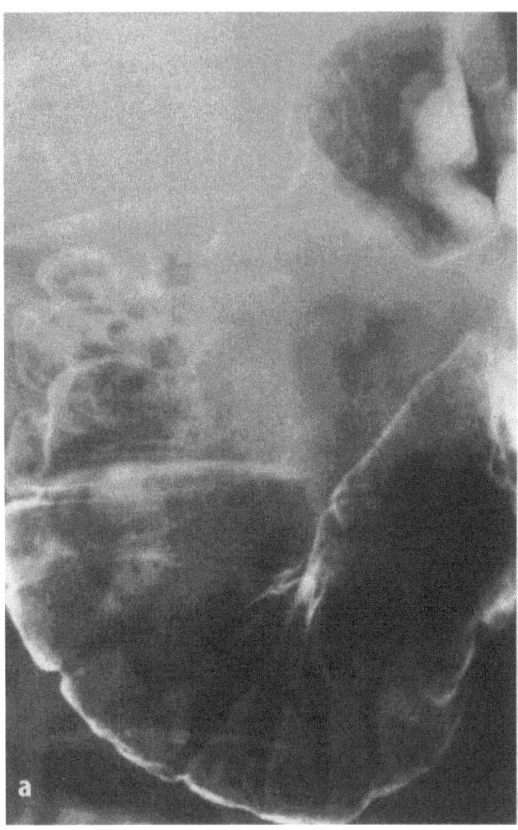

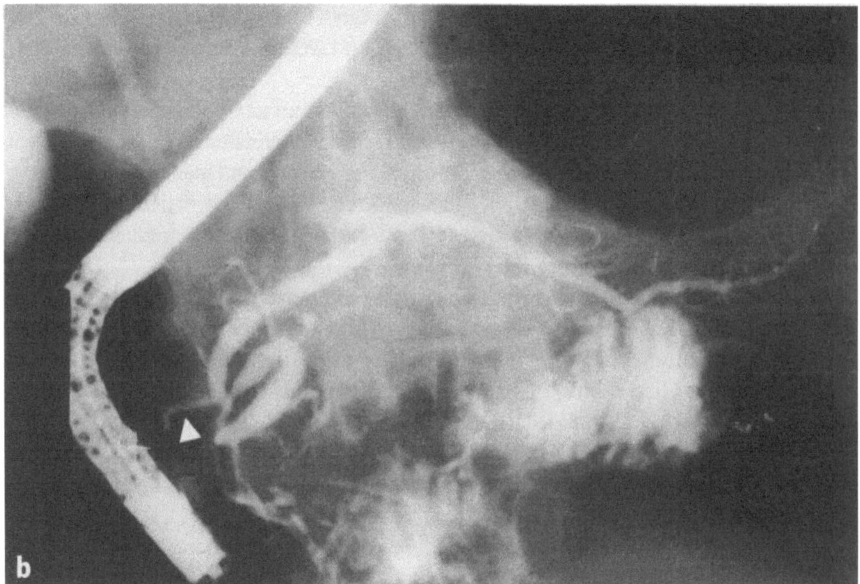

Fig. 1.6 a, b. a 66-year-old patient with abdominal pain occurring postprandially after 2–3 h for about 5 months. Gastroscopy and hypotonic duodenography showed a stenosis of the second portion of the duodenum. Intraoperatively, an annular pancreas was found to cause the stenosis. **b** 60-year-old female patient with unexplained abdominal pain. The ERCP showed an annular pancreas (arrow-head showing the duct beginning to encircle the duodenum)

1.2.4.3
Diagnosis

In neonates, plain abdominal X-ray films in the erect and supine position will show the classic *double bubble*, which is diagnostic of duodenal obstruction.

In older children and adults, plain abdominal X-ray is not helpful. Upper gastrointestinal studies will show the classic radiographic findings of an annular filling defect across the second portion of the duodenum, symmetrical dilatation of the proximal duodenum, and reverse peristalsis of the duodenal segment proximal to the annulus [50]. Gastroscopy and CT scan are helpful in diagnosing the stenosis of the descending duodenum, ERCP in demonstrating the characteristic, duodenum-encircling duct system. Interestingly, about one-third of the patients with annular pancreas also have pancreas divisum [44].

1.2.4.4
Treatment

Treatment of symptomatic annular pancreas is surgical, mostly in the form of a duodenojejunostomy or duodenoduodenostomy.

1.2.5
Congenital Cyst(s)

1.2.5.1
Definition

Congenital cysts may be solitary or multiple. True congenital cysts are distinctly unusual, with only 13 cases documented in infants and young children [62]. True cysts are lined by an epithelial layer that is backed by pancreatic acini. In contrast, the wall of a pancreatic pseudocyst is fibrotic, with granulation tissue and no epithelial lining. Multiple congenital cysts are also uncommon, are usually associated with other abnormalities, and have been described as *von Hippel-Lindau syndrome* (autosomal-dominant inherited syndrome with polytopic angioblastic abnormalities of the retina and the cerebellum and cysts in a number of organs) and *Meckel-Gruber's syndrome* (fatal autosomal-recessive inherited syndrome with encephalocele, polycystic kidneys, and abnormalities including pancreatic cysts). They are usually associated with multiple cysts of the kidneys, liver, lungs, or central nervous system, all of which are thought to be due to a common pathogenetic mechanism [22, 35, 68]. Recently, the first case of von Hippel-Lindau disease complicated by acute pancreatitis and Evan's syndrome has been described [69].

1.2.5.2
Clinical Presentation

Solitary congenital cysts are generally asymptomatic, but may become symptomatic secondary to abdominal distension or pressure effects on adjacent viscera [49, 65]. Recently, an adolescent with a congenital pancreatic cyst presenting as acute pancreatitis has been reported [62].

In multiple congenital cysts, associated other congenital abnormalities may lead to symptoms [22].

1.2.5.3
Diagnosis

The diagnosis is made by ultrasound and/or CT.

1.2.5.4
Treatment

Management of symptomatic solitary cysts is surgical, usually resection. In the case of multiple cysts, treatment is often unnecessary since the severity of associated abnormalities is often incompatible with life.

References

1. Alexander HC (1970) Annular pancreas in the adult. Am J Surg 119:702–704
2. Armstrong CP, King PM, Dixon JM, Macleod IB (1981) The clinical significance of heterotopic pancreas in the gastrointestinal tract. Br J Surg 68:384–387
3. Beachley MC, Lankau CA Jr (1973) Symptomatic adult annular pancreas. Am J Dig Dis 18:513–516
4. Benbow EW (1988) Simultaneous acute inflammation in entopic and ectopic pancreas. J Clin Pathol 41:430–434
5. Bernard JP, Sahel J, Giovannini M, Sarles H (1990) Pancreas divisum is a probable cause of acute pancreatitis: a report of 137 cases. Pancreas 5:248–254
6. Blair III AJ, Russell CG, Cotton PB (1984) Resection for pancreatitis in patients with pancreas divisum. Ann Surg 200:590–594
7. Bodian M, Sheldon W, Lightwood R (1964) Congenital hypoplasia of the exocrine pancreas. Acta Paediatr 53:282–293
8. Bozkurt T, Butsch B, Lederer PC, Lux G (1990) Pancreas anulare – Eine kongenitale Anomalie der Bauchspeicheldrüse. Z Gastroenterol 28:392–395
9. Bretagne J-F, Darnault P, Raoul JL, Gandon Y, Gosselin M, Cousin P, Gastard J (1987) Calcifying pancreatitis of a congenital short pancreas: a case report with successful endoscopic papillotomy. Am J Gastroenterol 82:1314–1317
10. Bühler H, Seefeld U, Deyhle P, Largiadèr F, Ammann R (1983) Klinische Bedeutung des Pancreas divisum. Schweiz Med Wochenschr 113:320–324
11. Claviez A, Heger S, Bohring A (1995) Annular pancreas in two sisters. Am J Med Genet 58:384
12. Cotton PB (1980) Congenital anomaly of pancreas divisum can cause obstructive pain and pancreatitis. Gut 21:105–114
13. Cotton PB, Kizu M (1977) Malfusion of dorsal and ventral pancreas; a cause of pancreatitis? Gut 18:A400 (abstr)
14. Dahm K, Grossner D, Knipper A, Soehendra N, Vogel H (1978) Zur Erkennung und Behandlung des Pancreas anulare. Zentralbl Chir 103:1349–1356
15. De Friend DJ, Saa-Gandi FW, Humphrey CS, Foster DN (1991) Symptomatic pancreatic heterotopia treated by local excision. Gut 32:332–333
16. DeBord JR, Majarakis JD, Nyhus LM (1981) An unusual case of heterotopic pancreas of the stomach. Am J Surg 141:269–273
17. Delhaye M, Engelholm L, Cremer M (1985) Pancreas divisum: congenital anatomic variant or anomaly? Contribution of endoscopic retrograde dorsal pancreatography. Gastroenterology 89:951–958
18. Delhaye M, Engelholm L, Cremer M (1988) Pancreas divisum: controversial clinical significance. Dig Dis 6:30–39
19. Dolan RV, ReMine WH, Dockerty MB (1974) The fate of heterotopic pancreatic tissue. A study of 212 cases. Arch Surg 109:762–765
20. Dowsett JF, Rode J, Russell RCG (1989) Annular pancreas: a clinical, endoscopic, and immunohistochemical study. Gut 30:130–135

21. England RE, Newcomer MK, Leung JWC, Cotton PB (1995) Case report: Annular pancreas divisum – a report of two cases and review of the literature. Br J Radiol 68:324–328
22. Fishman RS, Bartholomew LG (1979) Severe pancreatic involvement in three generations in von Hippel-Lindau disease. Mayo Clin Proc 54:329–331
23. Friedman AI (1957) Annular pancreas: a congenital abnormality manifest in the aged. Gastroenterology 32:1172–1177
24. Gamroth A, Fenn K (1989) Verkalkende Pankreasheterotopie im Bereich der kleinen Kurvatur des Magenkorpus. Fortschr Röntgenstr 150:738–739
25. Gilinsky NH, Del Favero G, Cotton PB, Lees WR (1985) Congenital short pancreas: a report of two cases. Gut 26:304–310
26. Gilinsky NH, Lewis JW, Flueck JA, Fried AM (1987) Annular pancreas associated with diffuse chronic pancreatitis. Am J Gastroenterol 82:681–684
27. Glazer GM, Margulis AR (1979) Annular pancreas: etiology and diagnosis using endoscopic retrograde cholangiopancreatography. Radiology 133:303–306
28. Green PHR, Barratt PJ, Percy JP, Cumberland VH, Middleton WRJ (1977) Acute pancreatitis occurring in gastric aberrant pancreatic tissue. Am J Dig Dis 22:734–740
29. Gregg JA (1977) Pancreas divisum: its association with pancreatitis. Am J Surg 134:539–543
30. Guillou L, Nordback P, Gerber C, Schneider RP (1994) Ductal adenocarcinoma arising in a heterotopic pancreas situated in a hiatal hernia. Arch Pathol Lab Med 118:568–571
31. Hayakawa T, Kondo T, Shibata T, Sugimoto Y, Kitagawa M, Suzuki T, Ogawa Y, Kato K, Katada N, Sano H (1989) Pancreas divisum. A predisposing factor to pancreatitis? Int J Pancreatol 5:317–326
32. Heiss FW, Shea JA (1978) Association of pancreatitis and variant ductal anatomy. Dominant drainage of the duct of Santorini. Am J Gastroenterol 70:158–162
33. Hendricks SK, Sybert VP (1991) Association of annular pancreas and duodenal obstruction – evidence for Mendelian inheritance? Clin Genet 39:383–385
34. Hill ID, Lebenthal E (1993) Congenital abnormalities of the exocrine pancreas. In: Go VLW, DiMagno EP, Gardner JD, Lebenthal E, Reber HA, Scheele GA (eds) The Pancreas: Biology, Pathobiology, and Disease, 2nd edn. Raven Press, New York, pp 1029–1040
35. Hough DM, Stephens DH, Johnson CD, Binkovitz LA (1994) Pancreatic lesions in von Hippel-Lindau disease: prevalence, clinical significance, and CT findings. Am J Roentgenol 162:1091–1094
36. Howard CP, Go VLW, Infante AJ, Perrault J, Gerich JE, Haymond MW (1980) Long-term survival in a case of functional pancreatic agenesis. J Pediatr 97:786–789
37. Itoh Y, Hada T, Terano A, Itai Y, Harada T (1989) Pancreatitis in the annulus of annular pancreas demonstrated by the combined use of computed tomography and endoscopic retrograde cholangiopancreatography. Am J Gastroenterol 84:961–964
38. Jackson LG, Apostolides P (1978) Autosomal dominant inheritance of annular pancreas. Am J Med Genet 1:319–321
39. Jeng K-S, Yang K-C, Kuo SHF (1991) Malignant degeneration of heterotopic pancreas. Gastrointest Endosc 37:196–198
40. Keith RG, Shapero TF, Saibil FG, Moore TL (1989) Dorsal duct sphincterotomy is effective long-term treatment of acute pancreatitis associated with pancreas divisum. Surgery 106:660–667
41. Kiernan PD, ReMine SG, Kiernan PC, ReMine WH (1980) Annular pancreas. Mayo Clinic experience from 1957 to 1976 with review of the literature. Arch Surg 115:46–50
42. Lai ECS, Tompkins RK (1986) Heterotopic pancreas. Review of a 26 year experience. Am J Surg 151:697–700
43. Lankisch PG, Creutzfeldt W (1986) Erythema ab igne (Livedo reticularis e calore): ein Hautzeichen für chronische Pankreaserkrankungen. Z Gastroenterol 24:119–120
44. Lehman GA, O'Connor KW (1985) Coexistence of annular pancreas and pancreas divisum – ERCP diagnosis. Gastrointest Endosc 31:25–28
45. Lindström E, Ihse I (1990) Dynamic CT scanning of pancreatic duct after secretin provocation in pancreas divisum. Dig Dis Sci 35:1371–1376
46. Liu HM, Potter EL (1962) Development of the human pancreas. Arch Pathol 74:439–452
47. Lowes JR, Lees WR, Cotton PB (1989) Pancreatic duct dilatation after secretin stimulation in patients with pancreas divisum. Pancreas 4:371–374
48. MacFadyen UM, Young ID (1987) Letter to the Editor: Annular pancreas in mother and son. Am J Med Genet 27:987–988
49. Mao C, Greenwood S, Wagner S, Howard JM (1992) Solitary true cyst of the pancreas in an adult. Int J Pancreatol 12:181–186
50. Mast WH, Telle MLD, Turek RO (1957) Annular pancreas. Errors in diagnosis and treatment of eight cases. Am J Surg 94:80–89
51. Mitchell CJ, Lintott DJ, Ruddell WSJ, Losowsky MS, Axon ATR (1979) Clinical relevance of an unfused pancreatic duct system. Gut 20:1066–1071

52. Nakajima H, Kambayashi M, Okubo H, Masuko Y, Yamada S, Hata Y, Oku T, Takahashi T, Takahashi T (1995) Annular pancreas accompanied by an ectopic pancreas in the adult: a case report. Endoscopy 27:713
53. Persson GE, Boiesen PT (1988) Cancer of aberrant pancreas in jejunum. Acta Chir Scand 154: 599–601
54. Richter JM, Schapiro RH, Mulley AG, Warshaw AL (1981) Association of pancreas divisum and pancreatitis, and its treatment by sphincteroplasty of the accessory ampulla. Gastroenterology 81: 1104–1110
55. Rose C, Kessaram RA, Lind JF (1980) Ectopic gastric pancreas: a review and report of 4 cases. Diagn Imag 49:214–218
56. Rösch W, Koch H, Schaffner O, Demling L (1976) The clinical significance of the pancreas divisum. Gastrointest Endosc 22:206–207
57. Rusnak CH, Hosie RT, Kuechler PM, McHattie JD, Piercey JR, Cameron RD (1988) Pancreatitis associated with pancreas divisum: results of surgical intervention. Am J Surg 155:641–643
58. Russell RCG, Wong NW, Cotton PB (1984) Accessory sphincterotomy (endoscopic and surgical) in patients with pancreas divisum. Br J Surg 71:954–957
59. Sahel J, Cros R-C, Bourry J, Sarles H (1982) Clinico-pathological conditions associated with pancreas divisum. Digestion 23:1–8
60. Schnedl WJ, Reisinger EC, Schreiber F, Pieber TR, Lipp RW, Krejs GJ (1995) Complete and partial agenesis of the dorsal pancreas within one family. Gastrointest Endosc 42:485–487
61. Seliger G, Goldman A (1973) Symptomatic annular pancreas in a 75-year old man. Am J Gastroenterol 60:185–190
62. Shich C-S, Eng HL, Huang S-C, Chuang J-H (1994) Congenital pancreatic cyst presenting as acute pancreatitis in an adolescent. J Pediatr Gastroenterol Nutr 18:490–493
63. Siegel JH, Ben-Zvi JS, Pullano W, Cooperman A (1990) Effectiveness of endoscopic drainage for pancreas divisum: endoscopic and surgical results in 31 patients. Endoscopy 22:129–133
64. Skandalakis JE, Gray SW, Rowe JS, Skandalakis LJ (1979) Anatomical complications of pancreatic surgery, part 2. Contemp Surg 15:21–50
65. Sperti C, Pasquali C, Costantino V, Perasole A, Liessi G, Pedrazzoli S (1995) Solitary true cyst of the pancreas in adults. Report of three cases and review of the literature. Int J Pancreatol 18:161–167
66. Staritz M, Meyer zum Büschenfelde KH (1988) Elevated pressure in the dorsal part of pancreas divisum: the cause of chronic pancreatitis? Pancreas 3:108–110
67. Strully LV, Schwartz DN, Nagaraj GS (1975) Pancreatoduodenectomy in annular pancreas for relief of duodenal obstruction. Am J Dig Dis 20:671–675
68. Tenner S, Roston A, Lichtenstein D, Sica G, Carr-Locke D, Banks P (1995) Von Hippel-Lindau syndrome (VHL) complicated by acute pancreatitis. Am J Gastroenterol 90:1708 (abstr)
69. Tenner S, Roston A, Lichtenstein D, Sica G, Carr-Locke D, Banks PA (1995) Von Hippel-Lindau disease complicated by acute pancreatitis and Evan's syndrome. Int J Pancreatol 18:271–275
70. Thomford NR, Knight PR, Pace WG, Madura JA (1972) Annular pancreas in the adult: selection of operation. Ann Surg 176:159–162
71. Thompson MH, Williamson RCN, Salmon PR (1981) The clinical relevance of isolated ventral pancreas. Br J Surg 68:101–104
72. Urayama S, Kozarek R, Ball T, Brandabur J, Traverso L, Ryan J, Wechter D (1995) Presentation and treatment of annular pancreas in an adult population. Am J Gastroenterol 90:995–999
73. Wang J-T, Lin J-T, Chuang C-N, Wang S-M, Chuang L-M, Chen J-C, Huang S-H, Chen D-S, Wang T-H (1990) Complete agenesis of the dorsal pancreas. A case report and review of the literature. Pancreas 5:493–497
74. Warshaw AL, Cambria RP (1984) False pancreas divisum. Acquired pancreatic duct obstruction simulating the congenital anomaly. Ann Surg 200:595–599
75. Warshaw AL, Richter JM, Schapiro RH (1983) The cause and treatment of pancreatitis associated with pancreas divisum. Ann Surg 198:443–452
76. Warshaw AL, Simeone J, Schapiro RH, Hedberg SE, Mueller PE, Ferrucci JT Jr (1985) Objective evaluation of ampullary stenosis with ultrasound and pancreatic stimulation. Am J Surg 149:65–72
77. Warshaw AL, Simeone JF, Schapiro RH, Flavin-Warshaw B (1990) Evaluation and treatment of the dominant dorsal duct syndrome (pancreas divisum redefined). Am J Surg 159:59–66
78. Wildling R, Schnedl WJ, Reisinger EC, Schreiber F, Lipp RW, Lederer A, Krejs GJ (1993) Agenesis of the dorsal pancreas in a woman with diabetes mellitus and in both her sons. Gastroenterology 104:1182–1186
79. Yasui A, Nimura Y, Kondou S, Kamiya J (1995) Duodenal obstruction due to annular pancreas associated with pancreatic head carcinoma. Hepatogastroenterology 42:1017–1022
80. Yorifuji T, Matsumura M, Okuno T, Shimizu K, Sonomura T, Muroi J, Kuno C, Takahashi Y, Okuno T (1994) Hereditary pancreatic hypoplasia, diabetes mellitus, and congenital heart disease: a new syndrome? J Med Genet 31:331–333

2 General Considerations: Anatomy

In the newborn, the wet organ weighs approximately 5 g, in adult females 85 g, and in adult males 100 g. In the adult, the pancreas is 14–18 cm long, 2–9 cm wide, and 2–3 cm thick. The gland is divided into head, neck, body, and tail [1]. The head of the pancreas forms the greatest mass of the gland and represents the structure which is derived in part from both dorsal and ventral pancreatic anlagen during the embryological development.

The fully developed pancreas contains endocrine (islet cells) and exocrine components (acini and excretory ducts). It appears distinctly lobulated to the unaided eye. The organ is divided into macroscopic lobules by connective tissue. The functional units of the exocrine gland consist of many microscopic lobules which form macroscopic lobules.

The organ is located in the retroperitoneum ventral to the second lumbar vertebra. The uncinate process projects from the lower portion of the head. The neck, body and tail extend in an oblique fashion upward to the level of the 12th thoracic vertebra (Figs. 2.1 a–c) [1].

The tail of the pancreas lies just anterior to the superior pole of the left kidney and is in close proximity to the spleen. The pancreas lies posterior to the stomach separated by the lesser sac. The mesocolon of the transverse colon extends from the anterior-inferior surface of the pancreas to the transverse colon.

During acute pancreatitis, inflammatory exudate may extend to the transverse colon by this route, and the lesser omental sac may fill with fluid displacing the stomach anteriorly and the transverse colon in a caudal direction (see Sects. 10.2.7.2, 18.3.1.2).

The pancreas lies directly anterior to the inferior vena cava and aorta near the midline. The splenic artery and vein lie immediately behind the neck and body of the pancreas in a horizontal position. The distal portion of the common bile duct usually passes through the substance of the head of the pancreas before entering the duodenum. During acute and chronic pancreatitis, thrombosis of the splenic vein may lead to varices of the lower esophagus and fundus of the stomach, and compression of the intrapancreatic portion of the common bile duct may cause jaundice (see Sects. 10.2.5, 18.3.2).

The arterial supply of the head of the pancreas occurs via a corona of anastomoses. The superior pancreaticoduodenal arteries start from the common hepatic artery. The inferior pancreaticoduodenal artery arises from the superior mesenterial pancreatic tributaries of the splenic artery. The veins running alongside of the arteries empty into the portal vein. Under physiological conditions, the lymphatics are not particularly

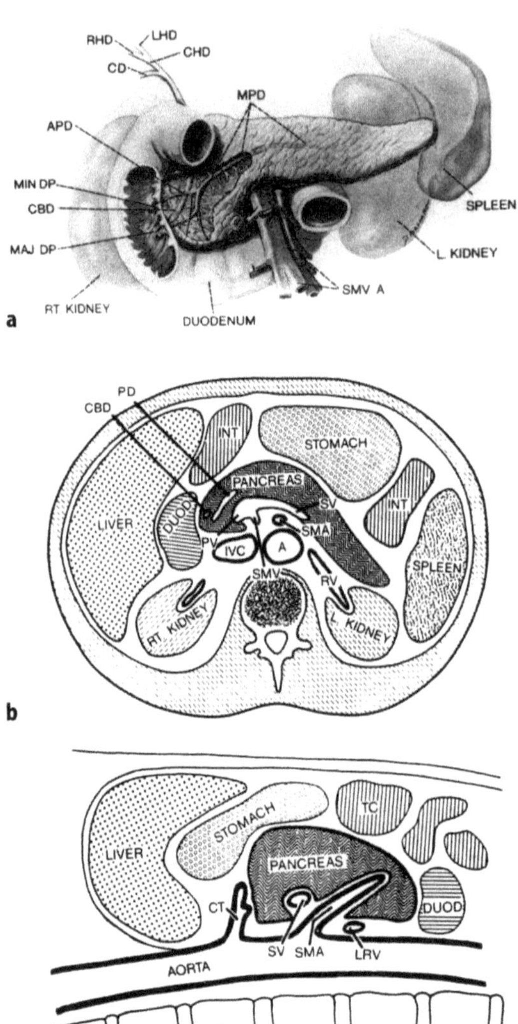

Fig. 2.1 a–c. a Frontal view of the pancreas to show its relationship with the duodenum and the relationship of pancreatic and bile ducts. The head of the pancreas is tucked into the curvature of the duodenum, overlapping somewhat both in front and behind. The main pancreatic duct (*MPD*) comes to lie to the left of the common bile duct (*CBD*) in the head, and they open into the duodenum at the major duonenal papilla (*MAJ DP*). The right hepatic duct (*RHD*) and left hepatic duct (*LHD*) unite after exiting from the liver to form the common hepatic duct (*CHD*), which in turn unites with the cystic duct (*CD*) to form the common bile duct, which is transmitted toward the pancreas and duodenum through the lesser omentum. An extension of the head, the uncinate process, is extended behind the emerging superior mesenteric vein and artery (*SMV A*). *APD*, accessory pancreatic duct; *MIN DP*, minor duodenal papilla. From [1]. **b** Representation of a cross section through the abdomen in the upper lumbar area. The relative locations of liver, stomach, spleen, kidneys, intestine (*INT*), and duodenum (*DUOD*) are shown. The pancreas lies immediately ventral to the aorta (*A*) and inferior vena cava (*IVC*). The superior mesenteric artery (*SMA*) lies between aorta and pancreas. The hepatic portal vein (*PV*) is represented where it is formed from the joining of the superior mesenteric vein (*SMV*) and splenic vein (*SV*). The left renal vein (*RV*) is shown as it proceeds toward its crossing the aorta posterior to the superior mesenteric artery to join the inferior vena cava. The main pancreatic duct (*PD*) and common bile duct (*CBD*) are shown in the head of the pancreas as they progress toward the major duodenal papilla. Compare with Figs. 2.1 a, c. From [1]. **c** Representation of a parasagittal section through the upper abdominal region, slightly to the left of the midline. The aorta is shown as it runs ventral to the vertebral column, giving off the celiac trunk (*CT*) or celiac artery, and the superior mesenteric artery (*SMA*) in the immediate area of the pancreas. The splenic vein (*SV*) is represented grooving the dorsal aspect of the pancreas as it proceeds to its junction with the superior mesenteric vein to form the portal vein. The left renal vein (*LRV*) is shown between superior mesenteric artery and aorta as it progresses to join the inferior vena cava. The relative locations of liver, stomach, horizontal duodenum (*DUOD*), and transverse colon (*TC*) are represented. Compare with Figs. 2.1 a, b. (From [1] with permission)

prominent. Their great potential for drainage of fluid and particulate material is evident, when edema, hemorrhage and cellular breakdown occur during pancreatitis [3].

The pancreas is supplied by branches from both parasympathetic and sympathetic divisions of the autonomic nervous system. In addition, visceral afferent fibers that run with each of these divisions supply the organ.

Pain is the most important symptom of chronic pancreatitis (see Sects. 17.1, 19.1). However, the mechanisms are still poorly understood. Recently, it has been shown that the perineurium, which normally forms a barrier within which the nerve fibers exist in a special microenvironment, is damaged in chronic pancreatitis. Inflammatory cells, mainly lymphocytes, but also granulocytes and macrophages, frequently are concentrated around nerves and ganglia in the pancreas of patients with chronic pancreatitis. Biologically active materials thus have direct access to the nerve fibers. The fact that nerves were found to be more numerous and their mean diameter was found to be greater than in normal pancreas, suggests that constriction due to fibrosis is not a stimulus for pain [2].

The approximately 12 cm long main pancreatic duct of Wirsung extends from the tail to the head, closer to the dorsal wall of the organ than the ventral surface. The accessory pancreatic duct of Santorini anastomoses with the main pancreatic duct and its branches in the head. It penetrates the wall of the duodenum via the minor duodenal papilla, which is approximately 2 cm superior to the major duodenal papilla (Fig. 2.1 a). Santorini's duct is not always functional [1].

Three basic forms of the orifice have been distinguished: in 60%–70% there is an Y-shaped orifice with a common final stretch between the pancreatic duct and the common bile duct (Fig. 2.2 c), in 20%–30% a V-shaped orifice of the neighboring ducts (Fig. 2.2 a), and in 10%–20% a U-shaped, separate orifice in the papilla (Fig. 2.2 b). The terminal stretch of the common bile duct runs through a ridge in the head of the pancreas in 40%, and in 15% it is completely surrounded by the pancreatic tissue. As a result, pancreatitis can lead to stenosis of the common bile duct (see Sects. 10.2.5, 18.3.2) [4].

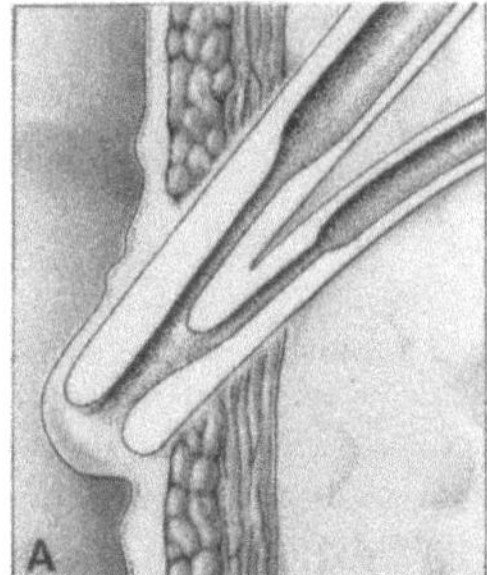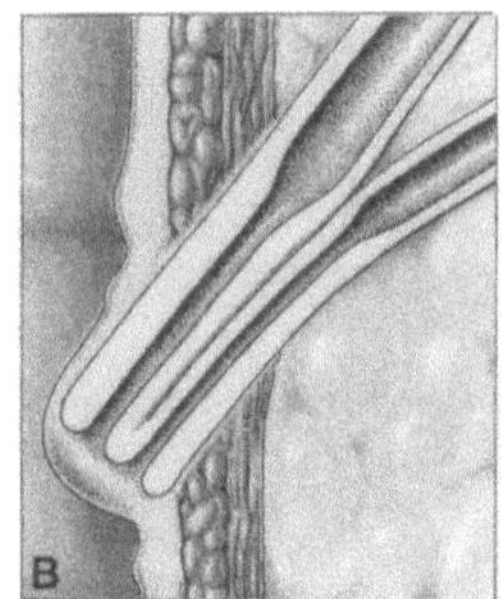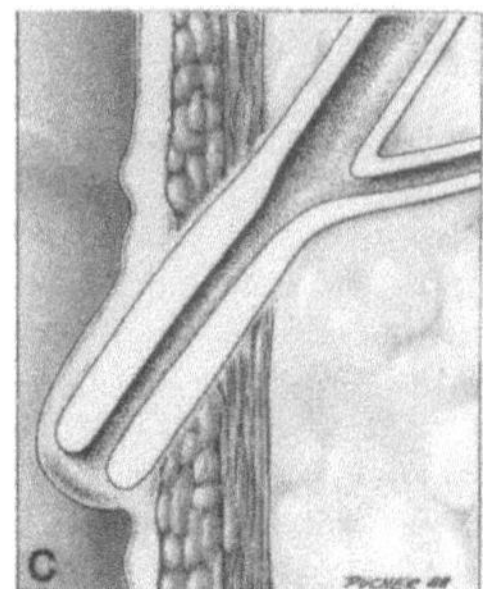

Fig. 2.2 A–C. Schematic presentation of the orifice of the ventral ductal system of the pancreas, the common bile duct and its variations. Three basic forms can be distinguished from one another. A V-shaped orifice of the neighboring ducts (20%–30%). B U-shaped separate orifices in the papilla (10%–20%). C Y-shaped orifice with common final stretch between the pancreatic duct and the common bile duct (60%–70%). (From [4] with permission)

Each microscopic pancreatic lobule is composed of a large proportion of cells that synthesize digestive enzymes and store them as zymogen granules (acinar cells) and a much smaller proportion of cells that comprises the ductal system (intralobular and intercalated ducts). Endocrine tissue, in the form of islets of Langerhans, occupies part of the lobules. Lobular arterioles supply a large proportion of blood to the islets and a smaller proportion directly to exocrine tissue. All the blood draining from the islets, however, passes through capillaries supplying exocrine tissue before exiting from the lobules via lobular venules. Thus, the exocrine tissue immediately surrounding islets normally is subjected to very high concentration of islet hormones [1].

References

1. Bockman DE (1993) Anatomy of the pancreas. In: Go VLW, DiMagno EP, Gardner JD, Lebenthal E, Reber HA, Scheele GA (eds) The Pancreas: Biology, Pathobiology, and Disease, 2nd edn. Raven Press, New York, pp 1–8
2. Bockman DE, Buchler M, Malfertheiner P, Beger HG (1988) Analysis of nerves in chronic pancreatitis. Gastroenterology 94:1459–1469
3. Bockman DE, Schiller WR, Suriyapa C, Mutchler JHW, Anderson MC (1973) Fine structure of early experimental acute pancreatitis in dogs. Lab Invest 28:584–592
4. Morgenroth K, Kozuschek W, Hotz J (1991) Pancreatitis. Walter de Gruyter, Berlin–New York

3 General Considerations: Physiology

The pancreas is composed of endocrine and exocrine elements. The endocrine pancreas is composed of only 2% of the mass of the pancreas. The exocrine pancreas comprises approximately 85%. The remainder of the pancreas is composed of connective tissue, nerves, and blood vessels. Recent studies have advanced our knowledge considerably regarding the physiology of the pancreas [1–16, 18–20, 22].

3.1
Function of the Exocrine Pancreas

The exocrine pancreas consists of clusters of acini and ducts. Acini are connected to small ductules termed *centroacinar cells*, which in turn are connected to progressively larger ducts that link up to the main pancreatic duct. Acinar cells synthesize, store, and secrete digestive enzymes at a higher rate than any other cell in the body (as much as 10 g of digestive enzymes each day). The amount that is synthesized daily generally equals the amount that is secreted such that the amount of digestive enzymes stored within acinar cells as zymogens is relatively constant.

3.2
Pancreatic Enzymes

Pancreatic acinar cells secrete many different digestive enzymes [19]. These include proteolytic enzymes, lipolytic enzymes, nucleases, amylolytic enzymes, and other enzymes including procolipase and trypsin inhibitors. The digestive enzymes capable of attacking pancreatic cell membranes are secreted as inactive proenzymes including trypsinogen, chymotrypsinogen, proelastase, procarboxypeptidase A and B, and phospholipase A_2. These enzymes require activation by trypsin. Lipase (without its substrate triglyceride) and amylase alone require no activation and do not appear to have the capability of damaging pancreatic tissue. In health, enterokinase in the duodenum activates trypsinogen to trypsin. Trypsin itself also has the capability of activating trypsinogen but is more effective in activating proteolytic enzymes and phospholipases. In terms of the total amount of protein secreted in pancreatic juice, proteolytic enzymes contribute approximately 80%. In comparison, amylase and lipase are present in small amounts but have very high enzymatic activities.

3.3
Enzyme Synthesis

Digestive enzymes and lysosomal hydrolases are synthesized on ribosomes attached to the rough endoplasmic reticulum and then migrate in a vectorial fashion [17] to the Golgi complex, where lysosomal hydrolases are packaged into lysosomes and separated from digestive enzymes [21]. In a process termed exocytosis, zymogen granules then fuse with the luminal plasma membrane and enzymes are released into the lumen (Fig. 3.1).

3.4
Protective Mechanisms to Prevent Autodigestion

The pancreas possesses a variety of protective mechanisms to prevent autodigestion. First, enzymes that are capable of attacking pancreatic cell membranes are synthesized and stored as inactive zymogens. Secondly, enzymes are separated from the cytoplasm within membrane-bound compartments. Third, the pancreas contains intra-

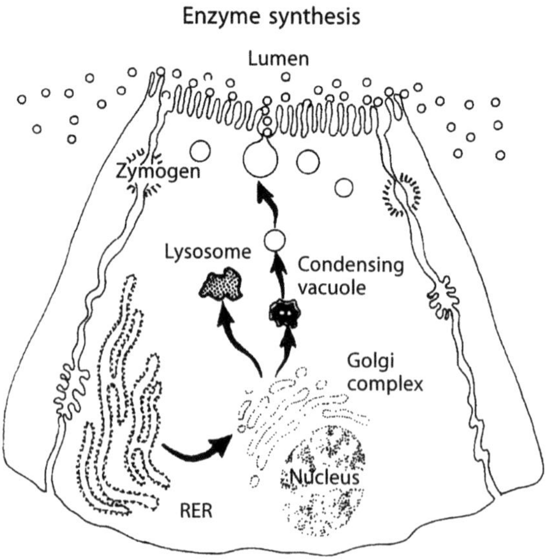

Fig. 3.1. Digestive enzymes and lysosomal hydrolases are synthesized on ribosomes, attached to the rough endoplasmic reticulum. From the endoplasmic reticulum, these newly synthesized proteins migrate within membrane-enclosed compartments to the Golgi complex. During the passage from the cis to the trans side of the Golgi complex, proteins are synthesized into either digestive enzymes or lysosomal hydrolases. Proteins that are synthesized as lysosomal hydrolases separate out from digestive enzymes as they pass through the Golgi complex and are eventually packaged in lysosomes. Zymogen granules fuse with the luminal plasma membrane, and enzymes are released into the lumen by a process termed exocytosis. *RER* = rough endoplasmic reticulum. From the American Gastroenterological Association: Clinical Teaching Project, Unit 5, Pancreatitis (with permission)

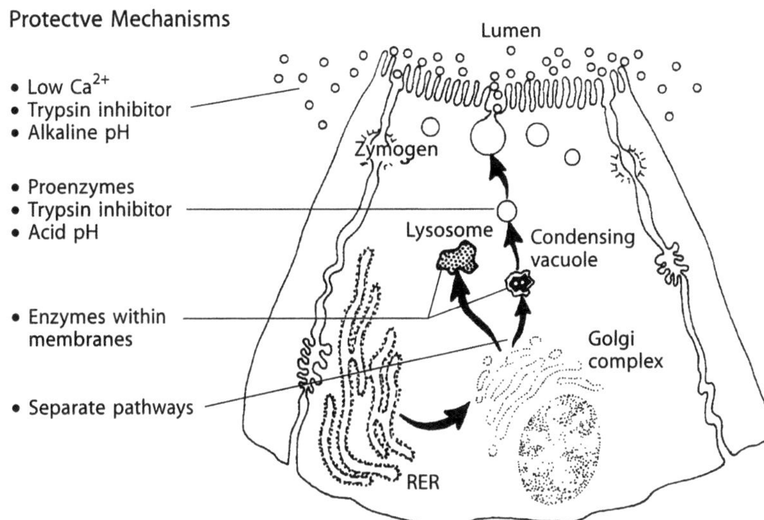

Fig. 3.2. Premature activation of pancreatic enzymes is prevented by a variety of mechanisms starting at the level of the Golgi complex: Digestive enzymes and lysosomal hydrolases mature along separate pathways; digestive enzymes and lysosomal hydrolases travel within membrane-enclosed compartments; digestive enzymes that would otherwise injure acinar cells are synthesized, transported and secreted as proenzymes; a trypsin inhibitor accompanies digestive enzymes and prevents a premature activation of trypsinogen from trypsin; and the acid pH within zymogens inactivates any trypsin that might be prematurely activated from trypsinogen. Within the lumen of pancreatic ducts, a low concentration of ionized calcium does not favor the activation of trypsin, and any trypsin that might be activated is either inhibited by the trypsin inhibitor or degraded in the alkaline pH. *RER* = rough endoplasmic reticulum. From the American Gastroenterological Association: Clinical Teaching Project, Unit 5, Pancreatitis (with permission)

cellular trypsin inhibitors. Fourth, the enzyme that is principally responsible for activating trypsinogen (namely, enterokinase) is in the small intestine rather than the pancreas (Fig. 3.2).

3.5
Pancreatic Secretagogues

3.5.1
Secretin

Secretin is a powerful stimulant of pancreatic fluid and bicarbonate from ductular cells. Secretin is also capable of stimulating a small amount of pancreatic enzymes. These actions can be inhibited by the intravenous administration of atropine [10]. Secretin is released from the duodenum by acid and to a lesser extent by bile and oleic acid [18, 19].

3.5.2
Cholecystokinin

Cholecystokinin (CCK) stimulates pancreatic enzyme secretion by two mechanisms. The first is by binding to its specific receptor on the acinar cell [1]. The second is by interacting with the cholinergic nervous system [1, 2, 11, 16, 20]. It appears that the second mechanism may be more important than the first. Atropine reduces enzyme output in response to CCK [16]. CCK is released in the duodenum in response to amino acids, oligopeptides, free fatty acids, 2-monoglyceride, glucose, and calcium. It would appear that neutral fat and complex protein are not effective stimulants of CCK. This apparent paradox that the products of fat and protein digestion are required to stimulate CCK for the purposes of digesting fat and protein is explained physiologically by the fact that the cephalic and gastric phases of pancreatic secretion ensure the presence of copious amounts of pancreatic enzymes in the duodenum in order to begin the digestion of complex fat and protein to their breakdown products that then create a powerful stimulus for the release of CCK and an enhancement of digestion [2].

Because the presence of acid ensures the release of secretin and the presence of food ensures the release of CCK, both hormones are in circulation simultaneously at least part of the time. The combination of secretin and CCK has been shown to potentiate bicarbonate secretion in man (that is, the amount of bicarbonate released by ductular cells in response to both hormones is in excess of an additive response) [2]. Atropine does not block potentiation [10]. As a result, there is a copious outpouring of bicarbonate in response to a meal. Thus far, the combination of secretin and CCK has not been shown to potentiate enzyme secretion.

3.5.3
Cholinergic Influence

Cholinergic pathways from the brain are important for the cephalic, gastric, and small intestinal phases of pancreatic secretion [19]. As mentioned, the effects of CCK on the acinar cell appear to be exhibited for the most part via the cholinergic nervous system. Anticholinergic agents block both the secretion of bicarbonate by secretin [10] and the secretion of enzymes by CCK [16].

3.6
Phases of Pancreatic Secretion

The cephalic phase contributes 25%–50%, gastric phase only 10%, and intestinal phase at least 50% of the total pancreatic enzyme output [19].

The cephalic phase of pancreatic enzyme secretion is represented almost entirely by the direct stimulation of acinar cells by the vagus nerve. There appears to be very little, if any, gastrin or CCK released by the cephalic phase.

The gastric phase is initiated by distention of the stomach and possibly also by the composition of the diet. These effects are mediated by vagal cholinergic mechanisms.

Gastrin appears to contribute very little in the stimulation of pancreatic enzyme secretion.

The intestinal phase is mediated by the release of secretin and CCK, and by vagal cholinergic stimulation. The release of secretin is mediated by hydrogen ions and to a lesser extent by oleic acid and bile salts [18]. The release of CCK is mediated primarily by products of fat and protein digestion. Hydrogen ion is also a stimulant of CCK release, albeit a weak one.

3.7
Ductular Secretion

Pancreatic ducts serve at least three very important functions. The first is as a conduit of bicarbonate to neutralize gastric acid. The maintenance of an alkaline milieu in the duodenum prevents the development of duodenal ulcers, increases the solubility of bile acids and fatty acids, and protects pancreatic and small intestinal brush border enzymes. The second is a conduit for pancreatic enzymes to reach the duodenum and aid in digestion of carbohydrate, fats, and proteins. The third is liquefaction of pancreatic enzymes and solubilization of pancreatic glycoprotein by bicarbonate-rich fluid secreted by ductular cells.

The centroacinar cells manufacture bicarbonate. Cells of the main pancreatic duct may also contribute to bicarbonate secretion [5]. Both bicarbonate and hydrogen ion are generated in the ductular cell by the action of carbonic anhydrase on CO_2 and H_2O. The hydrogen ion is extruded through the basolateral portion of the cell. The bicarbonate is secreted apically into the lumen in accordance with the following steps [13]. First, intracellular chloride is transported to the lumen by the cystic fibrosis transmembrane conductance regulator (CFTR). Secretin is thought to activate the CFTR by stimulating the production of cyclic adenosine monophosphate (AMP). Once chloride reaches the lumen by this step, it is then exchanged for intracellular bicarbonate, thereby providing the transport of bicarbonate into the lumen and chloride back into the cell.

By this mechanism, bicarbonate is secreted by ductular cells at a concentration of 154 mEq/l. At fast rates of flow, in response to a maximum stimulus by secretin, intraductal bicarbonate reaches the duodenum at a concentration that is close to 154 mEq/l. At slower rates of flow, the concentration of bicarbonate that reaches the duodenum is lower, presumably due to exchange of intraductal bicarbonate for interstitial chloride as bicarbonate-rich fluid travels through the pancreatic ductal system. In this way, the concentrations of bicarbonate and chloride are reciprocal. The intraductal concentrations of sodium and potassium remain constant in all rates of flow.

The threshold of pH in the duodenum for release of secretin is 4.0–4.5 [18]. This is a very sensitive mechanism since the amount of acid that is represented by a pH of 4.0 equals one-tenth of a milliequivalent per liter. As the pH is progressively lowered below the threshold of 4.0–4.5, there is an augmentation of release of secretin and a corresponding increase in the amount of bicarbonate that is secreted.

3.8
Acinar Secretion

The pathway of synthesis of pancreatic enzymes is, as follows [19]. Amino acids are incorporated on ribosomes of the rough endoplasmic reticulum. They travel via a series of membrane-bound compartments called cisternae and are eventually packaged as zymogen granules. These membane-bound compartments separate digestive enzymes from the remainder of the cell. The same membrane-bound compartments are shared by both digestive and lysosomal enzymes until the Golgi complex, where the pathways diverge. At this point, digestive and lysosomal enzymes are not yet capable of causing damage. The importance of diversion at this step is the fact that lysosomal enzymes (particularly cathepsin-β) can activate trypsinogen to trypsin.

The acinar cell has several receptors. First, there are receptors for neurons from the brain, stomach, and small intestine. Neurons release acetylcholine at their membrane receptors. The second is gastrin receptors. Gastrin is a very weak stimulant of pancreatic enzymes. The third is CCK receptors. CCK is the most potent stimulant of pancreatic enzymes. There are also receptors for secretin and vasoactive intestinal polypeptide (VIP).

The mechanism by which pancreatic enzymes contained within zymogens are extruded into the lumen in response to acetylcholine or CCK is called *exocytosis*. The steps that lead to exocytosis are complex and are poorly understood. Both acetylcholine and CCK convert a membrane phospholipid termed *phosphatidylinositol* to two breakdown products through a series of complex steps. One of these breakdown products mobilizes intracellular calcium (probably from the rough endoplasmic reticulum), and the release of calcium in some way impacts on zymogen cells to begin the process of exocytosis. The release of protein kinase C may also play a role in the instability of zymogen membranes.

Secretin and VIP cause the activation of adenylate cyclase with increase in intracellular cyclic AMP [5]. Through a series of intracellular steps, there is release of pancreatic enzymes. Neither secretin nor VIP is a strong stimulant of enzyme release.

3.9
Action of Pancreatic Lipase

Lipase acts in the interface of emulsified triglycerides to create two fatty acids, leaving intact 2-monoglyceride. The cleavage of the third fatty acid proceeds more slowly.

3.10
What Turns the Pancreas Off?

A variety of hormones may participate to reduce pancreatic secretion. One is pancreatic polypeptide [15]. Pancreatic polypeptide is located in the islets of Langerhans, is released postprandially, and is thought to play a physiologic role in the postprandial feedback inhibition of pancreatic secretion. Another is peptide YY [3, 7, 12]. This hormone is located in enteroendocrine cells in the distal small bowel, colon, and rectum. The presence of intraluminal fat is the most potent stimulant of peptide YY release. A third inhibitory hormone is somatostatin [4, 5, 9]. It appears that somatostatin is secreted from the gut during food intake and is possibly also released from D cells from islet cells. The release of this hormone from one or both sites inhibits pancreatic enzyme and bicarbonate secretion. The mechanism appears to be inhibition of intrapancreatic cholinergic pathways [4, 9]. A fourth hormone is glucagon, but the physiologic importance of this hormone in reducing pancreatic secretion has not been fully studied.

Another important mechanism for turning the pancreas off appears to be a phenomenon termed *negative feedback inhibition*. Both trypsin [9, 16] and bile salts [6, 14, 16, 22] appear to participate in negative feedback inhibition. The mechanisms appear to be, as follows.

Regarding negative feedback inhibition caused by trypsin, there is increasing evidence that the duodenum contains a trypsin-sensitive CCK-releasing peptide [8, 16]. During the basal state, a small quantity of pancreatic enzymes enters the duodenum. Trypsin denatures this peptide, thereby inhibiting CCK release substantially. As a result, the basal output of enzymes into the duodenum remains very low. Once food enters the duodenum, pancreatic trypsin apparently has a greater affinity for food than for the peptide itself. As a result, there is no further denaturing of the peptide, and CCK release is enhanced. Eventually, when all protein has been digested, trypsin is once again available to denature the peptide, thereby reducing serum levels of CCK and reducing the stimulation of the pancreas back to a basal condition.

Trypsin also appears to regulate pancreatic secretion of bicarbonate by a negative feedback mechanism. The presence of trypsin in the proximal jejunum results in inhibition of plasma secretin concentration and reduction in pancreatic bicarbonate output [8].

Regarding bile salts, it also appears that the presence of bile salts in the lumen of the duodenum inhibits pancreatic enzyme output. One mechanism appears to be the ability of bile salts to stabilize luminal trypsin and thereby inhibit CCK release [6, 14, 16]. A second mechanism appears to be inhibition of pancreatic enzyme release by a mechanism that is independent of luminal trypsin activity [14, 22].

References

1. Adler G, Beglinger C, Braun U, Reinshagen M, Koop I, Schafmayer A, Rovati L, Arnold R (1991) Interaction of the cholinergic system and cholecystokinin in the regulation of endogenous and exogenous stimulation of pancreatic secretion in humans. Gastroenterology 100:537–543
2. Adler G, Nelson DK, Katschinski M, Beglinger C (1995) Neurohormonal control of human pancreatic exocrine secretion. Pancreas 10:1–13
3. Brodish RJ, Kuvshinoff BW, McFadden DW, Fink AS (1995) Adrenergic pathways do not mediate peptide YY-induced inhibition of pancreatic exocrine secretion. Pancreas 10:187–193
4. Brodish RJ, Kuvshinoff BW, McFadden DW, Fink AS (1995) Somatostatin inhibits cholecystokinin-induced pancreatic protein secretion via cholinergic pathways. Pancreas 10:401–406
5. de Ondarza J, Hootman SR (1995) Regulation of cyclic AMP levels in guinea pig pancreatic ducts and cultured duct epithelial monolayers. Pancreas 11:261–270

6. Gomez G, Upp JR Jr, Lluis F, Alexander RW, Poston GJ, Greeley GH Jr, Thompson JC (1988) Regulation of the release of cholecystokinin by bile salts in dogs and humans. Gastroenterology 94: 1036–1046
7. Jin H, Cai L, Lee K, Chang T-M, Li P, Wagner D, Chey WY (1993) A physiological role of peptide YY on exocrine pancreatic secretion in rats. Gastroenterology 105:208–215
8. Jin HO, Song CW, Chang TM, Chey WY (1994) Roles of gut hormones in negative-feedback regulation of pancreatic exocrine secretion in humans. Gastroenterology 107:1828–1834
9. Kuvshinoff BW, Brodish RJ, James L, McFadden DW, Fink AS (1993) Somatostatin inhibits secretin-induced canine pancreatic response via a cholinergic mechanism. Gastroenterology 105: 539–547
10. Kuvshinoff BW, Demar AR, James L, McFadden DW, Fink AS (1993) Effect of pancreatic denervation and atropine on the pancreatic response to secretin. Pancreas 8:609–614
11. Li Y, Owyang C (1994) Endogenous cholecystokinin stimulates pancreatic enzyme secretion via vagal afferent pathway in rats. Gastroenterology 107:525–531
12. Lluis F, Gomez G, Fujimura M, Greeley GH Jr, Thompson JC (1988) Peptide YY inhibits pancreatic secretion by inhibiting cholecystokinin release in the dog. Gastroenterology 94:137–144
13. Marino CR (1993) Pancreatic duct cell physiology. Curr Opinion Gastroenterol 9:740–746
14. Miyasaka K, Sazaki N, Funakoshi A, Matsumoto M, Kitani K (1993) Two mechanisms of inhibition by bile on luminal feedback regulation of rat pancreas. Gastroenterology 104:1780–1785
15. Okumura T, Pappas TN, Taylor IL (1995) Pancreatic polypeptide microinjection into the dorsal motor nucleus inhibits pancreatic secretion in rats. Gastroenterology 108:1517–1525
16. Owyang C (1993) Neurohormonal control of the exocrine pancreas. Curr Opinion Gastroenterol 9:747–751
17. Palade G (1975) Intracellular aspects of the process of protein synthesis. Science 189:347–358
18. Rhodes RA, Skerven G, Chey WY, Chang T-M (1988) Acid-independent release of secretin and cholecystokinin by intraduodenal infusion of fat in humans. Pancreas 3:391–398
19. Solomon TE (1995) Physiology of the exocrine pancreas. In: Haubrich WS, Schaffner F, Berk JE (eds) Bockus Gastroenterology, 5th edn. W.B. Saunders Comp., Philadelphia-London etc, pp 2821–2834
20. Soudah HC, Lu Y, Hasler WL, Owyang C (1992) Cholecystokinin at physiological levels evokes pancreatic enzyme secretion via a cholinergic pathway. Am J Physiol 263:G102–G107
21. Steer ML, Meldolesi J (1987) The cell biology of experimental pancreatitis. N Engl J Med 316: 144–150
22. Tomita H, Miyasaka K, Matsumoto M, Funakoshi A (1994) Direct, concentration-dependent inhibition by taurocholate of pancreatic exocrine secretion and CCK release in conscious rats. Dig Dis Sci 39:1544–1549

4 General Considerations: Classification

4.1
Marseille Classification of 1963

At the Marseille Symposium in 1963, clinical definitions of pancreatitis, later known as the Marseille classification, were adopted. The different clinical manifestations of pancreatitis were classified into the following groups: (1) Acute pancreatitis; (2) Relapsing acute pancreatitis; (3) Chronic relapsing pancreatitis, defined as chronic pancreatitis with acute exacerbations; and (4) Chronic pancreatitis [13] (Table 4.1).

With respect to the two acute forms, it was believed that clinical and biological restitution of the pancreas would take place if the primary cause or factors were eliminated. Furthermore, development of acute into chronic pancreatitis was considered to be a rare occurrence. With respect to the two chronic forms, the opposite was stated, namely, pancreatic damage, either anatomical or functional, would persist, even if the primary cause or factors were eliminated. Chronic pancreatitis was said to develop from chronic relapsing pancreatitis, or it could even be chronic without prior attacks (i.e., painless).

The Marseille classification was primarily concerned with the pathological anatomy and the etiology of chronic pancreatitis. Correlation between the anatomical and functional changes was not explored.

Table 4.1. Classification of acute and chronic pancreatitis, proposed at different meetings

Marseille 1963	Cambridge 1983	Marseille 1984
Acute pancreatitis	Acute pancreatitis – Mild – Severe	Acute pancreatitis – Clinical – Morphological
Relapsing pancreatitis	—	—
Chronic relapsing pancreatitis	Chronic pancreatitis	Chronic pancreatitis – Clinical – Morphological
Chronic (primarily painless) pancreatitis	—	—
—	—	Obstructive chronic pancreatitis

4.2
Cambridge Classification of 1983

The development of modern laboratory and function tests as well as imaging procedures necessitated a reclassification of pancreatitis. The following definitions, later known as the Cambridge classification, were presented at an international workshop in Cambridge in 1983 (Table 4.1):

"Acute pancreatitis: This is defined as an acute condition typically presenting with abdominal pain, and usually associated with raised pancreatic enzymes in blood or urine, due to inflammatory disease of the pancreas.

Chronic pancreatitis: This is defined as a continuing inflammatory disease of the pancreas, characterised by irreversible morphological change, and typically causing pain and/or permanent loss of function.

Acute pancreatitis may recur. Many patients with chronic pancreatitis may have acute exacerbations but the condition may be completely painless" [16, 17].

The experts discussed two further main problems:

– A new classification was needed for comparing image findings of various centers. A classification based on grading of severity was adopted. The workshop defined such gradings for endoscopic retrograde cholangiopancreatography (ERCP), ultrasound and computed tomography (CT) findings (see Tables 17.8, 17.9) [2, 16, 17], but admitted that, despite a common classification, comparative interpretations would be difficult because techniques used by the different centers and groups remain so diverse. Gradations of severity of functional impairment have been devised since then for the secretin-pancreozymin test and fecal fat analysis and used successfully in subsequent studies (see Table 17.4) [8, 10].

– The second main problem discussed in Cambridge was the classification of patients who suffer pancreatic pain, but in whom unequivocal morphological or functional abnormalities have not yet been shown. Grouping their symptoms as intermediate, i.e., between acute and chronic pancreatitis, was finally rejected, and it was agreed that in practice the diagnosis for such patients would be "probably chronic pancreatitis" until further confirmation.

4.3
Revised Pancreatitis Classification of Marseille 1984

One year later, another group of experts, including some involved with the Cambridge classification, met at Marseille and revised the first Marseille classification (Table 4.1) [19].

"Acute Pancreatitis: Clinically acute pancreatitis is characterized by acute abdominal pain accompanied by increased pancreatic enzymes in blood or urine, or both. Though it usually runs a benign course, severe attacks may lead to shock with renal and pulmonary insufficiency that may prove fatal. Acute pancreatitis may be a single episode or it may recur.

Morphologically there is a gradation of lesions in acute pancreatitis. In the mild form peripancreatic fat necrosis and interstitial edema can be recognized, but as a rule

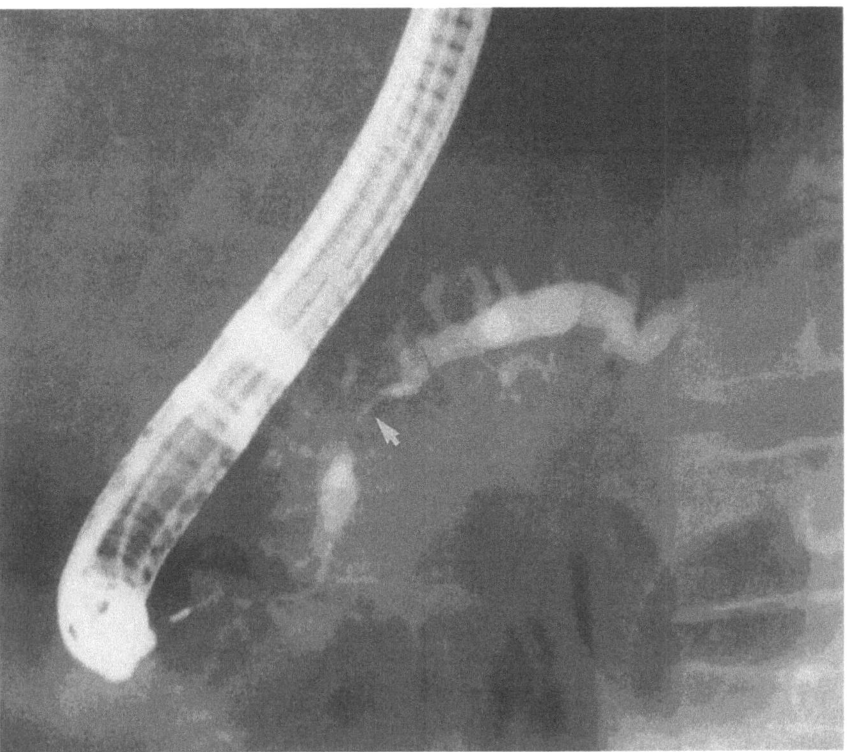

Fig. 4.1. ERCP in a 54-year-old woman with severe epigastric pain reveals marked stenosis of the pancreatic duct at the genu (*arrow*) with considerable dilatation of both the main pancreatic duct and side branches upstream. The findings are consistent with obstructive pancreatitis. At surgery, the patient was found to have unresectable adenocarcinoma at the head of the pancreas

pancreatic necrosis is absent. The mild form may develop into a severe form with extensive peripancreatic and intrapancreatic fat necrosis, parenchymal necrosis, and hemorrhage. The lesions may be either localized or diffuse. Occasionally, there may be little correlation between the severity of the clinical features and the morphologic findings.

Both exocrine and endocrine functions of the pancreas are impaired to a variable extent for a variable duration.

If the primary cause and complications such as pseudocysts are eliminated in acute pancreatitis, clinical, morphologic, and functional restitution to normal occurs. In some cases scarring and pseudocysts persist. Only rarely does acute pancreatitis lead to chronic pancreatitis.

Chronic Pancreatitis: Clinically chronic pancreatitis is characterized by recurrent or persisting abdominal pain, though chronic pancreatitis may present without pain. Evidence of pancreatic insufficiency, e.g., steatorrhoea or diabetes, may be present.

Morphologically, chronic pancreatitis is characterized by an irregular sclerosis, with destruction and permanent loss of exocrine parenchyma that may be either focal, seg-

mental, or diffuse. These changes may be associated with varying degrees of dilatation of segments of the duct system. Thus, dilatation of the duct of Wirsung and of its small ducts may occur together or independently. No obvious cause of the duct dilatation may be found, but most often it is associated with strictures of the ducts or intraductal protein plugs and calculi (calcification). All types of inflammatory cells may present in varying degrees, as well as edema and focal necrosis. Cysts and pseudocysts, with or without infection, which may or may not communicate with ducts, are not uncommon. Compared to the degree of acinar destruction, the islets of Langerhans are relatively well preserved. Based on the predominating structural features, the following descriptive terms can be used:
- Chronic pancreatitis with focal necrosis
- Chronic pancreatitis with segmental or diffuse fibrosis
- Chronic pancreatitis with or without calculi

A distinct morphologic form of chronic pancreatitis is obstructive chronic pancreatitis. It is characterized by dilatation of the ductal system proximal to the occlusion of one of the major ducts (e.g. by tumor or scars, Fig. 4.1), diffuse atrophy of the acinar parenchyma, and uniform diffuse fibrosis. Calculi are uncommon.

In chronic pancreatitis (with the exception of obstructive chronic pancreatitis), the irreversible morphologic changes in the pancreas may lead to a progressive or permanent loss of exocrine and endocrine pancreatic function. In obstructive chronic pancreatitis, both structural and functional changes tend to improve when the obstruction is removed" [19].

4.4
Pancreatitis Classification of Marseille-Rome 1988

Four years later, the supplemental pancreatitis classification of Marseille-Rome was created in 1988 [15]. The classification of chronic pancreatitis was expanded to include not only *chronic obstructive pancreatitis*, but also *chronic calcifying pancreatitis* and *chronic inflammatory pancreatitis*. It was noted, however, that intraductal calcifications do not appear in many patients with chronic calcifying pancreatitis at the initial examination; they develop later. In the experience of the authors of this book, the usual imaging procedures detect calcifications in about one-third of patients with chronic pancreatitis after observations of more than a decade.

Chronic inflammatory pancreatitis was said to occur in some cases, characterized by the loss of exocrine parenchyma replaced by a dense fibrosis infiltrated by mononuclear cells. These cases could represent lesions with a different origin and were considered to deserve further investigation.

Some, but not most, of the participants considered perilobular fibrosis, sometimes associated with some degree of intralobular fibrosis but without evident loss of exocrine parenchyma, also to be chronic pancreatitis.

In extension of the Marseille-Rome classification, Sarles [14] proposed another classification of pancreatic lithiasis (chronic calcifying or lithogenic pancreatitis):

- *Type I: hereditary pancreatitis*
  A dominant disease observed in children of both sexes and another possibly non-dominant form observed in adults and children. The exact biochemical composition of stones and the pathological lesions are not well known
- *Type II: transparent stones*
  This form of the disease was said to be observed in nonalcoholics of both sexes. Stones are composed of amorphous protein, not fibrillar and consisting of more degraded residues of pancreatic stone protein-secretory (PSP-S) than is seen in type III
- *Type III: nutritional pancreatitis*
  In this form of the disease, calculi are composed of more than 98% calcium carbonate and a small quantity of PSP-S1 or pancreatic thread protein, the 133 amino acid C terminal residue of PSP-S. *Type III-1* is due to alcohol consumption; high-protein, high-fat diets; and tobacco smoking. It is frequently observed in males aged 30–50 years at the onset of the disease. *Type III-2* is considered to be the tropical form observed in children and young adults, living in tropical countries and eating low-protein and very low fat diets
- *Type IV: hypercalcemic pancreatitis*
  The composition of stones in this condition is not known
- *Type V: pancreatic lithiasis (pure calcium salt stones)*
  This condition probably represents congenital absence of lithostatine (PSP) biosynthesis. Only one case has been described [14].

4.5
Pancreatitis Classification – Cambridge vs. Marseille: Features in Common and Differences

Both the Cambridge and the Marseille classifications stress that structural and functional damage in chronic pancreatitis is irreversible, and do away with the often difficult clinical distinction between chronic and chronic relapsing and acute and acute relapsing pancreatitis. Both classifications conclude that histological changes in chronic pancreatitis are irreversible, may be progressive, may lead to a loss of exocrine and endocrine pancreatic function, and are often associated with abdominal pain [4, 6]. Only the Marseille and later the Marseille-Rome classifications delineate subgroups, one of which, chronic obstructive pancreatitis, deserves special interest, as both structural and functional changes tend to improve if the ductal obstruction is removed.

The clinical description of acute pancreatitis is similar in both classifications, but there are differences concerning complications: the Cambridge group included necrosis, hemorrhage, phlegmon, pseudocyst and abscess; the Marseille classification, necrosis, hemorrhage, pseudocyst, but not abscess [4]. The Marseille classification goes beyond the description of the clinical picture of acute pancreatitis and defines mild acute pancreatitis morphologically as peripancreatitis, fat necrosis and interstitial edema; severe, as extensive peri- and intrapancreatic fat necrosis and hemorrhage. These lesions may be localized or diffuse.

The decision whether the initial attack should be labeled acute or chronic pancreatitis according to the Marseille classification has to be postponed until after recovery and subsequent function tests, or until material for histological examination becomes available at surgery or at autopsy. According to the Cambridge classification, such an attack would be labeled acute pancreatitis, and if subsequently structural damage were evidenced on ERCP or CT, it would be relabeled "exacerbation of chronic pancreatitis".

This result is certainly problematic because function may return to normal after acute pancreatitis, whereas ERCP findings do not [1], and calcifications may occur in patients with normal exocrine pancreatic function [9]. Furthermore, abnormal ERCP findings are frequent following acute pancreatitis and may persist without any clinical signs and symptoms of relapsing or chronic pancreatitis [11, 18].

A further difference between the two classifications is that the Cambridge group believed that the etiology of pancreatitis is pertinent to prognosis and management of the patient with either acute or chronic pancreatitis and should be noted, whereas the Marseille group did not.

According to both workshops and a reevaluation of both of their results by another group of experts, the following subjects should be investigated for improving classification.

- The significance of the synthesis and origin of stone protein, and its role in the pathogenesis of chronic pancreatitis
- The degree of stabilization or aggression of chronic pancreatitis after the primary cause is removed
- The degree and time for resolution or improvement of exocrine and endocrine dysfunction after an acute attack
- The pathophysiologic relationship between alcohol and acute and chronic pancreatitis
- The sensitivity and specificity of ultrasound and CT in identifying pancreatic inflammatory disease
- Development of criteria for defining irreversible morphologic change and loss of function
- The need for more sensitive markers of pancreatitis in patients with abdominal pain thought to be of pancreatic origin and in whom no functional or morphologic abnormalities can be detected with tests currently available [4]

Futhermore, it was recommended that definitions include as much pertinent information as possible in order to develop what may be termed as operational categories and definitions of pancreatitis. Only when patients who have similar clinical characteristics, etiologies, severity of disease, and complications are studied can meaningful data be generated. Only then are we able to compare data from one institution with another, develop prospective collaborative multicenter studies, and evaluate the costs of alternative methods of care.

Accordingly, it was suggested that a wide variety of components be covered in an operational classification (Table 4.2). This information could include etiologies, number of attacks, severity of attacks, complications, exocrine function, endocrine function, structural integrity based on CT scan, ultrasound, ERCP, and perhaps nuclear magnetic resonance, as well as morphology based on histology (whenever possible) [4, 6].

Table 4.2. Operational classification [4]

Patient name	Example
Etiology	Alcohol
Severity of attacks	Example: Ranson or Imrie criteria
Number of attacks	1
Complications	Example: Abscess Pseudocyst Phlegmon Duodenal obstruction Common bile duct obstruction
Exocrine function	Example: Pancreolauryl test abnormal
Endocrine function	Diabetes Glucose tolerance test
Morphology – Computed tomography	Mass in the body of the pancreas
– Endoscopic retrograde cholangio- pancreatography	Obstructed duct in the body of the pancreas
– Ultrasound	Dilated main pancreatic duct 3 mm
Nuclear magnetic resonance	Not available
Biopsy	Chronic pancreatitis
Treatment	Example: Incision and drainage 5/9/84
Status	Example: Pain free 8/10/84

4.6
Classification System for Acute Pancreatitis of Atlanta 1992

At a meeting in Atlanta in 1992, acute pancreatitis was again classified and the following definitions were made [5].

"Acute pancreatitis is an acute inflammatory process of the pancreas, with variable involvement of other regional tissues or remote organ systems.

Severe acute pancreatitis is associated with organ failure and/or local complications, such as necrosis, abscess, or pseudocyst. Abdominal findings include increased tenderness, rebound, distention, and hypoactive or absent bowel sounds. An epigastric mass may be present. Rarely, flank ecchymosis (Grey-Turner's sign), or periumbilical ecchymosis (Cullen's sign) may be seen.

Severe acute pancreatitis is further characterized by 3 or more Ranson criteria [12], or 8 or more APACHE-II (Acute Physiology and Chronic Health Evaluation) points [7].

Mild acute pancreatitis is associated with minimal organ dysfunction and an uneventful recovery, and it lacks the described features of severe acute pancreatitis.

Acute fluid collections occur early in the course of acute pancreatitis, are located in or near the pancreas, and always lack a wall of granulation or fibrous tissue. Acute fluid collections represent an earlier point in the development of acute pseudocysts or pancreatic abscesses. It is not known why most acute fluid collections regress while others progress to become pseudocysts or abscesses.

Pancreatic necrosis is a diffuse or focal area(s) of nonviable pancreatic parenchyma, which is typically associated with peripancreatic fat necrosis."

The clinical distinction between sterile pancreatic necrosis and infected pancreatic necrosis is critical, since development of infection in the necrotic tissues results in a 3-fold mortality risk.

"A pseudocyst is a collection of pancreatic juice enclosed by a wall of fibrous or granulation tissue, which arises as a consequence of acute pancreatitis, pancreatic trauma, or chronic pancreatitis."

When pus is present, the lesion is more correctly termed a pancreatic abscess.

"A pancreatic abscess is a circumscribed intraabdominal collection of pus, usually in proximity to the pancreas, containing little or no pancreatic necrosis, which arises as a consequence of acute pancreatitis or pancreatic trauma." A pseudocyst that becomes infected is also termed a pancreatic abscess.

4.7
Comment

Classification of different forms of a disease is necessary for comparison of interinstitutional data and follow-up examinations by clinicians and practioners. The Atlanta classification of acute pancreatitis is simple, noninvasive, objective, qualitative and accurate and should find entrance in general use of doctors taking care of patients with this disease and improve both patient care and quality of clinical research [3].

Regrettably, such a classification for chronic pancreatitis is currently not available.

References

1. Angelini G, Pederzoli P, Caliari S, Fratton S, Brocco G, Marzoli G, Bovo P, Cavallini G, Scuro LA (1984) Long-term outcome of acute necrohemorrhagic pancreatitis. A 4-year follow-up. Digestion 30:131–137
2. Axon ATR, Classen M, Cotton PB, Cremer M, Freeny PC, Lees WR (1984) Pancreatography in chronic pancreatitis: international definitions. Gut 25:1107–1112
3. Banks PA (1994) A new classification system for acute pancreatitis. Am J Gastroenterol 89:151–152
4. Banks PA, Bradley III EL, Dreiling DA, Frey CF, Go VLW, Ihse I, Imrie CW, Mallinson CN, McMahon MJ, Ranson JHC, Reber HA, Sarner M (1985) Classification of pancreatitis – Cambridge and Marseille. Gastroenterology 89:928–930
5. Bradley III EL (1993) A clinically based classification system for acute pancreatitis. Summary of the International Symposium on Acute Pancreatitis, Atlanta, Ga, September 11 through 13, 1992. Arch Surg 128:586–590
6. Frey CF (1986) Classification of pancreatitis: state-of-the-art, 1986. Pancreas 1:62–68
7. Knaus WA, Draper EA, Wagner DP, Zimmerman JE (1985) APACHE II: a severity of disease classification system. Critical Care Med 13:818–829
8. Lankisch PG, Andrén-Sandberg Å (1993) Standards for the diagnosis of chronic pancreatitis and for the evaluation of treatment. Int J Pancreatol 14:205–212
9. Lankisch PG, Otto J, Löhr A, Schirren C-A, Schuster R (1989) Pancreatic calcifications in patients with normal pancreatic function. Int J Pancreatol 5:281–293
10. Lankisch PG, Schreiber A, Otto J (1983) Pancreolauryl test. Evaluation of a tubeless pancreatic function test in comparison with other indirect and direct tests for exocrine pancreatic function. Dig Dis Sci 28:490–493

11. Lankisch PG, Seidensticker F, Otto J, Lübbers H, Mahlke R, Stöckmann F, Fölsch UR, Creutzfeldt W (1996) Secretin-pancreozymin test (SPT) and endoscopic retrograde cholangiopancreatography (ERCP): both are necessary for diagnosing or excluding chronic pancreatitis. Pancreas 12: 149–152

12. Ranson JHC, Rifkind KM, Roses DF, Fink SD, Eng K, Spencer FC (1974) Prognostic signs and the role of operative management in acute pancreatitis. Surg Gynecol Obstet 139:69–81

13. Sarles H (1965) Proposal adopted unanimously by the participants of the Symposium, Marseilles 1963. In: Sarles H (ed) Pancreatitis. Bibl. Gastroenterol. 7. Karger, Basel-New York, pp VII–VIII

14. Sarles H (1991) Definitions and classifications of pancreatitis. Pancreas 6:470–474

15. Sarles H, Adler G, Dani R, Frey C, Gullo L, Harada H, Martin E, Norohna M, Scuro LA (1989) The pancreatitis classification of Marseilles-Rome 1988. Scand J Gastroenterol 24:641–642

16. Sarner M, Cotton PB (1984) Classification of pancreatitis. Gut 25:756–759

17. Sarner M, Cotton PB (1984) Definitions of acute and chronic pancreatitis. Clin Gastroenterol 13: 865–870

18. Seidensticker F, Otto J, Lankisch PG (1995) Recovery of the pancreas after acute pancreatitis is not necessarily complete. Int J Pancreatol 17:225–229

19. Singer MW, Gyr K, Sarles H (1985) Revised classification of pancreatitis. Report of the Second International Symposium on the Classification of Pancreatitis in Marseille, France, March 28–30, 1984. Gastroenterology 89:683–685

5 Acute Pancreatitis: Etiology

The list of etiological factors of acute pancreatitis is long (Table 5.1). Most frequent etiologies of acute pancreatitis are biliary tract disease (38.1%) and alcoholism (35.4%) (Table 5.2). In about 10% of the patients, rare etiologies are responsible, but in 10%–30% of the patients, etiology remains unknown.

Percentage data on the different etiologies may differ considerably according to the individual hospital experience, location, and patient population. Geographical differences also play a role. Finally, the percentages shift over the years. In Germany, a shift

Table 5.1. Etiological factors for acute pancreatitis

- Biliary tract disease
- Alcoholism
- Obstruction of the pancreatic duct
  Tumors
  Duodenal disorders
  Pancreas divisum
  Helminthic obstruction
  Foreign body obstruction
- Infections
- Drugs
- Toxins
- Endocrine and metabolic disorders
  Primary hyperparathyroidism and hypercalcemia
  Pregnancy
  Hyperlipemia
  Hypothermia
- Vascular diseases
- Trauma
- Medical procedures
  Pancreatic biopsy
  Endoscopic retrograde cholangiopancreatography and endoscopic sphincterotomy
  Sphincter of Oddi manometry
- Surgical procedures
- Cystic fibrosis
- Inborn errors of metabolism
- Reye's syndrome
- Kawasaki disease
- Hereditary acute pancreatitis
- Unknown (idiopathic acute pancreatitis)

Table 5.2. Studies published during the last 3 decades with detailed data concerning gender distribution and the etiology of acute pancreatitis (first attack), including more than 100 patients each

Author(s)/ Place of the investigation	Period	Patients *n*	Men %	Women %	Etiology Biliary (%)	Alcoholism (%)
Renner et al. [167] Los Angeles	1949–1978	405	62.7	37.3	27.9	67.7
Trapnell and Duncan [208] Bristol	1950–1969	590	38.3	61.7	53.6	4.4
Edlund et al. [47] Göteborg	1956–1960	460	52.2	47.8	68.0	13.0
Imrie [82] Glasgow	1960–1970	140	47.8	52.2	50.0	12.2
Madsen and Schmidt [122] Copenhagen	1960–1970	122	68.8	31.2	14.0	40.0
Jacobs et al. [85] Boston	1963–1969	519	54.9	45.1	47.0	31.0
Satiani and Stone [182] Atlanta	1966–1975	389	59.9	40.1	3.1	91.8
Lukash [119] Bethesda	Not mentioned	100	82.0	18.0	23.0	66.0
Ong et al. [148] Hong Kong	1967–1976	311	39.5	60.5	52.4	15.1
Svensson et al. [196] Göteborg	1968–1969 1974–1975	105 204	83.0 77.0	17.0 23.0	20.0 26.0	68.0 66.0
Corfield et al. [37] Bristol	1968–1979	638	48.7	51.3	50.0	8.0
Thomson [204] Aberdeen	1968–1980	632	47.8	52.2	44.0	19.0
Ranson and Spencer [163] New York	1971–1977	450	78.0	22.0	16.0	70.0
Thomson et al. [205] Aberdeen	1983–1985	359	52.6	47.4	40.9	15.3
Fan et al. [52] Hong Kong	1983–1986	268	42.9	57.1	50.0	12.3
Fan et al. [51] Hong Kong	1988–1991	176	39.2	60.8	57.4	12.5
Beaux et al. [22] Edinburgh	1989–1993	279	61.6	38.4	41.6	34.8
Lankisch et al. [102] Göttingen-Lüneburg	1980–1994	602	55.6	44.4	37.7	29.4
Total	1949–1994	6749	57.4	42.6	38.1	35.4

from biliary tract disease to alcoholism as the major etiology has been reported [109]. Studies from England and Sweden reported a 3-fold [37] and 4-fold [196] increase of alcoholic pancreatitis.

5.1
Biliary Tract Disease

As the most common obstructive cause of acute pancreatitis, gallstones are associated with 30%–75% of all cases of the disease [17,192]. Obesity is frequent among these patients. The peak incidence of age is between 50 and 60 years and more women than men are affected [102,192]. However, acute pancreatitis seems to occur more frequently in male patients with gallstones than in women with gallstone disease [9,47,201]. In the majority of patients with so-called biliary pancreatitis, stones are found in the gallbladder, but not in the common bile duct, and stones impacted in the distal common bile duct are reported in only 3%–5% of patients with acute pancreatitis [214]. It is believed that gallstones cause acute pancreatitis by lodging temporarily in the sphincter of Oddi and then passing into the small intestine. The discussion is still controversial (see Sect. 6.5). The frequency of acute pancreatitis is inversely proportional to the size of stones. Houssin et al. [80] found that 20.2% of patients with microlithiasis (diameter <3 mm), 5% of patients with small stones (3–9 mm), 3% of patients with medium-sized stones (10–20 mm), and 1% of patients with larger stones (>20 mm) suffer from acute pancreatitis.

Choledochal cysts [59, 70, 88, 92, 144, 147, 198] are said to induce acute pancreatitis due to a long common channel with the risk of reflux of bile into the pancreatic duct. Juxtapapillary diverticula may also be associated with gallstones and acute pancreatitis [113, 158].

5.2
Alcoholism

Biliary tract disease is the predominant etiology in women, and excess alcohol consumption in men [89].

However, it is not clear whether an episode of acute pancreatitis associated with alcohol abuse represents an attack of acute or chronic pancreatitis. The diagnosis of acute pancreatitis implies that prior to the attack the pancreas was perfectly normal in all structural and functional aspects. With few exceptions, however, the antecedent state of the gland is unknown. Nevertheless, in the absence of signs of chronic pancreatitis, e.g., calcifications, at least the initial attacks of pancreatitis in an alcoholic are assumed to be "acute pancreatitis".

The typical case history of a patient with presumably alcohol-induced acute pancreatitis shows a consumption of large quantities of alcohol for 5–10 years prior to the first attack. Sometimes, acute pancreatitis occurs after a shorter exposure to alcohol. Recent work from the group of Ammann [7, 8] shows the progression of several attacks of acute pancreatitis to subsequent chronic pancreatitis. The mechanism by which alcohol might precipitate acute pancreatitis is unknown. Alcohol may exert a direct toxic effect on the acinar cells or influence exocrine pancreatic secretion and the sphincter of Oddi. Oral administration of alcohol causes transient stimulation of exocrine pancreatic secretion, followed by a later period of inhibition [139, 207], and causes contraction of the sphincter of Oddi [159]. The latter combined effect could explain acute pancreatitis after a drinking bout [191].

5.3
Obstruction of Pancreatic Ducts

5.3.1
Tumors

In animal experiments, simple occlusion of the pancreatic duct produces edema and, later on, atrophy and fibrosis of the pancreas but not actually pancreatitis [77].

Yet, partial or complete pancreatic outflow obstruction may facilitate the development of pancreatitis if other pathogenetic factors, such as vigorous stimulation of pancreatic secretion or vascular damage, are present [131].

Pancreatic carcinoma, either obstructing the duct system or involving the gland itself, or both, may induce acute pancreatitis [25, 65, 177]. Two studies – one on patients with all types of pancreatic carcinoma [100] and the other on ampullary carcinoma only [170] – reported an incidence of acute pancreatitis of 13.8% and 14.6%, respectively, and of hyperamylasemia in an additional 9.8% and 7.3%, respectively. Clinically, acute pancreatitis was mild to moderate, and modern imaging procedures soon revealed the underlying disease. Intraductal papillary-mucinous tumors may also cause acute pancreatitis (see Sect. 13.6).

A variety of nonpancreatic carcinoma, mainly bronchogenic carcinoma, but also tumors of the urogenital tract, gastric carcinoma, melanoma, tumors of the tonsillar glands and non-Hodgkin lymphoma, has been reported to metastasize into the pancreas and induce acute pancreatitis [15, 31, 73, 91, 104, 117, 121, 134, 140, 145, 165, 184, 197, 221]. The incidence rate may be as high as 7.5% of patients with oat cell lung cancer [221].

5.3.2
Duodenal Disorders

Periampullary duodenal diverticulae have been found with variable frequency in patients undergoing endoscopic retrograde cholangiopancreatography (ERCP): 23% [149], 5% [95], and 9% [113]. These duodenal disorders as well as obstruction of the ampulla of Vater by periampullary polyps of the duodenum [71], have been held responsible for recurrent pancreatitis and biliary tract disease.

Acute pancreatitis can complicate obstruction of the duodenum. This has been observed in cases of annular pancreas [5] (see Sect. 1.2.4), obstruction of an intraluminal duodenal diverticulum [81, 143], superior mesenteric artery syndrome, and obstructed afferent loop after gastrectomy [43, 136, 152].

Furthermore, involvement of the duodenum and especially of the papilla of Vater in Crohn's disease has been reported to induce acute pancreatitis [112].

5.3.3
Pancreas Divisum

Pancreas divisum results from incomplete fusion of the dorsal and ventral ductal systems (see Fig. 1.2). Whether pancreas divisum is related to acute and/or chronic pancreatitis is controversial. Authors in favor of an association have hypothesized that the accessory papilla and Santorini's duct are too small to accept total pancreatic secretion, resulting eventually in obstructive pain and pancreatitis (for details, see Sect. 1.2.2).

5.3.4
Helminthic Obstruction

Another form of obstructive acute pancreatitis, uncommon in the Western world, is ascariasis, the world's most common helminthic infection. It results from the migration of worms in and out of the biliary and pancreatic ductal system [93, 94, 115, 162, 192, 215]. Treatment includes various endoscopical procedures for removal of the worms [94, 115, 222].

5.3.5
Foreign Body Obstruction

Further curiosities obstructing the pancreatic duct and leading to acute pancreatitis include dental filaments, cornhusk bristles and vegetables [23, 39, 135].

5.4
Infections

The pancreas may be affected by several infectious diseases. In these cases, acute pancreatitis is usually mild, often subclinical, and tends to heal with disappearance of the infection.

Mumps is one such well known viral infection [56, 217]. Acute pancreatitis has also been reported in patients with infectious mononucleosis [74, 216]. Several studies have shown that acute pancreatitis is frequently associated with Coxsackie B virus [83], ECHO viruses, *Mycoplasma pneumoniae* infections [62, 128, 129], as well as varicella and measles [4, 83, 96]. Acute pancreatitis may also complicate fulminant viral hepatitis [2, 66, 107]. Proof that hepatitis virus may involve the pancreas has been strengthened by the finding of hepatitis B surface antigen in the pancreas [78]. However, acute pancreatitis has also been documented in liver failure of other origin [107,

151] so that the occurrence of acute pancreatitis may be the result of metabolic disturbances accompanying acute hepatic failure in general.

Furthermore, acute pancreatitis may occur in cases of salmonellosis and *Campylobacter* infection [41, 64, 161]. Involvement of the pancreas has also been described in tuberculosis and sarcoidosis [53, 130, 156, 175, 193, 220].

More recently, hyperamylasemia and acute pancreatitis in human immunodeficiency virus- (HIV-)infected patients have aroused considerable interest. However, it is not clear whether the HIV infection itself or concomitant opportunistic infections (cytomegalovirus, *Mycobacterium* tuberculosis, *Mycobacterium avium* complex or *Cryptococcus neoformans*), drugs (didanosine [ddI], pentamidine, trimethoprim-sulphamethoxazole or zalcitabine [ddC]), or neoplasm (Kaposi's sarcoma or lymphoma) are responsible for the induction of acute pancreatitis [27, 28, 32, 35, 142, 209, 213, 218].

5.5
Drugs

Ever since the first reports on cortisone [223] and thiazides [87] inducing acute pancreatitis, a large number of single case reports have been published on drug-induced acute pancreatitis. Subsequent review articles have noted deficiencies including inconsistency in the time interval between drug application and the onset of acute pancreatitis, and paucity of rechallenge trials. At present, the literature has identified about 30 drugs that definitely or possibly may be held responsible for inducing acute pancreatitis (Table 5.3) [42, 123, 124]. All drugs mentioned are given daily to thousands of patients all over the world without any signs and symptoms of acute pancreatitis. It is unknown, what precondition induces acute pancreatitis in a select few.

In the experience of the authors, drugs most frequently associated with acute pancreatitis are azathioprine, valproic acid, didanosine (ddI), pentamidine, and 5-ASA compounds.

A recent study on the incidence and severity of drug-induced acute pancreatitis included 1613 patients with acute pancreatitis treated in 45 German centers of gastroenterology. Drug-induced acute pancreatitis was diagnosed in 22 patients (incidence 1.4%). Laboratory investigations and imaging procedures showed that the disease usually takes a benign course. The mortality rate of 9% (2 patients) was due to the underlying disease and not to acute pancreatitis [103].

Despite epidemic levels of drug abuse in many industrial countries, very little is known about drug-related pancreatitis. Heffernon et al. [75] found that hyperamylasemia that occurs in 19% of heroin addicts, is probably caused by acute pulmonary complications ("heroin lung") rather than by the pancreas. There is a doubtful case of acute pancreatitis after marijuana smoking [40]. We recently reported on a case of acute pancreatitis following heroin intoxication [106]. Heroin (diacetyl morphine) is 6 times more potent than morphine and may have induced acute pancreatitis by causing temporary spasm or obstruction of the sphincter of Oddi. Further case reports would be of interest.

Table 5.3. Drugs held responsible for induction of acute pancreatitis [123]

1. **Drugs definitely associated with acute pancreatitis**

Azathioprine	Estrogens
Sulphonamides	Furosemide
Sulindac	6-mercaptopurine
Tetracycline	Pentamidine[a]
Valproic acid	5-ASA compounds
Didanosine (ddI)[a]	Corticosteroids[b]
Methyldopa	Octreotide[a]

2. **Drugs probably associated with acute pancreatitis**

Chlorothiazide and hydrochlorothiazide[c]	Colaspase
Hypercalcemia (iatrogenic)	Chlorthalidone
Methandienone	Combination cancer chemotherapy
Metronidazole	Cimetidine
Nitrofurantoin	Cisplatin
Phenformin	Cytosine arabinoside
Piroxicam	Diphenoxylate
Procainamide	Ethacrynic acid

3. **Drugs with a proposed association with pancreatitis, but evidence is contradictory or inadequate**

Amoxapine	Ibuprofen
Amphetamines	Lipid infusions
β-adrenergic blocking drugs	Mefenamic acid
BHI Regeneration tablets	Opiates
Carbamazepine	Paracetamol
Cholestyramine	Phenolphthalein
Colchicine	Rifampicin
Cyproheptadine	Salicylates
Diazoxide	Ticarcillin/clavulanic acid
Histamine	Warfarin
Indomethacin	

[a] Added to the original table from [123].
[b] Changed from group 2 to 1 according to the authors' opinion.
[c] Changed from group 1 to 2 according to the authors' opinion.

5.6
Toxins

Poisoning by a sting of *Tityus trinitatis* seems to be the most common cause of acute pancreatitis in Trinidad [19]. Subsequent intensive studies led to the scorpions' extinction on the island, but clarified the underlying mechanism of acute scorpion venom pancreatitis. The venom acted directly on the canine pancreas, on the one hand stimulating exocrine pancreatic enzyme secretion, and on the other hand contracting the sphincter of Oddi [20, 21, 181]. Other scorpion venoms are experimentally able to produce acute hemorrhagic pancreatitis [166].

Both painful and almost painless acute pancreatitis have been reported after cutaneous exposure to an organophosphate insecticide [126] and as a complication of organophosphate poisoning [105, 138].

5.7
Endocrine and Metabolic Disorders

5.7.1
Primary Hyperparathyroidism and Hypercalcemia

Clinical evidence of pancreatitis has been described in about 7% of patients with primary hyperparathyroidism [36, 183]. All types of acute and chronic pancreatitis have been described (see also Sect. 13.10). In a recent survey on 234 patients with primary hyperparathyroidism, diagnosis was made during acute pancreatitis [99].

The mechanism by which primary hyperparathyroidism induces acute pancreatitis is unknown. Hypercalcemia, which stimulates pancreatic enzyme secretion in man [69, 79] and animals [110], may play a role. Furthermore, hypercalcemia may cause acute pancreatitis by pancreatic secretory block, intracellular zymogen accumulation and acinar injury [63]. Patients treated with total parenteral nutrition (TPN) may develop hypercalcemia and pancreatitis [84]. Since TPN is used in severe acute pancreatitis, careful monitoring of serum calcium is recommended to prevent further damage to the pancreas.

5.7.2
Pregnancy

More than 100 cases of acute pancreatitis during pregnancy, especially in the last trimester, or in the postpartum period, have been reported [24]. More recent studies show that acute pancreatitis during pregnancy is mainly caused by some other coincident processes, most frequently gallstone disease [132, 202]. Therefore, pregnancy is probably not an etiological factor in acute pancreatitis.

5.7.3
Hyperlipemia

Patients with types I and V familial hyperlipoproteinemia may have attacks of acute pancreatitis. In these cases, hyperlipemia persists. In addition, hyperlipemia may occasionally occur as a sequela of acute pancreatitis. The preconditions of this complication and its incidence are unknown. Hyperlipemia vanishes with recovery.

In a recent study on the clinical assessment of hyperlipidemic pancreatitis, hypertriglyceridemia was the etiology in 1.3%–3.8% of patients discharged with a diagnosis of pancreatitis. The most common presentations were the following three: a poorly controlled diabetic with a history of hypertriglyceridemia, an alcoholic found to have hypertriglyceridemia or lactescent serum on admission, and nondiabetic, nonalcoholic, nonobese patients with drug- or diet-induced hypertriglyceridemia [60].

5.7.4
Uremia

In chronic uremia patients, chronic pancreatitis is frequent [1, 11, 12, 14]. Acute pancreatitis has been described with a 10-year incidence of 2.3% and an overall mortality of 20.8% in patients with end-stage renal disease without transplantation, more frequently associated with peritoneal dialysis than with hemodialysis [176]. In another series, the incidence was 6.4% and acute pancreatitis was more frequent in renal end-stage patients with alcohol abuse, systemic lupus erythematosus, and polycystic kidney disease [150]. Finally, a third series showed that acute pancreatitis occurred in 3.2% patients undergoing hemodialysis and 5.2% patients on chronic ambulatory peritoneal dialysis during a 4-year period [200].

5.7.5
Acute Intermittent Porphyria

Two cases of acute pancreatitis in acute intermittent porphyria have been described, the etiological link being unknown [98, 114].

5.7.6
Hypothermia

Acute pancreatitis is a common finding in adult patients with accidental hypothermia. Between 50% and 65% of hypothermic patients have raised serum amylase activity, and acute pancreatitis is found at necropsy in 20%–30% of the cases [44, 120]. Ischemia resulting from the microcirculatory shock of hypothermia is viewed as a likely operative factor in the causation of the pancreatic damage [61].

5.8
Vascular Disease

Because of the very efficient collateral blood supply of the pancreas, primary vascular disease is rarely the sole causative factor for pancreatitis. In most cases, local ischemia of the pancreas must be accompanied by other noxious factors in order to induce acute pancreatitis. So-called idiopathic pancreatitis has been attributed to a combination of stenosing atheromatosis in pancreatic vessels and shock [137]. Diffuse vascular injury to the pancreas as by necrotizing angiitis caused by amphetamines [34], malignant hypertension [133], periarteriitis nodosa [133, 146, 154], and systemic lupus erythematosus [29, 67, 125, 160, 169, 190, 219] may result in pancreatitis. The exact etiological links are unknown.

5.9
Trauma

Pancreatic injury occurs more frequently after a penetrating than after a blunt abdominal trauma [76]. Ryan et al. [179] reported elevated amylase and lipase levels in 17% and clinical acute pancreatitis in 5% of patients following abdominal trauma.

The degree of injury may range from mild contusion to fracture. Acute pancreatitis is the consequence of disruption of the ductular, vascular, and parenchymatous continuity and subsequent extravasation of enzymes. The incidence of pancreatic trauma as etiology of acute pancreatitis was 1.5% in a series of 5864 patients collected by Dürr [45].

About 40% of patients with large burns develop hyperamylasemia or hyperlipasemia. Most have symptoms of acute pancreatitis. Patients with high enzyme elevations and $\geq$ 50% body surface area burned were at severe risk of pancreatic pseudocyst or abscess development [178].

5.10
Medical Procedures

5.10.1
Pancreatic Biopsy

Severe and even fatal acute pancreatitis may occur following fine-needle (19–22 gauge) biopsies of the pancreas [46, 50, 116, 189]. In a series of 184 biopsies in 178 patients, severe acute pancreatitis developed in 5 (3%) patients usually within 24–48 h, independent of whether the pancreas was normal or diseased prior to biopsy [141]. Finally, percutaneous biopsy (20–22 gauge needles) of left adrenal masses via the anterior approach, routinely traversing the tail of the pancreas, led to acute pancreatitis in 6% of the cases [90].

5.10.2
Endoscopic Retrograde Cholangiopancreatography
and Endoscopic Sphincterotomy

Acute pancreatitis may occur after ERCP and endoscopic sphincterotomy (ES). During both procedures the pancreas is subjected to many types of potential injury: mechanical, chemical, hydrostatic, enzymatic, microbiological, allergic, and thermal. Incidence rates are low. In a retrospective survey of 25,299 patients who underwent ERCP, 229 (0.9%) patients developed acute pancreatitis, 6 (0.03%) required surgery and 4 (0.02%) died. Of 17,168 patients who underwent ES, 289 (1.7%) developed acute pancreatitis, 23 (0.13%) needed surgery and 35 (0.2%) died. Prospectively, the incidence of ERCP-related acute pancreatitis is 5% [186]. However, this was the combined result of 14 studies and definitions of post-ERCP pancreatitis may have differed among them

[186]. In general, post-ERCP pancreatitis should be diagnosed in patients with post-ERCP abdominal pain for > 24 h requiring narcotic administration plus elevated pancreatic enzymes. The diagnosis should be confirmed and the severity be assessed by an imaging procedure, e.g., CT scan.

Patient factors that increase the risk for pancreatitis in addition to inexperience of the endoscopist:
- Sphincter of Oddi disease or variant anatomy as manifested by abnormal manometry, prolonged contrast drainage time, dilated pancreatic duct, difficult cannulation
- ES performed in a setting of nondilated bile duct
- Recent or recurrent pancreatitis of any etiology
- Pseudocysts
- Pancreatic duct stricture
- Prior ERCP-induced pancreatitis [186]

5.10.3
Sphincter of Oddi Manometry

Acute pancreatitis may occur after sphincter of Oddi manometry with an overall risk between 6% and 14.5% [172, 187]. Acute pancreatitis seems to be mild in most patients; it occurs more frequently after catheterization of the pancreatic than of the bile duct and more frequently in patients with than without signs of chronic pancreatitis [172]. The frequency of acute pancreatitis caused by sphincter of Oddi manometry may be significantly decreased by using an aspiration manometry catheter which permits continuous aspiration of instilled fluid.

5.11
Surgical Procedures

Postoperative acute pancreatitis may occur after a variety of intraabdominal procedures including biliary tract operations, gastric resections, colectomies, and splenectomies [18, 30, 180, 185, 212]. How such surgical procedures lead to acute pancreatitis is unknown. Postoperative pancreatitis is rare with incidence rates of 0.6%–1.2% in large series [185, 210]. The condition is difficult to recognize and frequently not detected [108, 203]. The complication rate is significantly higher than in patients with acute pancreatitis of other etiologies [26] and mortality rate twice as high as in other etiologies [157].

Postoperative pancreatitis occurs also after operations in areas far away from the pancreas, e.g., after parathyroidectomy [118, 212].

Acute pancreatitis has also been reported following cardiac surgery including cardiopulmonary transplantation [3, 13, 55, 164, 174]. Risk factors for pancreatic cellular injury after cardiopulmonary bypass defined as hyperamylasemia with an increase in lipase or pancreatic isoamylase were preoperative renal insufficiency, valve surgery, postoperative hypotension, and perioperative administration of a considerable amount of calcium chloride [58].

Acute pancreatitis has also been described following liver transplantation [6, 101], and frequently after renal transplantation, ranging from 0.4%–7% [38, 48, 54, 57, 86, 155, 171, 199]. The mortality rate of this complication is distressingly high, varying from 20% in one small series [38] to 50%–70% [57, 86, 155]. Pancreatitis may occur within a few days after transplantation (true postoperative pancreatitis?) or, more commonly, several months or even years following surgery. Special medication given after renal transplanation, such as azathioprine, glucocorticoids, and L-asparaginase, may contribute to the development of pancreatitis [38]. Various infections, postoperative hyperparathyroidism and vasculitis have also been discussed as etiological factors [86, 206]. Pathologically, posttransplantation pancreatitis may be associated with marked destruction of the organ, including severe vasculitis [206], necrotizing pancreatitis [38], pancreatic abscess and pseudocyst [168]. Recently, acute pancreatitis has been observed also after marrow transplantation and was observed in 27% of autopsied marrow transplant patients [97].

5.12
Cystic Fibrosis

Shwachman et al. [188] reported acute pancreatitis in 0.5% of all cystic fibrosis patients. Other reports have also shown that acute pancreatitis may be a complication of cystic fibrosis and even be the initial presentation of the disease in the adult (see Sect. 21.1.1) [10, 72, 127].

5.13
Inborn Errors of Metabolism

Acute pancreatitis has been reported in single cases of patients with a variety of inborn errors of metabolism (see Sect. 21.2.3).

5.14
Reye's Syndrome

Acute pancreatitis has been found to be associated with Reye's syndrome and acute encephalopathy of other origin. Etiological connections are unclear [16, 33, 49, 68, 153, 195, 211].

5.15
Kawasaki Disease

Some patients with acute pancreatitis in Kawasaki disease (mucocutaneous lymph node syndrome) have been reported. The etiological connections are unclear [194].

5.16
Hereditary Acute Pancreatitis

For details see Sect. 21.2.1.

5.17
Idiopathic Acute Pancreatitis

Despite numerous actual and potential etiological factors that have been identified, the cause of acute pancreatitis is obscure in a number of cases. After gallstones and alcoholism, idiopathic etiology is the third main cause in most reported series. Recently, two studies indicated that the majority of cases of idiopathic pancreatitis were caused by biliary sludge and microlithiasis. No recurrence of acute pancreatitis occurred among patients following ES, gallbladder removal, or treatment with ursodeoxycholic acid [111, 173].

References

1. Abu-Alfa A, Ivanovich P, Mujais SK (1988) Uremic exocrine pancreopathy. Nephron 48:94–100
2. Achord JL (1968) Acute pancreatitis with infectious hepatitis. JAMA 205:129–132
3. Adiseshiah M, Wells FC, Cory-Pearce R, Wallwork J, English TAH (1983) Acute pancreatitis after cardiac transplantation. World J Surg 7:519–521
4. Adler JB, Mazzotta SA, Barkin JS (1991) Pancreatitis caused by measles, mumps, and rubella vaccine. Pancreas 6:489–490
5. Alexander HC (1970) Annular pancreas in the adult. Am J Surg 119:702–704
6. Alexander JA, Demetrius AJ, Gavaler JS, Makowka L, Starzl TE, Van Thiel DH (1988) Pancreatitis following liver transplantation. Transplantation 45:1062–1065
7. Ammann RW, Heitz PU, Klöppel G (1996) Course of alcoholic chronic pancreatitis: a prospective clinicomorphological long-term study. Gastroenterology 111:224–231
8. Ammann RW, Muellhaupt B (1994) Progression of alcoholic acute to chronic pancreatitis. Gut 35:552–556
9. Armstrong CP, Taylor TV, Jeacock J, Lucas S (1985) The biliary tract in patients with acute gallstone pancreatitis. Br J Surg 72:551–555
10. Atlas AB, Orenstein SR, Orenstein DM (1992) Pancreatitis in young children with cystic fibrosis. J Pediatr 120:756–759
11. Avram MM (1977) High prevalence of pancreatic disease in chronic renal failure. Nephron 18:68–71
12. Avram RM, Iancu M (1982) Pancreatic disease in uremia and parathyroid hormone excess. Nephron 32:60–62
13. Aziz S, Bergdahl L, Baldwin JC, Weiss LM, Jamieson SW, Oyer PE, Stinson EB, Shumway NE (1985) Pancreatitis after cardiac and cardiopulmonary transplantation. Surgery 97:653–661
14. Baggenstoss AH (1948) The pancreas in uremia: a histopathologic study. Am J Pathol 24:1003–1011
15. Balch CM (1985) Diagnostik und Prognose des malignen Melanoms. Dtsch Med Wochenschr 110:1783–1786
16. Banks PA (1981) Pancreatitis in Reye's syndrome? J Clin Gastroenterol 3:201–202
17. Banks PA (1995) Acute pancreatitis. In: Haubrich WS, Schaffner F, Berk JE (eds) Bockus Gastroenterology, vol. 4, 5th edn, W.B. Saunders Comp., Philadelphia-London-Toronto etc, pp 2888–2917

18. Bardenheier JA, Kaminski DL, Willman VL (1968) Pancreatitis after biliary tract surgery. Am J Surg 116:773–776
19. Bartholomew C (1970) Acute scorpion pancreatitis in Trinidad. Br Med J 1:666–668
20. Bartholomew C, McGeeney KF, Murphy JJ, FitzGerald O, Sankaran H (1976) Experimental studies on the aetiology of acute scorpion pancreatitis. Br J Surg 63:807–810
21. Bartholomew C, Murphy JJ, McGeeney KF, FitzGerald O (1977) Exocrine pancreatic response to the venom of the scorpion, Tytyus trinitatis. Gut 18:623–625
22. Beaux ACde, Palmer KR, Carter DC (1995) Factors influencing morbidity and mortality in acute pancreatitis; an analysis of 279 cases. Gut 37:121–126
23. Bedran K, Lucidarme D, Pollet E, Triboulet J-P, Lecomte-Houcke M, Filoche B (1994) Pancréatite aiguë récurrente secondaire à un corps étranger végétal dans le canal de Wirsung. Gastroenterol Clin Biol 18:1154–1156
24. Berk JE, Smith BH, Akrawi MM (1971) Pregnancy pancreatitis. Am J Gastroenterol 56:216–226
25. Bonetti A, Deyhle P, Largiadèr F, Nüesch HJ, Häcki WH, Satz N, Ammann R (1980) Pankreasmalignome, assoziiert mit Pankreatitis bzw. Pseudozysten. Schweiz Med Wochenschr 110:852–853
26. Bragg LE, Thompson JS, Burnett DA, Hodgson PE, Rikkers LF (1985) Increased incidence of pancreas-related complications in patients with postoperative pancreatitis. Am J Surg 150:694–697
27. Brivet F, Coffin B, Bedossa P, Naveau S, Petitpretz P, Delfraissy JF, Dormont J (1987) Pancreatic lesions in AIDS. Lancet 2:570–571
28. Brivet FG, Naveau SH, Lemaigre GF, Dormont J (1994) Pancreatic lesions in HIV-infected patients. Baillière Clin Endocrinol Metabol 8:859–877
29. Bruijn JA, van Albada-Kuipers GA, Smit VTHBM, Eulderink F (1986) Acute pancreatitis in systemic lupus erythematosus. Scand J Rheumatol 15:363–367
30. Burton CC, Eckman WG Jr, Haxo J (1957) Acute postgastrectomy pancreatitis. Am J Surg 94:70–79
31. Cameron-Strange A (1983) Acute pancreatitis associated with lymphosarcoma. Br J Surg 70:444
32. Cappell MS, Hassan T (1993) Pancreatic disease in AIDS – A review. J Clin Gastroenterol 17:254–263
33. Chaves-Carballo E, Menezes AH, Bell WE, Hernriquez EM (1980) Acute pancreatitis in Reye's syndrome: a fatal complication during intensive supportive care. South Med J 73:152–154
34. Citron BP, Halpern M, McCarron M, Lundberg GD, McCormick R, Pincus IJ, Tatter D, Haverback BJ (1970) Necrotizing angiitis associated with drug abuse. N Engl J Med 283:1003–1011
35. Clas D, Falutz J, Rosenberg L (1989) Acute pancreatitis associated with HIV infection. CMA J 140:823
36. Cope O, Culver PJ, Mixter CG Jr, Nardi GL (1957) Pancreatitis, a diagnostic clue to hyperparathyroidism. Ann Surg 145:857–863
37. Corfield AP, Cooper MJ, Williamson RCN (1985) Acute pancreatitis: a lethal disease of increasing incidence. Gut 26:724–729
38. Corrodi P, Knoblauch M, Binswanger U, Schölzel E, Largiadèr F (1975) Pancreatitis after renal transplantation. Gut 16:285–289
39. Danzi JT (1986) Two cases of acute pancreatitis due to a foreign body. Gastrointest Endosc 32:360–361
40. Darby V, Aach RA (1985) Acute pancreatitis after marijuana smoking: is there a relationship? JAMA 253:1791
41. De Bois MHW, Schoemaker MC, Van der Werf SDJ, Puylaert JBCM (1989) Pancreatitis associated with Campylobacter jejuni infection: diagnosis by ultrasound. Br Med J 298:1004
42. Dobrilla G, Felder M, Chilovi F (1985) Medikamentös induzierte akute Pankreatitis. Schweiz Med Wochenschr 115:850–858
43. Dreiling DA, Kirschner PA, Nemser H (1960) Chronic duodenal obstruction: a mechano-vascular etiology of pancreatitis. I. Report of 6 cases illustrating this clinical variety. Am J Dig Dis 5:991–1005
44. Duguid H, Simpson RG, Stowers JM (1961) Accidental hypothermia. Lancet 2:1213–1221
45. Dürr H-K (1979) Acute pancreatitis. In: Howat HT, Sarles H (eds) The Exocrine Pancreas. W.B. Saunders Comp., London–Philadelphia–Toronto, pp 352–401
46. Dzieniszewski GP, Neher M, Linhart P, Frank K (1982) Nekrotisierende Pankreatitis nach ultraschallgezielter Feinnadelpunktion. Dtsch Med Wochenschr 107:1438–1440

47. Edlund Y, Norbäck B, Risholm L (1968) Acute pancreatitis, etiology and prevention of recurrence. Follow-up study of 188 patients. Rev Surg 25:153–157
48. Eigler FW, Dostal G, Beersiek F, Medrano J, Bock K-D, Hartmann H, Kuwert EK (1979) Ergebnisse bei 200 Nierentransplantationen. Dtsch Med Wochenschr 104:1172–1176
49. Ellis GH, Mirkin LD, Mills MC (1979) Pancreatitis and Reye's syndrome. Am J Dis Child 133:1014–1016
50. Evans WK, Ho C-S, McLoughlin MJ, Tao L-C (1981) Fatal necrotizing pancreatitis following fine-needle aspiration biopsy of the pancreas. Radiology 141:61–62
51. Fan S-T, Lai ECS, Mok FPT, Lo C-M, Zheng S-S, Wong J (1993) Prediction of the severity of acute pancreatitis. Am J Surg 166:262–269
52. Fan ST, Choi TK, Lai CS, Wong J (1988) Influence of age on the mortality from acute pancreatitis. Br J Surg 75:463–466
53. Fan ST, Yan KW, Lau WY, Wong KK (1986) Tuberculosis of the pancreas: a rare cause of massive gastrointestinal bleeding. Br J Surg 73:373
54. Faro RS, Corry RJ (1979) Management of surgical gastrointestinal complications in renal transplant recipients. Arch Surg 114:310–312
55. Feiner H (1976) Pancreatitis after cardiac surgery. A morphologic study. Am J Surg 131:684–688
56. Feldstein JD, Johnson FR, Kallick CA, Doolas A (1974) Acute hemorrhagic pancreatitis and pseudocyst due to mumps. Ann Surg 180:85–88
57. Fernandez JA, Rosenberg JC (1976) Post-transplantation pancreatitis. Surg Gynecol Obstet 143:795–798
58. Fernández-del Castillo C, Harringer W, Warshaw AL, Vlahakes GJ, Koski G, Zaslavsky AM, Rattner DW (1991) Risk factors for pancreatic cellular injury after cardiopulmonary bypass. N Engl J Med 325:382–387
59. Forbes A, Leung JWC, Cotton PB (1984) Relapsing acute and chronic pancreatitis. Arch Dis Child 59:927–934
60. Fortson MR, Freedman SN, Webster PD (1995) Clinical assessment of hyperlipidemic pancreatitis. Am J Gastroenterol 90:2134–2139
61. Foulis AK (1982) Morphological study of the relation between accidental hypothermia and acute pancreatitis. J Clin Pathol 35:1244–1248
62. Freeman R, McMahon MJ (1978) Acute pancreatitis and serological evidence of infection with mycoplasma pneumoniae. Gut 19:367–370
63. Frick TW, Mithöfer K, Fernández-del Castillo C, Rattner DW, Warshaw AL (1995) Hypercalcemia causes acute pancreatitis by pancreatic secretory block, intracellular zymogen accumulation, and acinar cell injury. Am J Surg 169:167–172
64. Gallagher P, Chadwick P, Jones DM, Turner L (1981) Acute pancreatitis associated with campylobacter infection. Br J Surg 68:383
65. Gambill EE (1971) Pancreatitis associated with pancreatic carcinoma: a study of 26 cases. Mayo Clin Proc 46:174–177
66. Geokas MC, Olsen H, Swanson V, Rinderknecht H (1972) The association of viral hepatitis and acute pancreatitis. Calif Med 117:1–7
67. Giordano M, Gallo M, Chianese U, Maniera A, Tirri G (1986) Acute pancreatitis as the initial manifestation of systemic lupus erythematosus. Z Rheumatol 45:60–63
68. Glassman M, Tahan S, Hillemeier C, Rothstein P, Shaywith BA, Gryboski J (1981) Pancreatitis in patients with Reye's syndrome. J Clin Gastroenterol 3:165–169
69. Goebell H, Steffen C, Baltzer G, Bode C (1973) Stimulation of pancreatic secretion of enzymes by acute hypercalcaemia in man. Eur J Clin Invest 3:98–104
70. Goldberg PB, Long WB, Oleaga JA, Mackie JA (1980) Choledochocele as a cause of recurrent pancreatitis. Gastroenterology 78:1041–1045
71. Griffen WO Jr, Schaefer JW, Schindler S, Hyde G, Bryant LR (1968) Ampullary obstruction by benign duodenal polyps. Arch Surg 97:444–449
72. Gross V, Schoelmerich J, Denzel K, Gerok W (1989) Relapsing pancreatitis as initial manifestation of cystic fibrosis in a young man without pulmonary disease. Int J Pancreatol 4:221–228
73. Guttman FM, Ross M, Lachance C (1972) Pancreatic metastasis of renal cell carcinoma treated by total pancreatectomy. Arch Surg 105:782–784

74. Hedström SÅ, Belfrage I (1976) Acute pancreatitis in two cases of infectious mononucleosis. Scand J Infect Dis 8:124–126
75. Heffernon JJ, Smith WR, Berk JE, Fridhandler L, Glauser FL, Montgomery KA (1976) Hyperamylasemia in heroin addicts. Characterization by isoamylase analysis. Am J Gastroenterol 66:17–22
76. Heyse-Moore GH (1976) Blunt pancreatic and pancreaticoduodenal trauma. Br J Surg 63: 226–228
77. Hiatt N, Warner NE (1969) Serum amylase and changes in pancreatic function and structure after ligation of pancreatic ducts. Am Surg 35:30–35
78. Hohenberger P (1985) Das Pankreas als Zielorgan des Hepatitis B-Virus –Immunhistologischer Nachweis von HBsAg bei Pankreaskarzinom und chronischer Pankreatitis. Leber Magen Darm 15:58–63
79. Hotz J, Minne H, Ziegler R (1973) The influences of acute hyper- and hypocalcemia and of calcitonin on exocrine pancreatic function in man. Res Exp Med 160:152–165
80. Houssin D, Castaing D, Lemoine J, Bismuth H (1983) Microlithiasis of the gallbladder. Surg Gynecol Obstet 157:20–24
81. Howard JM, Wynn OB, Lenhart FM, Chandnani PC (1986) Intraluminal duodenal diverticulum: an unusual cause of acute pancreatitis. Am J Surg 151:505–508
82. Imrie CW (1974) Observations on acute pancreatitis. Br J Surg 61:539–544
83. Imrie CW, Ferguson JC, Sommerville RG (1977) Coxsackie and mumpsvirus infection in a prospective study of acute pancreatitis. Gut 18:53–56
84. Izsak EM, Shike M, Roulet M, Jeejeebhoy KN (1980) Pancreatitis in association with hypercalcemia in patients receiving total parenteral nutrition. Gastroenterology 79:555–558
85. Jacobs ML, Daggett WM, Civetta JM, Vasu MA, Lawson DW, Warshaw AL, Nardi GL, Bartlett MK (1977) Acute pancreatitis: analysis of factors influencing survival. Ann Surg 185:43–51
86. Johnson WC, Nabseth DC (1970) Pancreatitis in renal transplantation. Ann Surg 171:309–314
87. Johnston DH, Cornish AL (1959) Acute pancreatitis in patients receiving chlorothiazide. JAMA 170:1054–1056
88. Jones B (1977) Choledochocele demonstrated on percutaneous cholangiography: a patient with acute fulminant pancreatitis. Gastrointest Radiol 2:145–147
89. Kager L, Lindberg S, Ågren G (1972) Alcohol consumption and acute pancreatitis in men. Scand J Gastroenterol 7, Suppl. 15:1–38
90. Kane NM, Korobkin M, Francis IR, Quint LE, Cascade PN (1991) Percutaneous biopsy of left adrenal masses: prevalence of pancreatitis after anterior approach. Am J Roentgenol 157:777–780
91. Keller EHJ, Rückert K (1986) Metastasen im Pankreas. Chirurg 57:43–44
92. Khodkov K, Siech M, Beger HG (1996) Cyst of the common bile duct in combination with pancreas divisum as a cause of acute pancreatitis. Pancreas 12:105–107
93. Khuroo MS, Zargar SA, Yattoo GN, Dar MY, Alai MS (1992) Ascaris-induced acute pancreatitis. Br J Surg 79:1335–1338
94. Khuroo MS, Zargar SA, Yattoo GN, Javid G, Dar MY, Boda MI, Khan BA (1993) Worm extraction and biliary drainage in hepatobiliary and pancreatic ascariasis. Gastrointest Endosc 39:680–685
95. Kirk AP, Summerfield JA (1980) Incidence and significance of juxtapapillary diverticula at endoscopic retrograde cholangiopancreatography. Digestion 20:31–35
96. Kirschner S, Raufman J-P (1988) Varicella pancreatitis complicated by pancreatic pseudocyst and duodenal obstruction. Dig Dis Sci 33:1192–1195
97. Ko CW, Schoch HG, Lee SP, McDonald GB (1995) Acute pancreatitis in marrow transplant patients: prevalence at autopsy and risk factor analysis. Gastroenterology 108:A367 (abstr)
98. Kobza K, Gyr K, Neuhaus K, Gudat F (1976) Acute intermittent porphyria with relapsing acute pancreatitis and unconjugated hyperbilirubinemia without overt hemolysis. Gastroenterology 71:494–496
99. Koppelberg T, Bartsch D, Printz H, Hasse C, Rothmund M (1994) Die Pankreatitis beim primären Hyperparathyreoidismus (pHPT) ist eine Komplikation des fortgeschrittenen pHPT. Dtsch Med Wochenschr 119:719–724
100. Köhler H, Lankisch PG (1987) Acute pancreatitis and hyperamylasaemia in pancreatic carcinoma. Pancreas 2:117–119
101. Krokos NV, Karavias D, Tzakis A, Tepetes K, Ramos E, Todo S, Fung JJ, Starzl TE (1995) Acute pancreatitis after liver transplantation: incidence and contributing factors. Transplant Int 8:1–7

102. Lankisch PG, Burchard-Reckert S, Petersen M, Lehnick D, Schirren CA, Köhler H, Stöckmann F, Peiper HJ, Creutzfeldt W (1996) Morbidity and mortality in 602 patients with acute pancreatitis seen between the years 1980–1994. Z Gastroenterol 34:371–377
103. Lankisch PG, Dröge M, Gottesleben F (1995) Drug-induced acute pancreatitis: incidence and severity. Gut 37:565–567
104. Lankisch PG, Löhr A, Kunze E (1987) Metastasen-induzierte akute Pankreatitis beim Bronchialkarzinom. Dtsch Med Wochenschr 112:1335–1337
105. Lankisch PG, Müller C-H, Niederstadt H, Brand A (1990) Painless acute pancreatitis subsequent to anticholinesterase insecticide (parathion) intoxication. Am J Gastroenterol 85:872–875
106. Lankisch PG, Niederstadt H, Redlin-Kress E, Mahlke R, Brand A (1993) Acute pancreatitis: induced by heroin intoxication? Pancreas 8:123–126
107. Lankisch PG, Rahlf G, Schmidt H, Creutzfeldt W (1975) Pankreatitis bei Virushepatitis und Coma hepaticum. Z Gastroenterol 13:407–412
108. Lankisch PG, Schirren CA, Kunze E (1991) Undetected fatal acute pancreatitis: why is the disease so frequently overlooked? Am J Gastroenterol 86:322–326
109. Lankisch PG, Schirren CA, Schmidt H, Schönfelder G, Creutzfeldt W (1989) Etiology and incidence of acute pancreatitis: a 20-year study in a single institution. Digestion 44:20–25
110. Layer P, Hotz J, Schmitz-Moormann HP, Goebell H (1982) Effects of experimental chronic hypercalcemia on feline exocrine pancreatic secretion. Gastroenterology 82:309–316
111. Lee SP, Nicholls JF, Park HZ (1992) Biliary sludge as a cause of acute pancreatitis. N Engl J Med 326:589–593
112. Legge DA, Hoffman II HN, Carlson HC (1971) Pancreatitis as a complication of regional enteritis of the duodenum. Gastroenterology 61:834–837
113. Leinkram C, Roberts-Thomson IC, Kune GA (1980) Juxtapapillary duodenal diverticula. Association with gallstones and pancreatitis. Med J Aust 1:209–210
114. Leonhardt KF (1980) Acute pancreatitis in acute intermittent porphyria (AIP). Ital J Gastroenterol 12:91–92
115. Leung JWC, Chung SCS, King WWK (1986) Round worm pancreatitis: endoscopic worm removal without papillotomy. Br J Surg 73:925
116. Levin DP, Bret PM (1991) Percutaneous fine-needle aspiration biopsy of the pancreas resulting in death. Gastrointest Radiol 16:67–69
117. Levine M, Danovitch SH (1973) Metastatic carcinoma to the pancreas. Another cause for acute pancreatitis. Am J Gastroenterol 60:290–294
118. London NJM, Lloyd DM, Pearson H, Neoptolemos JP, Bell PRF (1986) Pancreatitis after parathyroidectomy. Br J Surg 73:766–767
119. Lukash WM (1967) Complications of acute pancreatitis. Unusual sequelae in 100 cases. Arch Surg 94:848–852
120. Maclean D, Murison J, Griffiths PD (1973) Acute pancreatitis and diabetic ketoacidosis in accidental hypothermia and hypothermic myxoedema. Br Med J 4:757–761
121. MacLennan AC, MacLeod IA (1993) Case report: Small cell carcinoma induced acute pancreatitis. Br J Radiol 66:161–162
122. Madsen OG, Schmidt A (1979) Acute pancreatitis. A study of 122 patients with acute pancreatitis observed for 5–15 years. World J Surg 3:345–352
123. Mallory A, Kern F (1988) Drug-induced pancreatitis. Baillière Clin Gastroenterol 2:293–307
124. Mallory A, Kern F Jr (1980) Drug-induced pancreatitis: a critical review. Gastroenterology 78:813–820
125. Marino C, Lipstein-Kresch E (1984) Pancreatitis in systemic lupus erythematosus. Arthritis Rheumatism 27:118–119
126. Marsh WH, Vukov GA, Conradi EC (1988) Acute pancreatitis after cutaneous exposure to an organophosphate insecticide. Am J Gastroenterol 83:1158–1160
127. Masaryk TJ, Achkar E (1983) Pancreatitis as initial presentation of cystic fibrosis in young adults. A report of two cases. Dig Dis Sci 28:874–878
128. Mårdh P-A, Ursing B (1973) Acute pancreatitis in mycoplasma pneumoniae infections. Br Med J 2:240–241
129. Mårdh P-A, Ursing B (1974) The occurrence of acute pancreatitis in mycoplasma pneumoniae infection. Scand J Infect Dis 6:167–171

130. McCormick PA, Malone D, Fitzgerald MX, FitzGerald O (1985) Pancreatitis in sarcoidosis. Br Med J 290:1472–1473
131. McCutcheon AD (1968) A fresh approach to the pathogenesis of pancreatitis. Gut 9:296–310
132. McKay AJ, O'Neill J, Imrie CW (1980) Pancreatitis, pregnancy and gallstones. Br J Obstet Gynaecol 87:47–50
133. McKay JW, Baggenstoss AH, Wollaeger EE (1958) Infarcts of the pancreas. Gastroenterology 35:256–264
134. McLatchie GR, Imrie CW (1981) Acute pancreatitis associated with tumour metastases in the pancreas. Digestion 21:13–17
135. Meltzer SJ, Goldberg MD (1986) Recurrent pancreatitis caused by vegetable matter obstruction. Am J Gastroenterol 81:1091–1092
136. Mithöfer K, Warshaw AL (1996) Recurrent acute pancreatitis caused by afferent loop stricture after gastrectomy. Arch Surg 131:561–565
137. Moberg A, Svenhamn K, Wågermark J (1968) Acute "idiopathic" pancreatitis. A post-mortem etiological study. Acta Chir Scand 134:369–372
138. Moore PG, James OF (1981) Acute pancreatitis induced by acute organophosphate poisoning? Postgrad Med J 57:660–662
139. Mott C, Sarles H, Tiscornia O, Gullo L (1972) Inhibitory action of alcohol on human exocrine pancreatic secretion. Am J Dig Dis 17:902–910
140. Mössner J, Wagner T, Wünsch PH, Schott H, Kujath P (1982) Zur Differentialdiagnose der Pankreatitis: Pankreasmetastasen. Leber Magen Darm 12:165–170
141. Mueller PR, Miketic LM, Simeone JF, Silverman SG, Saini S, Wittenberg J, Hahn PF, Steiner E, Forman BH (1988) Severe acute pancreatitis after percutaneous biopsy of the pancreas. Am J Roentgenol 151:493–494
142. Murthy UK, DeGregorio F, Oates RP, Blair DC (1992) Hyperamylasemia in patients with the acquired immunodeficiency syndrome. Am J Gastroenterol 87:332–336
143. Nance FC, Cocchiara J, Kinder JL (1967) Acute pancreatitis associated with an intraluminal duodenal diverticulum. Gastroenterology 52:544–547
144. Ng WD, Chan YT, Fung H (1987) Recurrent pancreatitis contributing to choledochal cyst formation. Br J Surg 74:206–208
145. Niccolini DG, Graham JH, Banks PA (1976) Tumor-induced acute pancreatitis. Gastroenterology 71:142–145
146. O'Neill PB (1961) Gastrointestinal abnormalities in the collagen diseases. Am J Dig Dis 6:1069–1083
147. Okada A, Higaki J, Nakamura T, Fukui Y, Kamata S (1995) Pancreatitis associated with choledochal cyst and other anomalies in childhood. Br J Surg 82:829–832
148. Ong GB, Lam KH, Lam SK, Lim TK, Wong J (1979) Acute pancreatitis in Hong Kong. Br J Surg 66:398–403
149. Osnes M, Myren J, Lötveit T, Swensen T (1977) Juxtapapillary duodenal diverticula and abnormalities by endoscopic retrograde cholangio-pancreatography (ERCP). Scand J Gastroenterol 12:347–351
150. Padilla B, Pollak VE, Pesce A, Kant KS, Gilinsky NH, Deddens JA (1994) Pancreatitis in patients with end-stage renal disease. Medicine 73:8–20
151. Parbhoo SP, Welch J, Sherlock S (1973) Acute pancreatitis in patients with fulminant hepatic failure. Gut 14:428 (abstr)
152. Paulino-Netto A, Dreiling DA (1960) Chronic duodenal obstruction: a mechano-vascular etiology of pancreatitis. II. Experimental observations. Am J Dig Dis 5:1006–1018
153. Pedal I, Oehmichen M, Raff G (1984) Reye-Syndrom mit Pankreatitis und hypoxischer Hirnschädigung. Dtsch Med Wochenschr 109:101–105
154. Pellegrini CA, Paloyan D, Acosta JM, Skinner DB (1977) Acute pancreatitis of rare causation. Surg Gynecol Obstet 144:899–902
155. Penn I, Durst AL, Machado M, Halgrimson CG, Booth AS Jr, Putman CW, Groth CG, Starzl TE (1972) Acute pancreatitis and hyperamylasemia in renal homograft recipients. Arch Surg 105:167–172
156. Peters MJ, Jones MG, Moulton J, Breslin ABX (1990) Sarcoidosis presenting as recurrent alcohol-induced pancreatitis. Med J Aust 153:104–107

157. Peterson LM, Collins JJ Jr, Wilson RE (1968) Acute pancreatitis occurring after operation. Surg Gynecol Obstet 127:23–28
158. Pinotti HW, Tacla M, Pontes JF, Bettarello A (1971) Juxta-ampullar duodenal diverticula as cause of bilio-pancreatic disease. Digestion 4:353–361
159. Pirola RC, Davis AE (1968) Effects of ethyl alcohol on sphincteric resistance at the choledocho-duodenal junction in man. Gut 9:557–560
160. Pollak VE, Grove WJ, Kark RM, Muehrcke RC, Pirani CL, Steck IE (1958) Systemic lupus erythematosus simulating acute surgical condition of the abdomen. N Engl J Med 259:258–266
161. Pönkä A, Kosunen TU (1981) Pancreas affection in association with enteritis due to campylobacter fetus ssp. jejuni. Acta Med Scand 209:239–240
162. Price J, Leung JWC (1988) Ultrasound diagnosis of Ascaris lumbricoides in the pancreatic duct: the "four-lines" sign. Br J Radiol 61:411–413
163. Ranson JHC, Spencer FC (1978) The role of peritoneal lavage in severe acute pancreatitis. Ann Surg 187:565–575
164. Rattner DW, Gu Z-Y, Vlahakes GJ, Warshaw AL (1989) Hyperamylasemia after cardiac surgery. Incidence, significance, and management. Ann Surg 209:279–283
165. Reinhard H, Hill K (1977) Tryptische Pankreatitis bei kleinzelligem Bronchialkarzinom. Dtsch Med Wochenschr 102:796–799
166. Renner IG, Pantoja JL, Abramson SB, Douglas AP (1979) The production of acute hemorrhagic pancreatitis in dogs using scorpion venom. Gastroenterology 76:1225 (abstr)
167. Renner IG, Savage III WT, Pantoja JL, Renner VJ (1985) Death due to acute pancreatitis. A retrospective analysis of 405 autopsy cases. Dig Dis Sci 30:1005–1018
168. Renning JA, Warden GD, Stevens LE, Reemtsma K (1972) Pancreatitis after renal transplantation. Am J Surg 123:293–296
169. Reynolds JC, Inman RD, Kimberly RP, Chuong JH, Kovacs JE, Walsh MB (1982) Acute pancreatitis in systemic lupus erythematosus: report of twenty cases and a review of the literature. Medicine 61:25–32
170. Robertson JFR, Imrie CW (1987) Acute pancreatitis associated with carcinoma of the ampulla of Vater. Br J Surg 74:395–397
171. Robinson DO, Alp MH, Grant AK, Lawrence JR (1977) Pancreatitis and renal disease. Scand J Gastroenterol 12:17–20
172. Rolny P, Anderberg B, Ihse I, Lindström E, Olaison G, Arvill A (1990) Pancreatitis after sphincter of Oddi manometry. Gut 31:821–824
173. Ros E, Navarro S, Bru C, García Pugés A, Valderrama R (1991) Occult microlithiasis in "idiopathic" acute pancreatitis: prevention of relapses by cholecystectomy or ursodeoxycholic acid therapy. Gastroenterology 101:1701–1709
174. Rose DM, Ranson JHC, Cunningham JN Jr, Spencer FC (1984) Patterns of severe pancreatic injury following cardiopulmonary bypass. Ann Surg 199:168–172
175. Rushing JL, Hanna CJ, Selecky PA (1978) Pancreatitis as the presenting manifestation of miliary tuberculosis. West J Med 129:432–436
176. Rutsky EA, Robards M, Van Dyke JA, Rostand SG (1986) Acute pancreatitis in patients with end-stage renal disease without transplantation. Arch Intern Med 146:1741–1745
177. Rückert K, Kümmerle F (1979) Das Papillencarcinom. Chirurg 50:308–312
178. Ryan CM, Sheridan RL, Schoenfeld DA, Warshaw AL, Tompkins RG (1995) Postburn pancreatitis. Ann Surg 222:163–170
179. Ryan S, Sandler A, Trenhaile S, Ephgrave K, Garner S (1994) Pancreatic enzyme elevations after blunt trauma. Surgery 116:622–627
180. Saidi F, Donaldson GA (1963) Acute pancreatitis following distal gastrectomy for benign ulcer. Am J Surg 105:87–92
181. Sankaran H, McGeeney FK, Bartholomew C, Raghupathy E (1987) Mechanism of scorpion toxin-induced pancreatitis in dogs. Biochem Arch 3:41–46
182. Satiani B, Stone HH (1979) Predictability of present outcome and future recurrence in acute pancreatitis. Arch Surg 114:711–716
183. Schmidt H, Creutzfeldt W (1970) Calciphylactic pancreatitis and pancreatitis in hyperparathyroidism. Clin Orthopaed 69:135–145

184. Schmitt JK (1985) Pancreatitis and diabetes mellitus with metastatic pulmonary oat-cell carcinoma. Ann Intern Med 103:638–639
185. Schwokowski CF, Albert H, Hartig W (1974) Erfahrungen bei der postoperativen Pankreatitis nach Magenresektionen. Zentralbl Chir 99:1233–1238
186. Sherman S, Lehman GA (1991) ERCP- and endoscopic sphincterotomy-induced pancreatitis. Pancreas 6:350–367
187. Sherman S, Troiano FP, Hawes RH, Lehman GA (1990) Sphincter of Oddi manometry: decreased risk of clinical pancreatitis with use of a modified aspirating catheter. Gastrointest Endosc 36:462–466
188. Shwachman H, Lebenthal E, Khaw K-T (1975) Recurrent acute pancreatitis in patients with cystic fibrosis with normal pancreatic enzymes. Pediatrics 55:86–95
189. Smith EH (1991) Complications of percutaneous abdominal fine-needle biopsy. Review. Radiology 178:253–258
190. Sparberg M (1967) Recurrent acute pancreatitis associated with systemic lupus erythematosus. Report of a case. Am J Dig Dis 12:522–526
191. Steer ML (1993) Etiology and pathophysiology of acute pancreatitis. In: Go VLW, DiMagno EP, Gardner JD, Lebenthal E, Reber HA, Scheele GA (eds) The Pancreas: Biology, Pathobiology, and Disease, 2nd edn. Raven Press, New York, pp 581–591
192. Steinberg W, Tenner S (1994) Acute pancreatitis. N Engl J Med 330:1198–1210
193. Stock K-P, Riemann JF, Stadler W, Rösch W (1981) Tuberculosis of the pancreas. Endoscopy 13:178–180
194. Stoler J, Biller JA, Grand RJ (1987) Pancreatitis in Kawasaki disease. Am J Dis Child 141:306–308
195. Stover SL, Wanglee P, Kennedy C (1968) Acute hemorrhagic pancreatitis and other visceral changes associated with acute encephalopathy. Report of three cases. J Pediatr 73:235–241
196. Svensson J-O, Norbäck B, Bokey EL, Edlund Y (1979) Changing pattern in aetiology of pancreatitis in an urban Swedish area. Br J Surg 66:159–161
197. Swensen T, Osnes M, Serck-Hanssen A (1980) Endoscopic retrograde cholangio-pancreatography in primary and secondary tumours of the pancreas. Br J Radiol 53:760–764
198. Swisher SG, Cates JA, Hunt KK, Robert ME, Bennion RS, Thompson JE, Roslyn JJ, Reber HA (1994) Pancreatitis associated with adult choledochal cysts. Pancreas 9:633–637
199. Taft PM, Jones AC, Collins GM, Halasz NA (1978) Acute pancreatitis following renal allotransplantation. A lethal complication. Am J Dig Dis 23:541–544
200. Tayeb G, Mitra S, Karras P, Michalos A (1995) Acute pancreatitis in chronic dialysis patients. Gastroenterology 108:A395 (abstr)
201. Taylor TV, Rimmer S, Holt S, Jeacock J, Lucas S (1991) Sex differences in gallstone pancreatitis. Ann Surg 214:667–670
202. Tegenfeldt EG, Kirtland HB, Brown RG (1967) Gallstones, pancreatitis and pregnancy. Am Surg 33:88–90
203. Thompson JS, Bragg LE, Hodgson PE, Rikkers LF (1988) Postoperative pancreatitis. Surg Gynecol Obstet 167:377–380
204. Thomson HJ (1985) Acute pancreatitis in North and North-East Scotland. J R Coll Surg Edinburgh 30:104–110
205. Thomson SR, Hendry WS, McFarlane GA, Davidson AI (1987) Epidemiology and outcome of acute pancreatitis. Br J Surg 74:398–401
206. Tilney NL, Collins JJ Jr, Wilson RE (1966) Hemorrhagic pancreatitis. A fatal complication of renal transplantation. N Engl J Med 274:1051–1057
207. Tiscornia O, Gullo L, Sarles H (1973) The inhibition of canine exocrine pancreatic secretion by intravenous ethanol. Digestion 9:231–240
208. Trapnell JE, Duncan EHL (1975) Patterns of incidence in acute pancreatitis. Br Med J 2:179–183
209. Vendrell J, Nubiola A, Goday A, Bosch X, Muñoz A, Esmatjes E, Gomis R (1987) HIV and the pancreas. Lancet 2:1212–1213
210. Wagner E, Irfanoglu ME (1971) Die postoperative Pankreatitis. Ihre Erkennung und Behandlung. Chirurg 42:162–167
211. Weizman Z, Durie PR (1988) Acute pancreatitis in childhood. J Pediatr 113:24–29
212. White TT, Morgan A, Hopton D (1970) Postoperative pancreatitis. A study of seventy cases. Am J Surg 120:132–137

213. Wilcox CM, Forsmark CE, Grendell JH, Darragh TM, Cello JP (1990) Cytomegalovirus-associated acute pancreatic disease in patients with acquired immunodeficiency syndrome. Report of two patients. Gastroenterology 99:263–267
214. Wilson C, Imrie CW, Carter DC (1988) Fatal acute pancreatitis. Gut 29:782–788
215. Winters C Jr, Chobanian SJ, Benjamin SB, Ferguson RK, Cattau EL Jr (1984) Endoscopic documentation of Ascaris-induced acute pancreatitis. Gastrointest Endosc 30:93–84
216. Wislocki LC (1966) Acute pancreatitis in infectious mononucleosis. N Engl J Med 275:322–323
217. Witte CL, Schanzer B (1968) Pancreatitis due to mumps. JAMA 203:1068–1069
218. Wolf P, Reiser JR, Fellow JE, Haghighi P (1989) Pancreatitis in patients with AIDS presumptively due to CMV. J Clin Lab Analysis 3:152–155
219. Wolman R, de Gara C, Isenberg D (1988) Acute pancreatitis in systemic lupus erythematosus: report of a case unrelated to drug therapy. Ann Rheum Dis 47:77–79
220. Wu CS, Wang SH, Kuo TT (1994) Pancreatic tuberculosis mimicking pancreatic head carcinoma: a case report and review of the literature. Infection 22:287–289
221. Yeung K-Y, Haidak DJ, Brown JA, Anderson D (1979) Metastasis-induced acute pancreatitis in small cell bronchogenic carcinoma. Arch Intern Med 139:552–554
222. Yi-sheng C, Ben-xian D, Bi-la H, Ling-zhen X (1986) Endoscopic diagnosis and management of ascaris-induced acute pancreatitis. Endoscopy 18:127–128
223. Zion MM, Goldberg B, Suzman MM (1955) Corticotrophin and cortisone in the treatment of scleroderma. Quart J Med 24:215–227

6 Acute Pancreatitis: Pathophysiology

Our knowledge of the pathophysiology of acute pancreatitis is limited. Clinical and postmortem studies of the early stages in acute pancreatitis are almost impossible. What knowledge we do have, is based on experimental models only, the relevance of which is questionable [31].

6.1
Mechanisms of Pancreatic Injury

Events preceding pancreatic necrosis can be investigated only in experimental animal models. Most models have started with blockage of pancreatic enzyme secretion (Fig. 6.1) [19, 26, 28]. In experimental models using mechanical outflow obstruction [28],

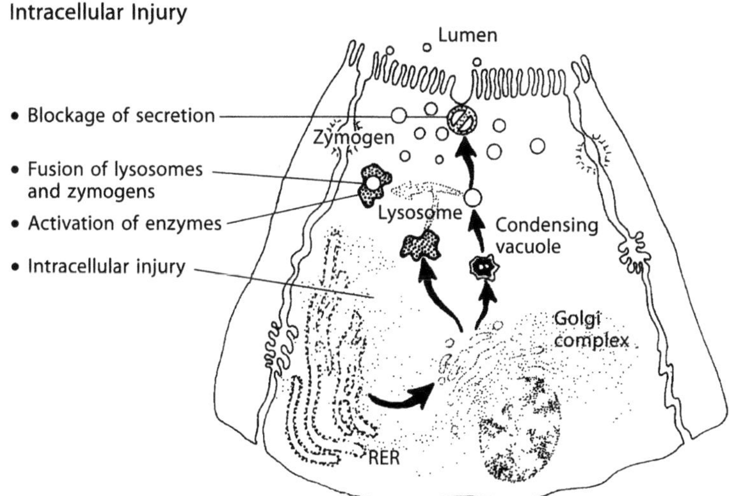

Fig. 6.1. One hypothesized mechanism of acute pancreatitis culminates in intracellular injury. The initiating event is a blockage of secretion, leading to accumulation of zymogen granules within acinar cells. Once blockage occurs, there is a fusion of lysomones and zymogens within large vacuoles (a process termed *crinophagy*). There is then an activation of enzymes and acute intracellular injury. *RER* = rough endoplasmatic reticulum. From the American Gastroenterological Association: Clinical Teaching Project, Unit 5, Pancreatitis (with permission)

supramaximal secretagogue stimulation [3, 28] or a choline-deficient ethionine-supplemented (CDE) diet [16] for induction of acute experimental pancreatitis, acinar cells fail to discharge their digestive enzymes. In all models, large vacuoles appear containing both digestive enzymes and lysosomal hydrolases. In diet-induced pancreatitis, the large vacuoles appear to result from fusion between zymogen granules and lysosomes (crinophagy), whereas in the hyperstimulation model the vacuoles appear to reflect an arrest of the processes involved in condensing vacuole maturation that normally results in the segregation of lysosomal hydrolases away from digestive enzymes [12, 21, 28, 32, 33].

Whether or not similar events occur in clinical pancreatitis remains to be established [31].

6.2
Gallstone-induced Acute Pancreatitis

The association between gallstones and acute pancreatitis was first demonstrated almost 100 years ago [22–24]. However, the risk of acute pancreatitis in patients with gallstones is low. Only 3.4% of these will develop an acute inflammation of the pancreas [18].

Nevertheless, in the majority of patients with acute abdominal pain suggesting acute pancreatitis and an appropriate elevation of pancreatic enzymes in serum, the diagnosis of acute biliary pancreatitis is made when gallstones are found in the gallbladder by ultrasound or computed tomography (CT). Little is known about the exact pathogenetic mechanism.

Gallstones have been found in feces in 95% of patients with acute pancreatitis associated with gallstones (without acute biliary conditions), but only in 8% of patients suffering from acute biliary conditions associated with gallstones but not acute pancreatitis [1]. These findings suggest that somehow smaller gallstones induce acute pancreatitis on their passage to the duodenum.

However, data on the frequency of impacted gallstones vary considerably. In one surgical series [9], they were found in 2.9%, but in another [2] in 33% of patients with acute biliary pancreatitis. However, in the latter study, the frequency of impacted gallstones decreased with increasing time interval between the onset of pancreatitis and surgery. The frequency was 73% in patients who were operated within the first 48 h, and 25% in patients who were operated after 4 or more days, thus indicating that an impacted stone eventually found its way into the duodenum. In fatal acute biliary pancreatitis, an impacted gallstone was found only in 5% of the cases [35].

6.3
Alcohol-induced Acute Pancreatitis

Acute pancreatitis per definition is the first acute inflammation of the pancreas. However, as we never know the status of the gland prior to the first attack, this first attack in a previously asymptomatic patient is considered to be "acute" pancreatitis, unless evidence of chronic pancreatitis (e.g., calcifications) or prior attacks of silent acute pancreatitis (e.g., pancreatic pseudocysts) can be shown by ultrasound or CT (see also Sect. 5.2). Previously it was believed that excessive alcohol abuse would lead to a maximal release of pancreatic enzymes which once activated would cause acute inflammation. Rarely does an excessive consumption of alcohol lead to acute pancreatitis. In a prospective study, in 300 drunken drivers, only 1% had serum amylase levels exceeding twice the upper limit of normal [20]. None of them clinically had acute pancreatitis.

Clinically, alcohol-induced acute and chronic pancreatitis are usually dealt with separately. However, since the first attack of acute pancreatitis is frequently considered also to be the first of chronic pancreatitis, the pathophysiology of alcohol-induced acute pancreatitis is dealt with in the Chronic Pancreatitis section (see Sect. 14.2).

6.4
Concept of Oxidative Stress

Recently, Braganza and colleagues [6] postulate from animal studies that acute pancreatitis always starts with a blockage in the regulated secretory pathway in acinar cells, a process which they termed pancreastasis. They suggest the following pathogenetic sequence in acute pancreatitis:
- Oxidative stress in pancreatic acinar cells, i.e., an excess of oxygen-free radicals over available antioxidants in the gland, subsequently
- Compensatory fusion of lysosomal and zymogen compartments, together with a reversal in secretory polarity
- Lipid oxidation fragments in the interstitium
- Mast cell degranulation
- Platelet activation
- Potent inflammatory response with or without the activation of pancreatic zymogens

Recurrent pancreatitis seems to indicate recurrent oxidative stress in acinar cells, with a higher degree or longer duration of the problem in chronic pancreatitis [6].

6.5
Theories Explaining the Pathogenetic Mechanism
of Acute Biliary Pancreatitis

Among the first to study the pathogenetic mechanism was Eugene Lindsay Opie, a pathologist at the Johns Hopkins University in Baltimore [22]. He reported a patient in whom a gallstone in the common bile duct had occluded the orifice of the pancreatic duct. Opie believed that the impairment of pancreatic secretion triggered acute pancreatitis (first hypothesis). Shortly afterwards, he reported another patient in whom a gallstone had been found impacted at the duodenal papilla. Behind the stone, there was a communication between the pancreatic and the biliary duct which Opie named the *common channel*. It was believed that in presence of a common channel bile would enter the pancreatic duct inducing acute pancreatitis once the papilla was blocked (second hypothesis).

A third hypothesis is based on observations from animal models. Seidel [29] and later Pfeffer et al. [25] ligated the duodenum above and below the papilla of Vater, creating a closed duodenal loop with increasing duodenal pressure. Duodenal content was forced through the sphincter of Oddi inducing acute pancreatitis. In contrast to the common channel hypothesis, in this *duodenal reflux theory* the contact of pancreatic juice with the duodenal brush border would assure activation of pancreatic proteases.

A fourth theory is that of combined bile and pancreatic duct obstruction. The American opossum is ideal for testing the pathogenesis of acute biliary pancreatitis because it has a single pancreatic and common bile duct with a long communication in between allowing a common channel situation after surgical ligation of the papilla. Senninger et al. [30] ligated both the pancreatic duct and the common bile duct. Pancreatic ductal obstruction alone was associated with only mild interstitial pancreatitis, biliary obstruction alone led to no histological evidence of pancreatic inflammation. Only the combined obstruction of both ducts led to necrotizing pancreatitis. The possible mechanism could be the stimulation of exocrine pancreatic secretion that is known to occur after bile duct ligation or diversion of bile from the duodenum [13].

6.6
The Pros and Cons of the Theories

The connection between the pancreatic duct and the common bile duct is much too short in most humans to allow for a common channel to form in the presence of an impacted gallstone at the papilla [8]. Nevertheless, a common channel can be demonstrated on intraoperative cholangiography in 67% of patients with gallstone pancreatitis as compared to 32% of patients with cholelithiasis or choledocholithiasis without pancreatic disease [11]. Pancreatic duct reflux in operative cholangiographies is much more frequent in patients who had a previous attack of acute pancreatitis (62.3%) as compared to patients with no history of pancreatic disease (14.6%) [4].

An impacted stone would most likely obstruct both ducts. However, pancreatic secretory pressure exceeds biliary secretory pressure [7, 17], and reflux of pancreatic juice into the biliary tract rather than vice versa would occur. The pressure gradient is maintained until long after the initial pancreatic damage has already developed [14]. When during the development of pancreatic necrosis the pancreatic duct has lost its barrier function, bile could probably flow into the necrotic pancreas if the stone at the papilla is still present and a common channel is present [13]. However, by that time, most stones will have passed into the duodenum.

But even if bile regurgitates into the pancreas before necrosis develops, it would probably be harmless. When sterile bile is perfused to the pancreas at physiological pressure, it does not induce acute pancreatitis [27, 34]. However, when the pancreatic duct in cats is exposed to specific bile salts at physiological concentrations and pressures, it undergoes marked structural alterations, and becomes permeable to molecules at least as large as 20 000 daltons, whereas it is normally impermeable to molecules as small as 3000 daltons [10]. Finally, most studies in the opossum model of pancreatitis show that a common channel, although present, is not critical for the development of pancreatitis [13].

The *duodenal reflux theory* is based on animal experiments only. In man, acute pancreatitis rarely occurs on the basis of duodenal obstruction [5]. Moreover, in man, the passage of gallstones through the duodenal papilla constantly produces stenosis of the sphincter rather than sphincter insufficiency.

Concerning Opie's [24] hypothesis that pancreatic secretion is blocked, further studies are required. It is supported by a recent case report on a male patient in whom biliary reflux or biliary obstruction was effectively prevented by the surgical insertion of a T-drain into the common bile duct. He developed acute pancreatitis due to a residual stone in the papilla of Vater and recovered after the stone had been removed and pancreatic flow restored [15].

References

1. Acosta JM, Ledesma CL (1974) Gallstone migration as a cause of acute pancreatitis. N Engl J Med 290:484–487
2. Acosta JM, Pelligrini CA, Skinner DB (1980) Etiology and pathogenesis of acute biliary pancreatitis. Surgery 88:118–125
3. Adler G, Hupp T, Kern HF (1979) Course and spontaneous regression of acute pancreatitis in the rat. Virchows Arch [Pathol Anat] 382:31–47
4. Armstrong CP, Taylor TV (1986) Pancreatic-duct reflux and acute gallstone pancreatitis. Ann Surg 204:59–64
5. Bradley III EL, Clements JL Jr (1981) Idiopathic duodenal obstruction. An unappreciated complication of pancreatitis. Ann Surg 193:638–648
6. Braganza JM (1991) Evolution of pancreatitis. In: Braganza JM (ed) The Pathogenesis of Pancreatitis: Based on a Symposium Held on 15 November 1990 at the University of Manchester under the Auspices of the Pancreatic Society of Great Britain and Ireland. Manchester University Press, Manchester-New York, pp 19–33
7. Carr-Locke DL, Gregg JA (1981) Endoscopic manometry of pancreatic and biliary sphincter zones in man. Basal results in healthy volunteers. Dig Dis Sci 26:7–15
8. DiMagno EP, Shorter RG, Taylor WF, Go VLW (1982) Relationships between pancreaticobiliary ductal anatomy and pancreatic ductal and parenchymal histology. Cancer 49:361–368
9. Dzieniszewski GP, Neher M, Schmidt H-D, Kümmerle F (1984) Cholelithiasis und akute Pankreatitis. Dtsch Med Wochenschr 109:1349–1355
10. Farmer RC, Tweedie J, Maslin S, Reber HA, Adler G, Kern H (1984) Effects of bile salts on permeability and morphology of main pancreatic duct in cats. Dig Dis Sci 29:740–751
11. Jones BA, Salsberg BB, Bohnen JMA, Mehta MH (1987) Common pancreaticobiliary channels and their relationship to gallstone size in gallstone pancreatitis. Ann Surg 205:123–125
12. Koike H, Steer ML, Meldolesi J (1982) Pancreatic effects of ethionine: blockade of exocytosis and appearance of crinophagy and autophagy precede cellular necrosis. Am J Physiol 242:G297–G307
13. Lerch MM, Adler G (1994) Pathophysiology of acute pancreatitis. Dig Surg 11:186–192
14. Lerch MM, Saluja AK, Dawra R, Ramarao P, Saluja M, Steer ML (1992) Acute necrotizing pancreatitis in the opossum: earliest morphological changes involve acinar cells. Gastroenterology 103:205–213
15. Lerch MM, Weidenbach H, Hernandez CA, Preclik G, Adler G (1994) Pancreatic outflow obstruction as the critical event for human gall stone induced pancreatitis. Gut 35:1501–1503
16. Lombardi B, Estes LW, Longnecker DS (1975) Acute hemorrhagic pancreatitis (massive necrosis) with fat necrosis induced in mice by DL-ethionine fed with a choline-deficient diet. Am J Pathol 79:465–480 (abstr)

17. Menguy RB, Hallenbeck GA, Bollman JL, Grindlay JH (1958) Intraductal pressures and sphincteric resistance in canine pancreatic and biliary ducts after various stimuli. Surg Gynecol Obstet 106:306–320
18. Moreau JA, Zinsmeister AR, Melton III LJ, DiMagno EP (1988) Gallstone pancreatitis and the effect of cholecystectomy: a population-based cohort study. Mayo Clin Proc 63:466–473
19. Niederau C, Niederau M, Lüthen R, Strohmeyer G, Ferrell LD, Grendell JH (1990) Pancreatic exocrine secretion in acute experimental pancreatitis. Gastroenterology 99:1120–1127
20. Niederau C, Niederau M, Strohmeyer G, Bertling L, Sonnenberg A (1990) Does acute consumption of large alcohol amounts lead to pancreatic injury? A prospective study of serum pancreatic enzymes in 300 drunken drivers. Digestion 45:115–120
21. Ohshio G, Saluja AK, Leli U, Sengupta A, Steer ML (1989) Esterase inhibitors prevent lysosomal enzyme redistribution in two noninvasive models of experimental pancreatitis. Gastroenterology 96:853–859
22. Opie (1901) The relation of cholelithiasis to disease of the pancreas and to fat-necrosis. Johns Hopkins Hosp Bull 12:19–21
23. Opie EL (1901) The etiology of acute hemorrhagic pancreatitis. Johns Hopkins Hosp Bull 12:182–188
24. Opie EL (1970) The theory of retrojection of bile into the pancreas. Rev Surg 27:1–7
25. Pfeffer RB, Stasior O, Hinton JW (1957) The clinical picture of the sequential development of acute hemorrhagic pancreatitis in the dog. Surg Forum 8:248–251
26. Powers RE, Saluja AK, Houlihan MJ, Steer ML (1986) Diminished agonist-stimulated inositol triphosphate generation blocks stimulus-secretion coupling in mouse pancreatic acini during diet-induced experimental pancreatitis. J Clin Invest 77:1668–1674
27. Robinson TM, Dunphy JE (1963) Continuous perfusion of bile and protease activators through the pancreas. JAMA 183:530–533
28. Saluja A, Saluja M, Villa A, Leli U, Rutledge P, Meldolesi J, Steer M (1989) Pancreatic duct obstruction in rabbits causes digestive zymogen and lysosomal enzyme colocalization. J Clin Invest 84:1260–1266
29. Seidel H (1910) Bemerkungen zu meiner Methode der experimentellen Erzeugung der akuten hämorrhagischen Pankreatitis. Zentralbl Chir 37:1601–1604
30. Senninger N, Moody FG, Coelho JCU, Van Buren DH (1986) The role of biliary obstruction in the pathogenesis of acute pancreatitis in the oppossum. Surgery 99:688–693
31. Steer ML (1993) Etiology and pathophysiology of acute pancreatitis. In: Go VLW, DiMagno EP, Gardner JD, Lebenthal E, Reber HA, Scheele GA (eds) The Pancreas: Biology, Pathobiology, and Disease, 2nd edn. Raven Press, New York, pp 581–591
32. Steer ML, Meldolesi J, Figarella C (1984) Pancreatitis. The role of lysosomes. Dig Dis Sci 29:934–938
33. Watanabe O, Baccino FM, Steer ML, Meldolesi J (1984) Supramaximal caerulein stimulation and ultrastructure of rat pancreatic acinar cell: early morphological changes during development of experimental pancreatitis. Am J Physiol 246:G457–G467
34. White TT, Magee DF (1960) Perfusion of the dog pancreas with bile without production of pancreatitis. Ann Surg 151:245–250
35. Wilson C, Imrie CW, Carter DC (1988) Fatal acute pancreatitis. Gut 29:782–788

7 Acute Pancreatitis: Pathology

The histopathological evaluation of acute pancreatitis depends on the severity of the disease. We have no histologic information on lesions of the pancreas in clinically very mild acute pancreatitis, since these patients do not require surgery or die of the disease. It may be even difficult to distinguish mild acute (interstitial) pancreatitis from severe acute (necrotizing) pancreatitis because of the progressive changes seen in both forms. The two terms do not define two separate disease entities, rather only severity grades of acute autodigestive pancreatitis. Morphologically, differentiation of acute pancreatitis into mild and severe largely depends on the extension and site of fat necrosis.

In the mild form, fat necrosis is minimal and scattered in the edematously enlarged gland. In the severe form, the pancreas displays large confluent foci of fat necrosis around the pancreas associated with intrapancreatic fat necrosis, focal hemorrhage, and parenchymal necrosis [6].

7.1
Gross Pathology

At the time of operation or post mortem, in patients with the clinical diagnosis of acute necrotizing pancreatitis, necrosis is seen predominantly in peripancreatic fatty tissue while the parenchyma of the gland is usually less affected. At surgery, overestimation of the extent of pancreatic necrosis is not uncommon [9–11, 13, 14]. Characteristically, the necrosis on the surface of the gland shows an extremely variegated pattern with areas of white fat necrosis and hemorrhages (Fig. 7.1). Fat necrosis may be scattered in the bursa omentalis, omentum, and mesentery as well as deep in the retroperitoneum. The peritoneal cavity contains turbid or hemorrhagic fluid. In severe necrotizing pancreatitis, the gland may be partly or totally transformed into a hemorrhagic-necrotic mass. Necrosis involving the main pancreatic duct may cause rupture [6].

In some patients there is a striking discrepancy between a high degree of extraperitoneal necrosis and the comparative normality of residual portions of the pancreas. It has been suggested that in these cases the duct system is disrupted and the secretions of the surviving pancreas cause progressive enzymatic destruction of extrapancreatic tissues and thus contribute to the mortality of the disease (Fig. 7.2) [12].

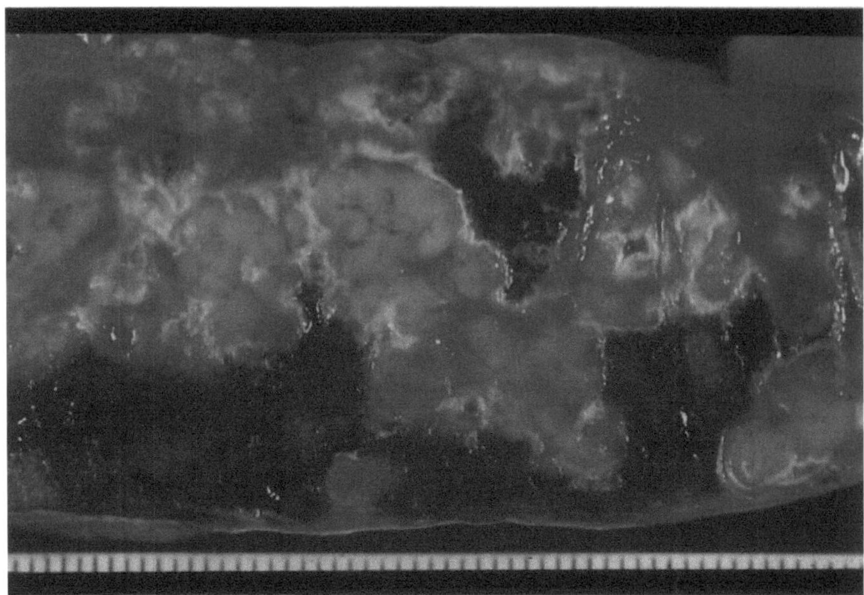

Fig. 7.1. Coexistence of necrosis on the surface of the gland with areas of white fat necrosis and hemorrhage in severe hemorrhagic pancreatitis

In pancreatitis caused by infectious agents, the gland may be swollen but does not show autodigestive changes such as fat necrosis [6].

7.2
Histopathology

No histological differences exist between the various etiological groups [13].

Necrosis mainly involves the interlobular fatty tissue. Fat necrosis particularly involves small veins, leads to swelling and granulocytic infiltration of the wall, followed by thrombosis, necrosis, rupture, and eventual hemorrhage. Arterial thrombosis leads to panlobular ischemic necrosis [6].

A few, notably elderly, patients with severe extrapancreatic disease may develop a special type of acute pancreatitis, which is characterized by disseminated and periductal necrosis, which outnumber the foci of fat necrosis and may even present without any fat necrosis [3, 5]. It seems that these patients may easily develop purulent peritonitis [5].

In infectious pancreatitis, induced by certain viruses such as mumps or Coxsackie virus, a scattered acinar cell necrosis without any fat necrosis or ductal necrosis is found [4, 6, 15].

Fig. 7.2. Striking discrepancy in a patient who died of acute hemorrhagic pancreatitis showing a high degree of extraperitoneal necrosis along the ribs, at the pleura (upper part of the figure), and especially along ribs and at the pleura (middle part of the figure), but comparative normality of the pancreas (cross section) with only necrotic areas around the gland (lower part of the figure)

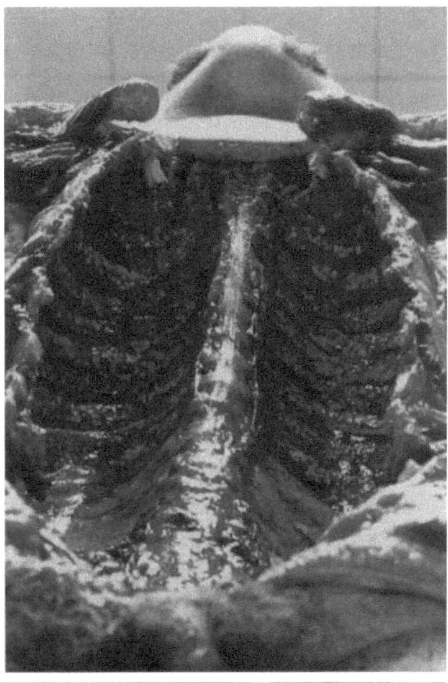

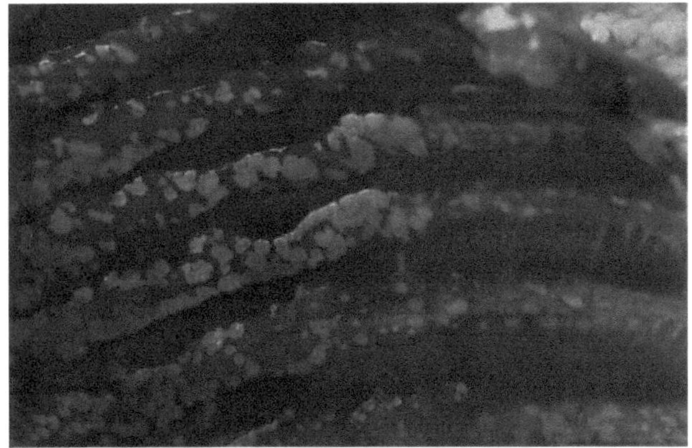

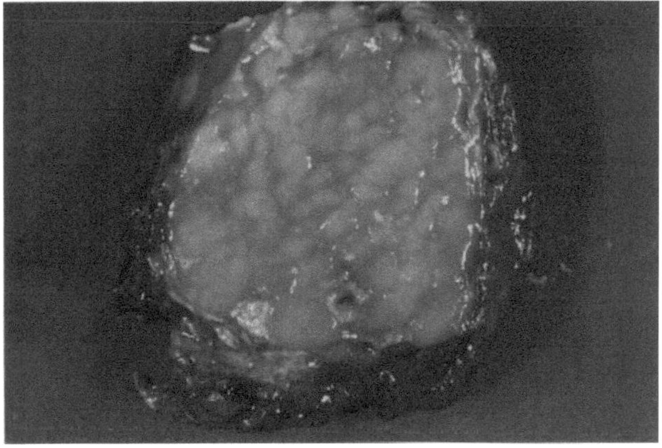

7.3
Sequential Changes and Outcome

The resolution and outcome of fat necrosis depends on its localization and size. Small peripancreatic fat necrosis (<1 cm) resolves entirely. The liquefied necrotic content of larger peripancreatic fat necrosis (diameter 2–4 cm) is demarcated by a rim of macrophages which may eventually absorb the contents (mostly activated enzymes and often degraded blood). In larger areas (diameter ≥5 cm) that do not spontaneously dissolve, the macrophages are replaced by a thin layer of granulation tissue within 10–20 days after the onset of the disease. After 20–30 days the granulation tissue produces a fibrotic capsule that gradually increases in thickness and forms a grossly visible wall.

Pancreatic pseudocysts contain enzyme-rich pancreatic juice, a finding which suggests that a connection persists to a pancreatic duct following a rupture of the duct during the acute phase of inflammation. Some cysts may increase in size, causing compression of and/or perforation into structures such as the bile duct, duodenum, stomach, vessels, and peritoneum. Infection occurs mostly during day 4 to 20, i.e., early during the development of the pseudocyst, when the liquefied necrotic areas are demarcated only by a rim of macrophages or a thin layer of granulation tissue (Fig. 7.3). According to the Atlanta classification [2], an infected pancreatic pseudocyst shall be termed an abscess. Other pancreatic pseudocysts with or without connection with the pancreatic duct may persist without expanding or leading to symptoms.

Necrotic areas within the pancreas originating from intralobular fat necrosis with hemorrhage usually resolve slowly and may induce interlobular fibrosis. This process has been named by Klöppel and his group as the *necrosis-fibrosis sequence* [8] (see Fig. 14.1). If it takes place repeatedly, acute pancreatitis may evolve into chronic pancreatitis [1, 7].

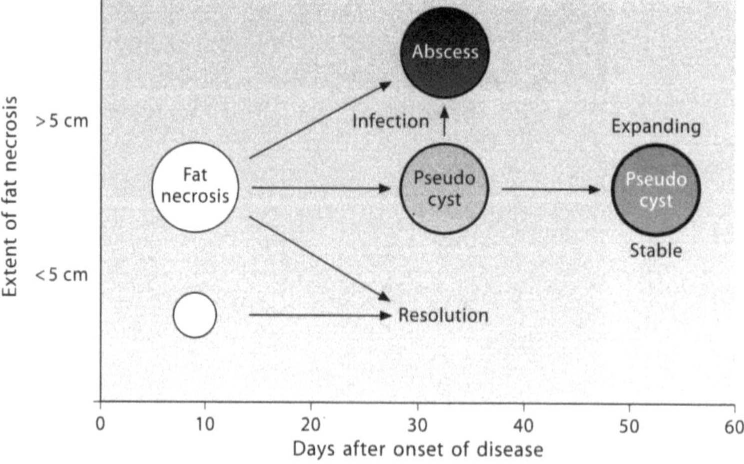

Fig. 7.3. Natural history of fat necrosis in acute pancreatitis. (From [6] with permission)

References

1. Ammann RW, Heitz PU, Klöppel G (1996) Course of alcoholic chronic pancreatitis: a prospective clinicomorphological long-term study. Gastroenterology 111:224–231
2. Bradley III EL (1993) A clinically based classification system for acute pancreatitis. Summary of the International Symposium on Acute Pancreatitis, Atlanta, Ga, September 11 through 13, 1992. Arch Surg 128:586–590
3. Foulis AK (1980) Histological evidence of initiating factors in acute necrotising pancreatitis in man. J Clin Pathol 33:1125–1131
4. Jenson AB, Rosenberg HS, Notkins AL (1980) Pancreatic islet-cell damage in children with fatal viral infections. Lancet 2:354–358
5. Kimura W, Ohtsubo K (1989) Clinical and pathological features of acute interstitial pancreatitis in the aged. Int J Pancreatol 5:1–10
6. Klöppel G (1994) Pathology of severe acute pancreatitis. In: Bradley III EL (ed) Acute Pancreatitis: Diagnosis and Therapy. Raven Press, New York, pp 35–46
7. Klöppel G, Maillet B (1991) Chronic pancreatitis: evolution of the disease. Hepatogastroenterology 38:408–412
8. Klöppel G, Maillet B (1992) The morphological basis for the evolution of acute pancreatitis into chronic pancreatitis. Virchows Arch [Pathol Anat] 420:1–4
9. Leger L, Chiche B, Louvel A (1977) La nécrose dans les pancréatites aiguës. Confrontations opératoires et anatomo-pathologiques. 7 observations. Nouv Presse Med 6:337–340
10. Leger L, Chiche B, Louvel A (1981) Pancreatic necrosis and acute pancreatitis. World J Surg 5:315–317
11. Leger L, Chiche B, Moullé P, Louvel A (1978) Pancreatic necrosis and acute pancreatitis. Int Surg 63:41–45
12. Maclean N (1977) The role of the surviving pancreas in late fatalities of acute pancreatitis. Br J Surg 64:345–346
13. Nordback I, Lauslahti K (1986) Clinical pathology of acute necrotising pancreatitis. J Clin Pathol 39:68–74
14. Nordback I, Pessi T, Auvinen O, Autio V (1985) Determination of necrosis in necrotizing pancreatitis. Br J Surg 72:225–227
15. Sibert JR (1975) Pancreatitis in children. A study in the North of England. Arch Dis Child 50:443–448

8 Acute Pancreatitis: Epidemiology

Although epidemiology in acute pancreatitis has attracted more interest than in chronic pancreatitis (see Chap. 16), the data obtained vary considerably. This may be explained by several factors:
- The diagnosis of acute pancreatitis is not always easy even though direct diagnosis has been improved in recent years by the introduction of imaging procedures such as ultrasound and computed tomography (CT). For example, in several series, in 30%–42% of fatal cases, the diagnosis was first made at autopsy [6, 10, 16]. Furthermore, epidemiological evaluations do not identify all cases when based only on the first listed diagnosis in hospital records. The first diagnosis may be, for example, biliary tract disease, but without mention that this was associated with an acute inflammation of the pancreas.
- Despite the availability of a number of prognostic scores and classification systems for imaging procedures in acute pancreatitis, these are not widely used, with the result that the different epidemiological studies contain little information on the severity of acute pancreatitis.
- Diagnoses for purposes of death certificates are not helpful sources for exact statistical analysis. Since post mortem examinations are declining in most countries, the true incidence of the disease and its severity is not known.

Nevertheless, the data available on epidemiology of acute pancreatitis show interesting findings among different centers:
- The incidence rate of acute pancreatitis per 100 000 inhabitants/year differs considerably: comparatively low figures for England [6, 7, 15] and the Netherlands [14], medium high figures for Scotland [12, 13] and Germany [1] and high figures for the United States of America [8] and Finland [9] (Table 8.1).
- Comparative studies within the United Kingdom (Bristol area: Trapnell and Duncan [15], Corfield et al. [6]; Nottingham: Giggs et al. [7]), in Denmark [18], Scotland [17], and the Netherlands [14] showed distinct increased incidence of acute pancreatitis (Fig. 8.1), which was also seen in Göttingen [11].

The increased incidence of acute pancreatitis derived from an increase in male patients [9, 17, 18], whereas there was no significant increase in female patients, and in the Netherlands [14] and in Finland [9] was significantly correlated with alcohol consumption.

However, it has to be taken into account, both for the figures given for the incidence of acute pancreatitis and its increase, that all the studies were not published at the

Table 8.1. Overall incidence of acute pancreatitis in different parts of the world

Authors	Localization	Period	Incidence (10^5) population/year
Trapnell and Duncan [15]	Bristol	1961–1967	5.4
Corfield et al. [6]	Bristol	1968–1979	7.3
Giggs et al. [7]	Nottingham	1977–1983	11.7
Thomson [12]	North and North-East Scotland	1968–1980	9.4
Thomson et al. [13]	North-East Scotland	1983–1985	24.2
Tran and Schilfgaarde [14]	Netherlands	1971	6.5
	Netherlands	1990	10.2
Assmus et al. [1]	Lüneburg	1989–1994	15.6
Worning [18]	Denmark	1981	26.8
		1990	35.4
Go [8]	United States of America	1987	49.5[a]
			79.8[b]
Jaakkola and Nordback [9]	Finland	1970	46.6
		1989	73.4

Includes [a] all first-listed and [b] all subsequent-listed diagnoses from the National Hospital discharge data base.

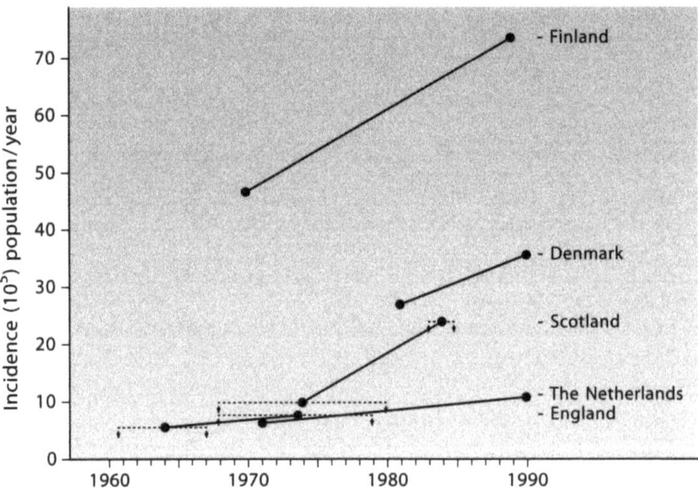

Fig. 8.1. Increase of incidence of acute pancreatitis in different parts of the world

same time, i.e., available diagnostic tests were not comparable. Therefore, to some extent, higher figures of incidence could be due to the development of better diagnostic procedures

- Concerning severity, two studies can be mentioned. In Denmark, only about 5% of all registered cases of acute pancreatitis between 1981 and 1990 were necrotic; however, data on the basis of this diagnosis were not given [18]. In Lüneburg, where a Municipal Hospital serves a defined population of 150000, of whom slightly more than half live in the country-side, 141 patients received on admission a CT examination scored according to Balthazar [2, 3]. Only 16% of them scored 5–10 points, which means that they had necrosis, whereas in 13% the CT on admission was normal [1].

– A very interesting epidemiological finding over several decades was reported from Nottingham. The spatial distribution of patients revealed the highest cluster of incidence rates of acute pancreatitis in an area of the city center which is supplied with particularly hard water. Thus, the chemical composition of the domestic water supply may play a role in the manifestation of acute pancreatitis [4, 5, 7]. Further studies are required.

References

1. Assmus C, Petersen M, Gottesleben F, Dröge M, Lankisch PG (1996) Epidemiology of acute pancreatitis in a defined German population. Digestion 57:217 (abstr)
2. Balthazar EJ, Ranson JHC, Naidich DP, Megibow AJ, Caccavale R, Cooper MM (1985) Acute pancreatitis: prognostic value of CT. Radiology 156:767–772
3. Balthazar EJ, Robinson DL, Megibow AJ, Ranson JHC (1990) Acute pancreatitis: value of CT in establishing prognosis. Radiology 174:331–336
4. Bourke JB (1975) Variation in annual incidence of primary acute pancreatitis in Nottingham, 1969–74. Lancet 2:967–969
5. Bourke JB, Giggs JA, Ebdon DS (1979) Variations in the incidence and the spatial distribution of patients with primary acute pancreatitis in Nottingham 1969–76. Gut 20:366–371
6. Corfield AP, Cooper MJ, Williamson RCN (1985) Acute pancreatitis: a lethal disease of increasing incidence. Gut 26:724–729
7. Giggs JA, Bourke JB, Katschinski B (1988) The epidemiology of primary acute pancreatitis in Greater Nottingham: 1969–1983. Soc Sci Med 26:79–89
8. Go VLW (1994) Etiology and epidemiology of pancreatitis in the United States. In: Bradley III EL (ed) Acute Pancreatitis: Diagnosis and Therapy. Raven Press, New York, pp 235–239
9. Jaakkola M, Nordback I (1993) Pancreatitis in Finland between 1970 and 1989. Gut 34:1255–1260
10. Lankisch PG, Schirren CA, Kunze E (1991) Undetected fatal acute pancreatitis: why is the disease so frequently overlooked? Am J Gastroenterol 86:322–326
11. Lankisch PG, Schirren CA, Schmidt H, Schönfelder G, Creutzfeldt W (1989) Etiology and incidence of acute pancreatitis: a 20-year study in a single institution. Digestion 44:20–25
12. Thomson HJ (1985) Acute pancreatitis in North and North-East Scotland. J R Coll Surg Edinb 30:104–110
13. Thomson SR, Hendry WS, McFarlane GA, Davidson AI (1987) Epidemiology and outcome of acute pancreatitis. Br J Surg 74:398–401
14. Tran DD, Van Schilfgaarde R (1994) Prevalence and mortality from acute pancreatitis in the Netherlands during 1971–1990. Digestion 55:342–343 (abstr)
15. Trapnell JE, Duncan EHL (1975) Patterns of incidence in acute pancreatitis. Br Med J 2:179–183
16. Wilson C, Imrie CW (1988) Deaths from acute pancreatitis: why do we miss the diagnosis so frequently? Int J Pancreatol 3:273–282
17. Wilson C, Imrie CW (1990) Changing patterns of incidence and mortality from acute pancreatitis in Scotland, 1961–1985. Br J Surg 77:731–734
18. Worning H (1994) Acute interstitial (edematous) pancreatitis in Denmark. In: Bradley III EL (ed) Acute Pancreatitis: Diagnosis and Therapy. Raven Press, New York, pp 265–269

9 Acute Pancreatitis: Diagnosis

9.1
Clinical Manifestation

9.1.1
Signs and Symptoms

Abdominal pain is the most frequently reported symptom in acute pancreatitis and occurs in almost every case. The patient experiences pain either in the epigastrium alone or in the epigastrium and left upper abdomen, or throughout the entire upper abdomen. Pain radiates through to the back in about half of the patients. Sometimes, it radiates into the left anterior chest, the left shoulder, or the lower abdomen. Pain reported in the right or left lower abdomen is probably caused by pancreatic exudate spreading via the transverse mesocolon to the cecum or along the left colon. Pain is usually more intensive in the upper than in the lower abdomen [16, 17].

According to Paxton and Payne [150], clinical presentation of acute pancreatitis may be divided into the following five categories:

Those in category 1 fit the standard text book description of "an elderly, obese, florid individual who has eaten a large meal preceded by several highballs. A few hours later he is seized with excruciating upper abdominal pain followed immediately by nausea and profuse vomiting". Indeed, acute pancreatitis follows a large meal and/or alcohol excess in 22%–29% of patients [150, 168, 204]. Thus, this form of acute pancreatitis resembles the cerulein-induced experimental pancreatitis caused by overstimulation of the gland [1].

In category 2, the pancreatic attack simulates acute cholecystitis. The onset is usually sudden, with moderately severe epigastric or right upper abdominal pain.

In category 3, the pancreatic attack imitates mechanical obstruction of the small intestine.

Category 4 symptoms resemble acute alcoholism combined with acute gastritis, and patients in category 5 present with a mass either in the epigastrium or the left upper abdomen.

Pancreatic abdominal pain is commonly characterized by violent onset. In some patients it increases gradually and reaches maximum intensity after several hours, but in most cases it starts suddenly and reaches its maximum intensity within 10–30 min.

The intensity of pain rarely fluctuates and, when not treated, persists for several hours or even days. On a scale of 1–10 (10 equals intolerable, agonizing pain), the severity of pain in acute pancreatitis is often described as 10 [17].

A comparative study of the duration of abdominal pain during first attacks of acute pancreatitis showed that pain associated with alcoholic pancreatitis usually lasts longer than pain associated with biliary pancreatitis (mean 6.1 compared to 3.4 days [167]).

Although pain is the leading symptom in acute pancreatitis, it is by no means universal. Cases of painless acute pancreatitis have been described [59, 60, 67, 119, 120, 181]. In patients with postoperative pancreatitis pain may be unappreciated due to sedation. Cases like these contribute to the high rate of undetected acute pancreatitis [123, 199].

Nausea and, in severe cases, vomiting occur often in acute pancreatitis. Both may be caused by abdominal pain, by anterior extension of the retroperitoneal inflammation to the region of the posterior wall of the stomach, or by the development of a significant fluid collection in the lesser sac compressing the body of the stomach and causing obstruction. Another cause may be gastric dilatation, which can be relieved by insertion of a nasogastric tube [17].

9.1.2
Physical Examination

In mild pancreatitis, vital signs may be relatively stable, and the patient may not appear severely ill. In severe pancreatitis, the patient appears seriously ill on first view.

Most patients have difficulty finding a position that provides pain relief. Blood pressure may be low, but hypertension has also been reported [80], the pulse is frequently rapid, and the temperature up to 38.5 °C. Due to abdominal pain, many patients breath shallowly, and due to temperature or pulmonary involvement, most are tachypneic.

General physical examination may show scleral icterus due to compression of the common bile duct by acute inflammation of the head of the pancreas. This has been more frequently observed in patients with biliary than alcoholic acute pancreatitis [33, 167]. In the rare event of hypertriglyceridemia as the underlying etiology, an arcus lipoides may be found or eruptive xanthoma of the skin. In pancreatitis caused by hypercalcemia, band keratopathy, an infiltration on the lateral margins of the cornea, has been described [17]. Visual disturbances due to Purtscher's retinopathy is a very rare event [42, 73, 105, 137, 171, 173, 194].

Tetany is a very rare but usually fatal complication in acute pancreatitis [107]. Psychosis, as reported in older papers, is also rare [170]; however, it remains unclear whether transient hallucinations in alcoholics are due to the withdrawal of alcohol or to the disease itself.

In severe acute pancreatitis cyanosis may be apparent on the face and the extremities. In the event of retroperitoneal hemorrhage there may be dissection of blood causing ecchymosis in the flanks (Grey-Turner's sign, Fig. 9.1) or the umbilicus (Cullen's sign). These *skin signs* are rarely seen (3%), but are associated with a poor prognosis and a fatal outcome in 35% (Table 9.1) [55].

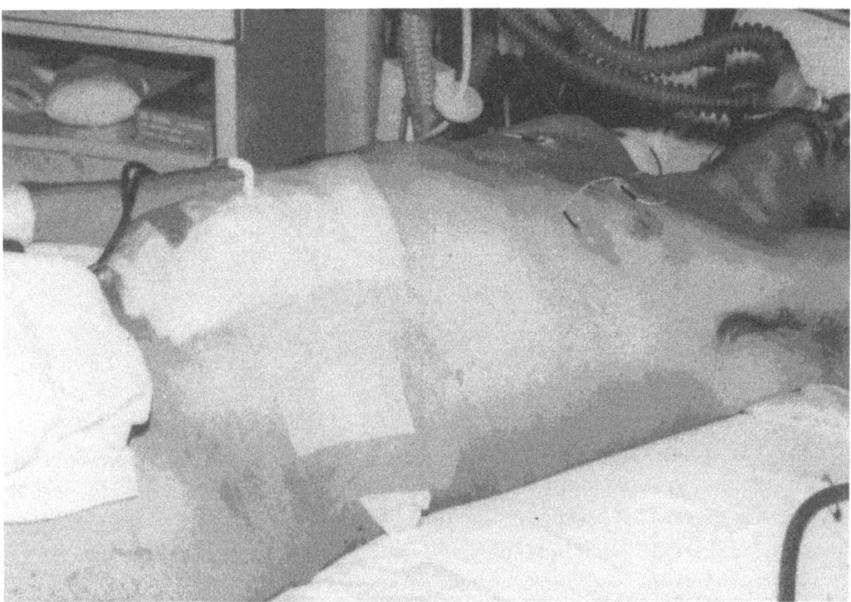

Fig. 9.1. Grey-Turner's sign in a patient with subsequent fatal acute hemorrhagic pancreatitis

Table 9.1. Prognosis of body wall ecchymosis in acute pancreatitis [55]

Sign	Patients	Fatal outcome
Grey-Turner's plus Cullen's	5	1
Grey-Turner's	9	3
Cullen's	9	4
All	23	8 (35%)

On very rare occasions, patients present with discolored swelling of the scrotum or the penis [53, 79, 98, 103], or with subcutaneous fat necrosis (small tender red nodules usually less than 2 cm in size located predominantly over the distal extremities and occasionally over the trunk, buttock, and even the scalp). Sometimes, the necrosis occurs over a joint or even into the joint space, thus producing arthritis as a symptom [23, 29, 45, 54, 96, 132, 135, 152, 155, 169, 201].

Examination of the chest may reveal limited diaphragmatic excursions if there is splinting of the diaphragm as a result of abdominal pain. Dullness to percussion and decreased breath sounds at either side may indicate the presence of a pleural effusion, which is a sign of severe pancreatitis [83, 115]. Cardiac examination will usually only reveal tachycardia; pericarditis and cardiac tamponades are very rare events [141, 142, 172, 185].

Palpation of the abdomen reveals epigastric tenderness in almost all patients with acute pancreatitis. In mild pancreatitis the tenderness may be moderate, and muscular rigidity may be absent.

Table 9.2. Correct prediction of severity of acute pancreatitis [138]

Final assessment	Time after admission	Clinical assessment (%)	Predictors by multiple criteria	
			Ranson et al. [158] (%)	Imrie et al. [101] (%)
Mild acute pancreatitis	8 h	100	—	—
	24 h	98	—	—
	48 h	100	79	83
Severe acute pancreatitis	8 h	39	—	—
	24 h	73	—	—
	48 h	83	82	71

In severe pancreatitis, epigastric tenderness is also severe and may be present throughout the abdomen, usually accompanied by muscular rigidity (i.e., voluntary guarding). Ascites may be present, and especially in alcoholics an enlargement of the liver and the spleen may be found. On auscultation, the bowel sounds may be absent. An ileus is found in 25% of interstitial and in 95% of necrotizing pancreatitis [144].

Now that imaging procedures such as ultrasound and computed tomography (CT) are more available, the diagnosis of acute pancreatitis has become somewhat easier. It is worthwhile to remember that good clinical evaluation alone as early as 8 h after admission to the hospital will correctly predict the final assessment of the disease as mild in 100% but as severe in only 39% of the cases. When compared to assessment of the disease by multiple criteria according to Ranson [158] and Imrie [101] after 48 h, clinical assessment is superior in evaluating mild, and just as good for severe acute pancreatitis (Table 9.2) [138].

9.2
Laboratory Investigations

9.2.1
Enzymes

9.2.1.1
Serum Amylase

Amylase is an enzyme with a molecular weight of 50000 daltons that hydrolyzes the internal α-1,4 linkages of starch. Amylase hydrolyzes this α-1,4 bonds only when there are at least two glucose molecules on either side of the linkage, and it has no effect on the branching α-1,6 linkages. Therefore, the endproducts of digestion are maltose, maltotriose, and larger fragments (dextrins) that contain the branching α-1,6 linkages. With one possible exception (hypertriglyceridemic serum), there appear to be no clinically important inhibitors of amylase in serum or urine.

The pancreas and salivary glands have amylase concentrations that are several orders of magnitude higher than those in other tissues. Low levels of poorly characterized amylases are also present in the Fallopian tube, lung, tears, sweat, and human milk. The small bowel contains maltase as well as adherent pancreatic isoamylase; however, the bowel does not appear to synthetize a true α-amylase. However, in patients with extended gut infarction, luminal amylase may be reabsorbed and levels may reach the diagnostic range of acute pancreatitis [198].

With obstruction and/or inflammation of the salivary glands or the pancreas, amylase enters the blood directly or via the lymphatics, thus accounting for the elevated serum amylase levels in acute pancreatitis or parotitis [129].

Amylase is cleared from the serum with a half-life time of up to 10 h [147]. Thus, even very high serum amylase levels will return to normal within 24 h if this enzyme is not continuously added to the serum. As a result, it is important to determine serum amylase concentration as soon as possible. Post mortem reports of normal serum amylase levels in patients with necrotizing pancreatitis may reflect inability of the destroyed gland to continue to synthesize amylase [129].

Wohlgemuth [203] in 1910 was the first to describe an increase of urinary amylase in patients with acute pancreatitis. Elman et al. [66] began in 1929 to measure serum amylase to diagnose the disease. As the result of detection of other pancreatic enzymes and the development of more sophisticated measuring techniques, numerous studies have compared the increase of enzyme levels and their significance for diagnosing acute pancreatitis.

Sensitivity and specificity of serum amylase estimation probably comprise the gold standard for diagnosing acute pancreatitis. In two studies in which diagnosis of acute pancreatitis was ascertained by imaging procedures, laparotomy, or post mortem examinations, sensitivity of amylase estimation was between 81% and 88.9% [47, 178]. Of all pancreatic enzymes, serum amylase is the first to return to normal [90, 114, 187, 188]. Winslet et al. [202] showed that the sensitivity of amylase estimation decreases to 33% after 48 h, and Ventrucci et al. [188] found that on day 4 after admission only 67% of patients had elevated serum amylase levels as compared to 90% with elevated lipase levels. In another study [114] where enzyme elevation was correlated with clinical recovery (i.e., relief of pain and start of oral food intake), amylase and pancreatic isoamylase were found to be normal, whereas lipase (12% of the patients) and especially trypsin (52% of the patients) were still 3 times above the upper limit of normal. Thus, serum amylase reflects the clinical condition of the patients best.

Concerning the day-by-day decrease of pancreatic enzymes following acute pancreatitis, the majority of studies show that amylase returns quicker to normal levels than lipase [37, 64, 112, 175]. In proportion to amylase, the decrease of pancreatic isoamylase, trypsin, and elastase-1 is also slower [30, 64, 74, 112, 143, 186]. This nonparallel decrease may be of clinical importance in patients with a long interval between the onset of symptoms and the admission to hospital. In these cases, amylase may be in the nondiagnostic range or even normal on admission, whereas lipase levels are still significantly elevated.

Serum amylase levels vary depending on the etiology of pancreatitis. Many investigators found lower amylase levels on admission in patients with alcohol-induced acute pancreatitis as compared to other etiological groups, but due to large overlap, this difference cannot be used for an early etiological differentiation [50, 95, 121, 148, 149, 179, 202]. Recently, serum carbohydrate-deficient transferrin (CDT) estimation has been used to detect alcoholic etiology for acute pancreatitis and has been found to have a sensitivity of 75% and a specificity of 100% [104].

Another reason for nonelevated serum amylase levels in acute pancreatitis may be hyperlipidemia [182]. Hyperlipidemia associated with acute pancreatitis may be primary or secondary to alcohol abuse [56]. In about 50% of patients with abdominal pain and hypertriglyceridemia clinically believed to have acute pancreatitis, serum or urinary amylase, or lipase levels, are not elevated. This may occur even when CT has confirmed obvious pancreatic inflammation [182]. Further proof of the presence of acute pancreatitis is that a urinary amylase-creatinine clearance ratio is abnormal in this setting [128, 191]. Also, dilution of the serum permits demonstration of elevated enzyme levels suggesting the presence of an inhibitor in the blood. However, neither the presence of an inhibitor [78] nor the abnormal clearance ratio have been confirmed by others [182].

In patients with abdominal pain typical for acute pancreatitis and an amylase elevation above 3 times the upper limit of normal, the diagnosis of acute pancreatitis is usually clear. In comparison, the significance of less than 3-times elevation is unclear. This may be due to a long interval between the onset of symptoms and first measurement of amylase at the time of admission to hospital. In this case, other enzymes, especially lipase, usually will still be in the diagnostic range. Furthermore, in alcoholics, pain may represent a relapsing attack of chronic pancreatitis. At this stage, the destroyed gland may not be able to synthetize enough amylase.

A variety of other conditions (Table 9.3) may cause or be associated with hyperamylasemia, and in these cases, the differential diagnosis may be difficult and requires separation of serum amylase into the pancreatic and salivary isoamylase components, especially if imaging and endoscopic procedures and the case history do not explain the reason for extrapancreatic hyperamylasemia [153, 166].

9.2.1.2
Macroamylasemia

In 1964, Wilding et al. [195] described in one patient a prolonged hyperamylasemia, ascribed to binding of amylase with serum globulin. Three years later, Berk et al. [28] described 3 more patients and suggested the term *macroamylasemia* for the peculiar form of hyperamylasemia. Today, it is known that macroamylases are large molecules ranging in molecular weight from 150 000 to 2 000 000 compared with 50 000 to 55 000 for normal human amylase [27]. Macroamylasemia occurs in 0.1% of the population [102], but in up to 2.7% of hospitalized patients [24, 38, 93]. Three types have been identified by a number of diagnostic procedures:

Type I is the classic form initially described [28, 195]. It is characterized by persistent hyperamylasemia, reduced urinary amylase levels and a relative high concentration of serum macroamylase complex.

Type II is also associated with hyperamylasemia, but the urinary amylase concentration is not uniformly diminished, and the ratio of macroamylase to normal-sized serum amylase is much less than in *type I*.

In *type III*, urinary and serum amylases are normal, and usually a low ratio of macroamylase to normal-sized serum amylase exists. The condition may be considered as

Table 9.3. Conditions that cause or are associated with hyperamylasemia according to Salt and Schenker [166], modified by Pieper and Bigelow [153]

Disease	Likely predominant type of serum amylase
● Pancreatic diseases	
Pancreatitis – acute or chronic	P
– Pseudocyst	P
– Pancreatic ascites	P
Pancreatic trauma	
– Blunt trauma	P
– Abdominal or retroperitoneal surgery	P
– Endoscopic retrograde pancreatography	P
Choledocholithiasis	P
Pancreatic cancer	P
Early cystic fibrosis	P
● Salivary diseases	
Parotitis	S
Trauma/surgery	S
Radiation	S
Calculi	S
● Gut diseases	
Perforated bowel	P
Mesenteric infarction	P
Intestinal obstruction	P
Appendicitis	P
Peritonitis	P
● Liver diseases	
Hepatitis	S and P
Cirrhosis	S and P
● Alcoholism	S or P
● Ectopic amylase production by malignancies	S
● Acidosis	
Ketoacidosis	S or P
Nonketotic	S
● Renal failure	S and P
● Macroamylasemia	M
● Female genital tract	
Ruptured ectopic pregnancy	S
Fallopian or ovarian cysts	S
Salpingitis	S
● Postoperative	
Extracorporeal circulation	S or P
Nonabdominal surgery	S or P
● Miscellaneous	
Pneumonia	S
Cerebral trauma	[a]
Burns	[a]
Abdominal aortic aneurysm	P
Drugs	S or P
Anorexia nervosa and/or bulimia	S

P, pancreatic isoamylase; S, salivary type amylase; M, macroamylase.

[a] No data given on the source of amylase.

a benign biochemical alteration and may persist for many years without obvious ill effects and may spontaneously disappear.

However, the possibility of this condition has to be remembered in cases of unexplained hyperamylasemia, because otherwise the patient may be subject to an enormous amount of unnecessary diagnostic and therapeutic procedures. However, this applies only for types I and II both associated with hyperamylasemia, and not for type III, where serum and urine amylases are normal.

Of further importance is that macroamylasemia can be induced by hydroxyethyl starch as a plasma substitute [62, 140].

9.2.1.3
Pancreatic Isoamylase

Since total serum amylase levels are influenced by changes in either the salivary (S) type or pancreatic (P) type component, different methods such as chromatography, electrophoresis, isoelectric focusing or a biochemical method using a salivary isoamylase inhibitor have been used to separate these two components [113]. Because these methods are time-consuming, they are not part of common clinical practice. Nonetheless, measurement of pancreatic isoamylase may be helpful for differential diagnosis of unexplained hyperamylasemia (Table 9.3) and in patients with normal serum amylase who are suspected of having acute pancreatitis. As a curiosity, normal serum amylase activity due to pancreatic isoamylase deficiency has been described in severe acute pancreatitis [36].

9.2.1.4
Urinary Amylase

Since considerable amount of amylase is excreted in the urine, urinary amylase estimation has been used for the diagnosis of acute pancreatitis. Estimation in spontaneously passed urine seems to show the same results as a 2-h urinary collection [88]. Comparative studies have shown that estimation of serum and urinary amylases shows similar results [51, 87, 88, 92, 180]. The development of urinary amylase test tape has much simplified the estimation of urinary amylase [51, 92, 180], but has not been widely used.

In patients with unexplained abdominal pain and hyperamylasuria in the absence of hyperamylasemia, Münchhausen's syndrome should be suspected. At least one patient with personality disorders has been described who added his saliva to his urine resulting in hyperamylasuria [162].

9.2.1.5
Amylase-Creatinine Clearance Ratio

Renal clearance of amylase from the blood expressed as a proportion of simultaneous creatinine clearance has been claimed to increase regularly and significantly in acute pancreatitis, enabling a differential diagnosis between patients with acute pancreatitis and those with hyperamylasemia due to diseases other than pancreatitis [192]. Numerous studies [63, 71, 89, 118, 139, 190] have failed to confirm this. Also, renal insufficiency interferes with the accuracy and specificity of the clearance. Even in moderate renal insufficiency, amylase-creatinine clearance ratio is close enough to values characteristic of acute pancreatitis to cause potential diagnostic confusion [22].

9.2.1.6
Serum Lipase

Lipase is an enzyme with a molecular weight of 58 000 daltons that catalyzes hydrolysis of triglycerides into diglycerides and fatty acids. It is not found exclusively in the pancreas. Other sources of lipase include the stomach, the tongue and the liver. Serum lipase, however, appears mainly to be of pancreatic origin [84]. Until recently, most of the lipase assays were technically demanding, thus preventing the wide use of this enzyme estimation.

The sensitivity of serum lipase test ranges from 85%–100% (for review see Agarwal [4]). Whereas Steinberg et al. [178] found that serum lipase levels were not as accurate as amylase levels, several others have found that serum lipase levels are more sensitive than serum amylase levels [8, 180]. The specificity of lipase estimation in acute pancreatitis is considered to be excellent [178]. In normoamylasemic pancreatitis [47], confirmed by CT, more than two-thirds of the patients had elevated lipase levels. Finally, in a large study of patients with either nonpancreatic abdominal pain or acute pancreatitis, the sensitivity of serum lipase levels >3 times of normal in detecting acute pancreatitis was 100%, and the specificity was 99% as compared with 72% and 99% for serum amylase, respectively [86].

Since patients with acute episodes of alcoholic pancreatitis have high serum lipase levels, whereas patients with gallstone pancreatitis have high serum amylase levels, a prospective study was undertaken to determine whether this ratio of serum lipase to serum amylase would discriminate between these two etiologies. Gumaste et al. [85] reported that sensitivity of such a ratio of >2 in detecting alcoholic acute pancreatitis was 91% and the specificity 76%. Tenner and Steinberg [179] found that the higher the lipase-amylase ratio, the greater the specificity of alcohol as etiology of acute pancreatitis. Only patients with alcoholic acute pancreatitis had a ratio of >5 (sensitivity 31%, specificity 100%). However, subsequent studies showed that lipase-amylase ratio is not good enough for differentiation [94, 121].

Thus, measurement of serum lipase levels seem to have three distinctive advantages over measurement of serum amylase levels:
- Increased sensitivity in detecting acute alcoholic pancreatitis
- Ability to detect pancreatitis in patients who present after several days
- Usefulness in detecting pancreatitis in patients with normal amylase levels

Since amylase levels seem to correlate best with the clinical symptoms [114, 117], it is recommended to measure both enzymes simultaneously, at least on admission of patients suspected to suffer from acute pancreatitis.

9.2.1.7
Macrolipasemia

There are two reports on female patients, one with non-Hodgkin's lymphoma and one with liver cirrhosis who had persistently elevated lipase but normal amylase levels. Imaging procedures showed no evidence of acute pancreatitis. Further investigation revealed a complex formation of lipase with IgA [35, 176].

9.2.1.8
Other Enzymes: Trypsin, Elastase-1, Phospholipase A

Trypsin is a protease present exclusively in the pancreas. Therefore, serum trypsin levels would ideally fulfil the criterion of organ specificity. Serum elastase-1 is a pancreatic enzyme that has specific elastolytic action and plays a key role in the development of vascular complications in acute pancreatitis. Phospholipase A_2 is a lipolytic enzyme that hydrolyzes phospholipids to their corresponding lysocompounds. This enzyme, too, probably plays a decisive role in the development of acute pancreatitis.

Thus, the 3 enzymes increase in acute pancreatitis, and at least trypsin and elastase-1 decrease more slowly than amylase and lipase [74, 114]. However, since all estimation procedures are time-consuming and expensive, none of these has been utilized widely.

Trypsinogen activation can be quantified by measurement of released activation peptides (TAP assay). Urinary TAP concentration correlated significantly with subsequent disease severity [82]. However, due to the difficult estimation (radioimmunoassay) of TAP, this test is not yet measured routinely.

9.2.2
Other Laboratory Investigations

The following laboratory investigations should be made for evaluation of the severity of acute pancreatitis according to prognostic laboratory scores (see Sect. 12.4.3). These tests include:
- C-reactive protein (CRP) and complete blood count (leukocytes, hemoglobin, hematocrit) for evaluation of the inflammatory process and the state of dehydration
- Electrolytes (potassium, sodium, calcium) for evaluation of the state of dehydration and fluid balance

In acute pancreatitis with hyperlipemia, the latter may lead to hyponatremia. Therefore, serum sodium should be measured before and after removing the creamy layer to obtain reliable sodium levels [61].

A reduction in total serum calcium is sometimes severe enough to cause tetany [107]. For the most part, the decrease merely is a reflection of the hypoalbuminia that occurs, and in these cases, ionized, i.e., nonprotein-bound, calcium levels remain at normal or near normal levels [5]. A reduction in the level of ionized calcium may occur for a variety of reasons. A loss of calcium may be due to precipitation of calcium salts into areas of fat necrosis [65], a decrease in parathormone release from the parathyroid glands [48, 161], failure of bony tissues to respond to release parathormone [193] and/or enhanced release of thyrocalcitonin [9]. However, Imrie et al. [100] have shown a rise in parathormone in hypocalcemic patients with acute pancreatitis

- Parameters indicating cholestasis due to compression of the common bile duct by an inflammatory process of the head of the pancreas (alkaline phosphatase, serum glutamic-alanine transaminase (ALT/SGPT), bilirubin)
- Renal function parameters (serum creatinine, blood urea nitrogen (BUN)) for evaluation of renal failure
- Blood coagulation parameters (thrombocytes, Quick's test, partial thrombin time, fibrinogen) for evaluation of blood coagulation disorders
- Blood glucose for evaluation of endocrine failure
- Blood gas analysis (arterial pO_2, base deficit) for evaluation of shock and acute respiratory failure
- Serum albumin, ALT/SGPT, serum glutamic-aspartatic transferase (AST/SGOT), lactate dehydrogenase, and creatine kinase for further evaluation of severity of the disease

9.3
Imaging Procedures

9.3.1
Survey Film of the Abdomen

A preliminary roentgenogram of the abdomen may reveal important radiologic features associated with pancreatitis, including changes involving the colon, small bowel, and stomach.

Colon cut-off sign in acute pancreatitis has been applied to a variety of abnormalities involving the colon. The precise abnormality depends on the pattern of spread of pancreatic exudation. If pancreatitis is confined to the head of the pancreas, pancreatic exudate may extend to the proximal transverse colon, causing intense spasm of this segment, and resulting in dilatation of the ascending colon. If the pancreas is more uniformly inflamed, the pancreatic exudation may extend diffusely from the anterior surface of the pancreas to the lower border of the transverse colon within the mesocolon causing diffuse spasm and irregularity of the haustral pattern of the transverse colon. A third variety of the colon cut-off sign takes place if pancreatic exudate from the tail of the pancreas near the splenic flexure becomes trapped in the phrenicocolic ligament and permeates the descending colon below the splenic flexure. This leads to spasm of the descending colon with secondary dilatation of the transverse colon.

Abnormalities of the small intestine caused by the flow of pancreatic exudation to the mesentery of the small bowel include an ileus of one or more loops of jejunum (the so-called *sentinel loop*), an ileus involving the distal ileum, and at times the cecum as well, or an ileus of the duodenum. The descending duodenum may also be displaced and stretched by an inflamed head of the pancreas.

Abnormalities involving the stomach occur if pancreatic exudate extends from the anterior pararenal space to the lesser sac. When this occurs, there is anterior displacement of the stomach with separation of the contour of the stomach from that of the transverse colon.

On occasion, additional features may be seen on plain roentgenogram of the abdomen. One is the presence of calcified gallstones. This finding would suggest the possibility of acute pancreatitis secondary to passage of gallstones. The second finding is calcification of the pancreas. This finding would suggest that a patient with chronic pancreatitis has experienced a bout of acute inflammation.

9.3.2
Chest Radiography

Radiologic abnormalities involving the chest in acute pancreatitis include elevation of the diaphragms, plate-like atelectasis caused by limited respiratory excursion, or a pleural effusion which may occur bilaterally, on the left side, or on rare occasion on the right side alone [83, 115]. During the first week, there may be evidence of congestive heart failure or acute respiratory distress syndrome. A pericardial effusion is rarely visualized.

9.3.3
Barium Studies

Barium meal study is rarely utilized in evaluation of acute pancreatitis. During evaluation of severe abdominal pain in which the differential diagnosis includes acute pancreatitis, perforated ulcer, or mesenteric infarction, abdominal CT scan is more commonly obtained. In acute pancreatitis, a barium meal examination may show anterior displacement of the stomach and duodenum by an enlarged pancreas, widening of the duodenal loop by an edematous head of the pancreas, and inflammatory changes on the inner aspect of the duodenum caused by adjacent pancreatic inflammation. There may also be mucosal irregularity and pleating of duodenal mucosal folds. If there is a duodenal ileus, barium may remain static in the duodenal loop. Pancreatic inflammation may cause depression of the ligament of Treitz, a jejunal ileus or slow transit (especially if a narcotic agent is administered for relief of pain).

Barium enema is rarely utilized. If there is a colon cut-off sign, a barium enema may reveal spasm in either the descending colon or transverse colon with dilatation of the more proximal segment.

9.3.4
Abdominal Ultrasound

Abdominal ultrasound is an important procedure in the initial evaluation of acute pancreatitis and should be performed within the initial 24 h of hospitalization. Unless bowel gas obscures the pancreas, there may be evidence of acute pancreatitis including enlargement of the gland and loss of normal internal echoes (Fig. 9.2 a–c). However, the severity of pancreatitis can rarely be ascertained by ultrasound. Additional factors that may be of importance include the presence of gallstones and dilatation of

Fig. 9.2a. 26-year-old male patient, no abdominal complaints, routine abdominal ultrasound. *1* liver, *2* pancreas, *3* confluence, *4* splenic vein, *5* vena cava inferior, *6* left renal vein, *7* aorta, *8* stomach, *9* acoustic shadow due to air in the stomach

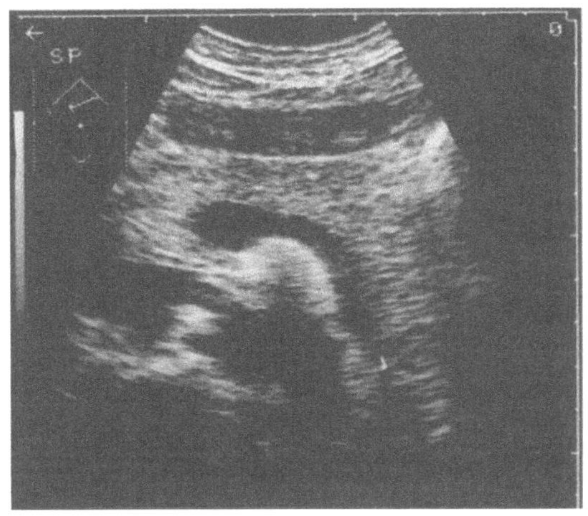

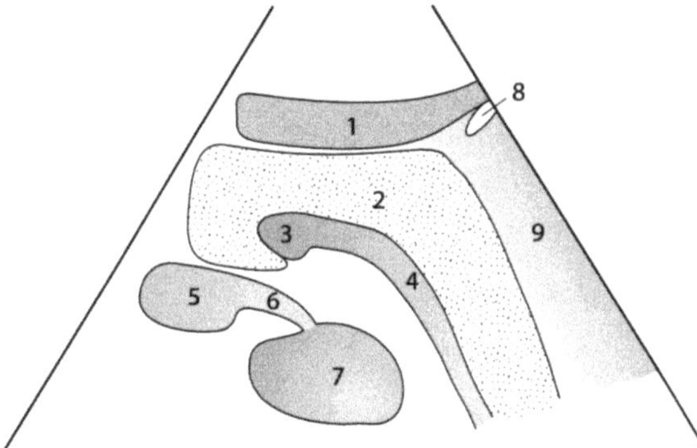

the common bile duct secondary to choledocholithiasis. In addition, an ultrasound examination may reveal the presence of ascites or evidence of prior pancreatic damage in the form of pancreatic ductal calculi. In time, ultrasound can be utilized to monitor the size of a pancreatic pseudocyst.

9.3.5
Endoscopic Ultrasound

Endoscopic ultrasound has not been shown to play an important role in the early evaluation of acute pancreatitis. However, there is recent evidence that endoscopic ultrasound is more sensitive than abdominal ultrasonography and CT in the diagnosis of choledocholithiasis [6]. It will be important to determine whether endoscopic ultrasound is as accurate as the more invasive endoscopic retrograde cholangiopancreatography (ERCP) in determining the presence of gallstones within the common bile duct. If its accuracy can be confirmed, patients with severe gallstone pancreatitis who otherwise would undergo urgent ERCP [68, 145] should undergo the less invasive endoscopic ultrasound.

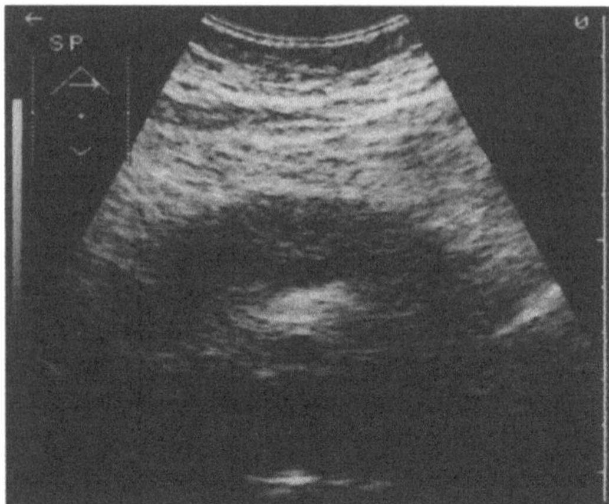

Fig. 9.2 b. 44-year-old female patient with biliary-induced interstitial acute pancreatitis. Diffuse echo-poor swelling of the total gland. *1* head of the pancreas, *2* body of the pancreas, *3* tail of the pancreas, *4* arteria mesenterica superior

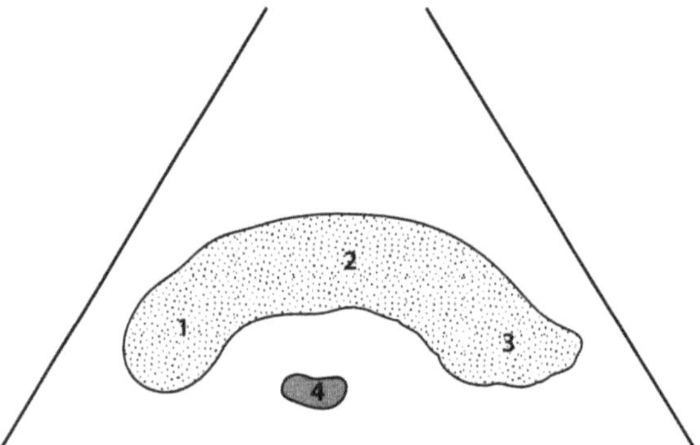

9.3.6
Computed Tomography

Computed tomographic (CT) scan has been of enormous benefit in the care of patients with acute pancreatitis [10, 12, 14, 34, 41, 76, 124, 130]. There are three principle indications for obtaining a CT scan in acute pancreatitis. The first is to establish the diagnosis if other serious intraabdominal conditions such as a perforated ulcer or mesenteric infarction cannot be excluded. Since severe abdominal pain and tenderness associated with acute pancreatitis are caused by the spread of pancreatic inflammatory exudate out of the pancreas, CT scan that demonstrates these changes provides convincing evidence for this diagnosis. The second indication is to stage the severity of acute pancreatitis. As will be noted, severity can be gauged by the presence or absence of pancreatic parenchymal necrosis and by the extent of spread of pancreatic inflammation beyond the confines of the pancreas [12–14, 76]. The third is to define the presence of complications of pancreatitis including involvement of nearby blood vessels, the gastrointestinal tract, and nearby solid organs such as liver, spleen, and kidney [76].

Fig. 9.2c. Same patient as 9.2b, cross section scan. Echo-poor swelling of the pancreas at the border between head and body of the gland. *1* pancreas, *2* vena mesenterica superior

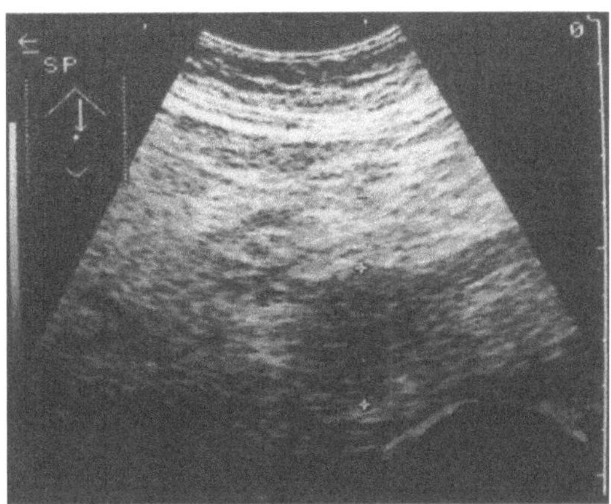

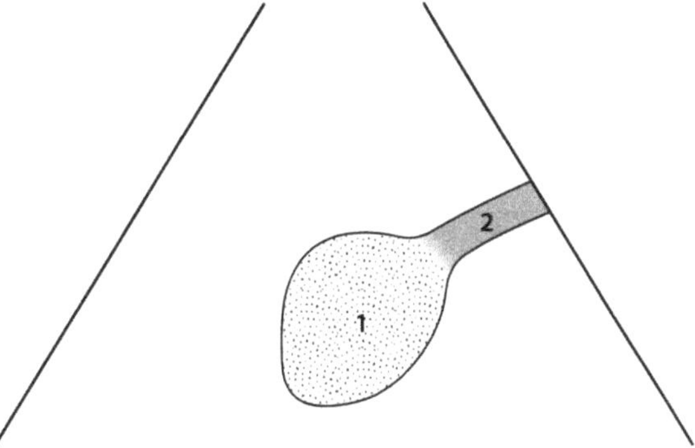

Spiral CT is the most common technique utilized to visualize the pancreas and peripancreatic inflammatory changes. The patient is instructed in breath-holding for 24–30 sec. With this technique, a scan can be obtained from the lower chest to the iliac crest, with continuous data acquisition and computer-generated reconstruction that ensure that there is no gap in visualization. Each tissue slice is typically 5 mm. An oral contrast agent should be administered to opacify the bowel. This step is important to recognize complications of pancreatitis that involve bowel and to be sure that unopacified bowel is not interpreted as a pancreatic fluid collection. Intravenous contrast is also administered when it is important to distinguish interstitial from necrotizing pancreatitis. There are several methods for the rapid intravenous administration of contrast material. One is to infuse 100–150 ml of 60% iodinated contrast agent at a constant rate of 3 ml/sec. Another is to administer the first portion of intravenous contrast at a faster rate and the second portion at a slower rate. Following the rapid administration of intravenous contrast, there is normally an increase in attenuation of pancreatic parenchyma of 40–60 Hounsfield units above baseline attenuation [12, 41, 76]. Nearby vessels are also enhanced, thereby permitting the identification of vascular complications.

If there is suspicion of bleeding as a consequence of pancreatitis, a nonenhanced CT scan should be obtained first. The reason is that blood following a recent bleed is high attenuation material and the prior use of intravenous contrast may hamper its recognition.

There are several contraindications to the use of intravenous contrast. One contraindication is a history of prior severe allergy (such as anaphylaxis or respiratory difficulties) caused by iodinated contrast material. Another is the presence of significant renal impairment, such as a serum creatinine >2 mg%. Some authorities have suggested that when there is total renal shutdown requiring dialysis, intravenous contrast is then permitted [76].

If an allergic reaction is less severe, such as hives, a nonionic contrast agent can be utilized, and the patient can receive an intravenous injection of 200 mg of hydrocortisone intravenously every 6 h for 4 doses prior to the scan plus 25–50 mg of Benadryl intramuscularly 30 min prior to the scan [76]. If renal impairment is less pronounced and the contrast-enhanced CT scan is considered to be necessary, some radiologists prefer to administer a nonionic rather than an ionic agent [76] although the benefit of a nonionic agent has not as yet been clearly demonstrated. In addition, patients should be hydrated intravenously with 0.45% saline 3–6 h prior to and following the CT [174], and if considered necessary, should receive 25–50 g of mannitol intravenously

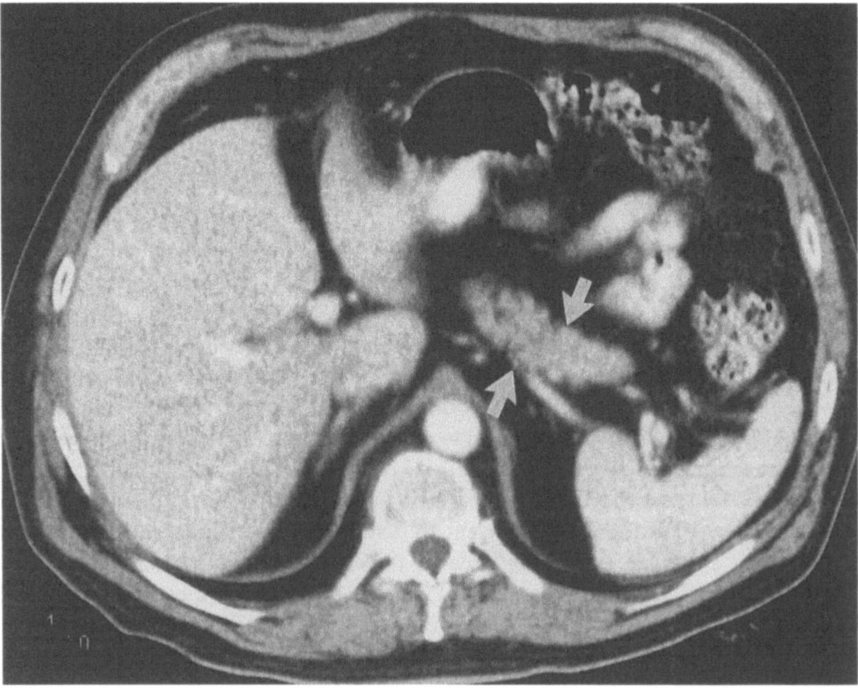

Fig. 9.3 a. Normal CT scan. Dynamic contrast-enhanced CT scan through the body and tail of the pancreas shows normal uniform enhancement and size of the pancreatic parenchyma (*arrows*). The peripancreatic fat is well preserved

immediately after the contrast bolus [76]. In addition, the volume of contrast can be reduced to 75 ml.

Some concern has also been expressed that the use of intravenous contrast early in the course of acute pancreatitis might intensify pancreatic necrosis. In one animal model of acute pancreatitis utilizing the rat, pancreatic necrosis became more extensive following the use of intravenous contrast [75]. The explanation was that the contrast material accentuated tissue hypoxemia. However, in a second animal model of pancreatitis utilizing the opossum, intravenous contrast did not increase the amount of pancreatic necrosis [108]. Several radiologists have expressed confidence that contrast-enhanced CT is not harmful early in acute pancreatitis [11].

CT scan clearly demarcates the extraperitoneal region into 3 spaces: the anterior pararenal space, the perirenal space, and the posterior pararenal space [130]. The anterior pararenal space contains the pancreas and retroperitoneal portions of the alimentary tract, including descending duodenum and colon (Fig. 9.3a, b). The perirenal space is confined by the anterior and posterior renal (Gerota) fascia and contains the kidney, adrenal gland, proximal renal collecting system, renal vessels, and some fat. The perirenal space is rarely involved in acute pancreatitis. The posterior pararenal space contains no organs. Fluid from the anterior pararenal space may extend into the posterior pararenal space.

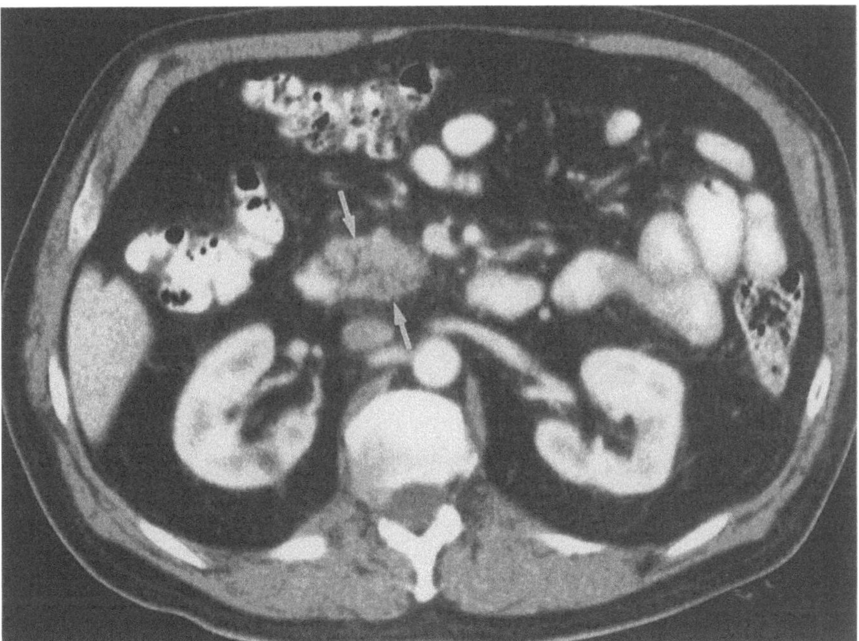

Fig. 9.3 b. Normal CT scan. Dynamic contrast-enhanced CT scan through the head of the pancreas reveals normal enhancement and size of pancreatic parenchyma (*arrows*) with well-preserved peripancreatic fat

In mild acute pancreatitis, inflammatory changes are confined primarily to the pancreas; in severe pancreatitis, pancreatic enzymes and other toxic materials may extravasate out of the pancreas into the anterior pararenal space, posterior pararenal space, and into other locations including the peritoneal cavity.

When intravenous contrast is used, a distinction can usually be made between interstitial and necrotizing pancreatitis. In interstitial pancreatitis, there is an increase in the attenuation of the gland of 40–60 Hounsfield units above baseline [12, 41, 76]. If the enhancement is homogenous, the process is termed *interstitial pancreatitis* (Fig. 9.4 a, b). However, if following intravenous contrast there is a well-marginated zone of unenhanced parenchyma, consideration must be given to the possibility that this zone represents an area of pancreatic necrosis (Fig. 9.5 a, b). According to the conclusions reached at the Atlanta symposium (an international symposium on acute pancreatitis held in Atlanta, Georgia, on September 11–13, 1992 [19]), a well-marginated zone of unenhanced parenchyma > 3 cm in diameter is considered strong evidence in favor of pancreatic necrosis. Presumably, a zone that is < 3 cm in diameter could represent displacement of viable parenchyma by intrapancreatic fluid. At times, more than 90% of the pancreas is completely necrotic yielding a widespread homogenous low attenuation configuration sometimes called *central cavitary necrosis* [21, 46].

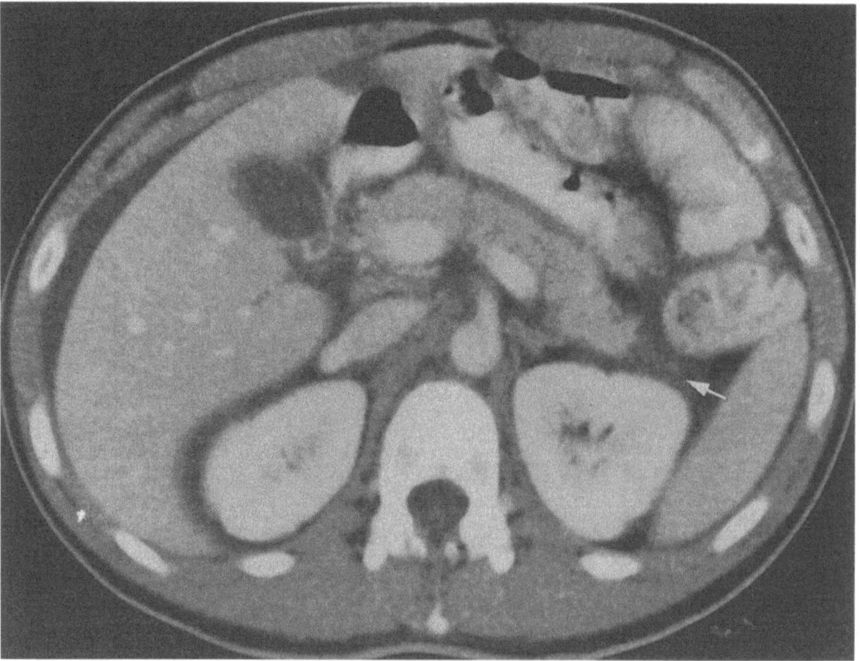

Fig. 9.4 a. Interstitial pancreatitis. Dynamic contrast-enhanced CT scan during an acute episode of pancreatitis in a 46-year-old woman with recurrent idiopathic pancreatitis reveals a normal appearing pancreas. There are inflammatory changes near the tail of the pancreas (*arrow*). The patient made an uneventful recovery within 4 days

When there is pancreatic necrosis, there invariably is also peripancreatic necrosis [110]. However, it is not usually possible to determine by CT scan whether low attenuation areas in the peripancreatic area contain fat necrosis or fluid [106].

The Atlanta symposium also recognized that acute fluid collections are a frequent occurrence early in the course of acute pancreatitis. Acute fluid collections are typically located near the pancreas and regress spontaneously in approximately one-half of cases (Figs. 9.4 a, b, 9.5 a, b). In comparison, a pseudocyst was defined as a collection of pancreatic juice enclosed by a wall of fibrous or granulation tissue that requires at least 4 weeks to form (Fig. 9.6). A pseudocyst may increase in size, remain stable in configuration, or regress spontaneously. A pancreatic abscess was defined as a loculated intraabdominal collection of pus close by the pancreas that contains little if any pancreatic necrosis. In most instances, a pancreatic abscess is a late phenomenon and appears to be caused by either liquefaction of an area of pancreatic necrosis or secondary infection within a pancreatic pseudocyst [19, 31, 39, 72].

Several grading systems have been advanced in an effort to quantitate the severity of pancreatitis as evidenced by CT scan [12–14, 76]. One CT system developed by Balthazar et al. [13] assesses severity in acute pancreatitis into five categories (Table 9.4): grade A is represented by a normal appearing pancreas; grade B by focal or diffuse

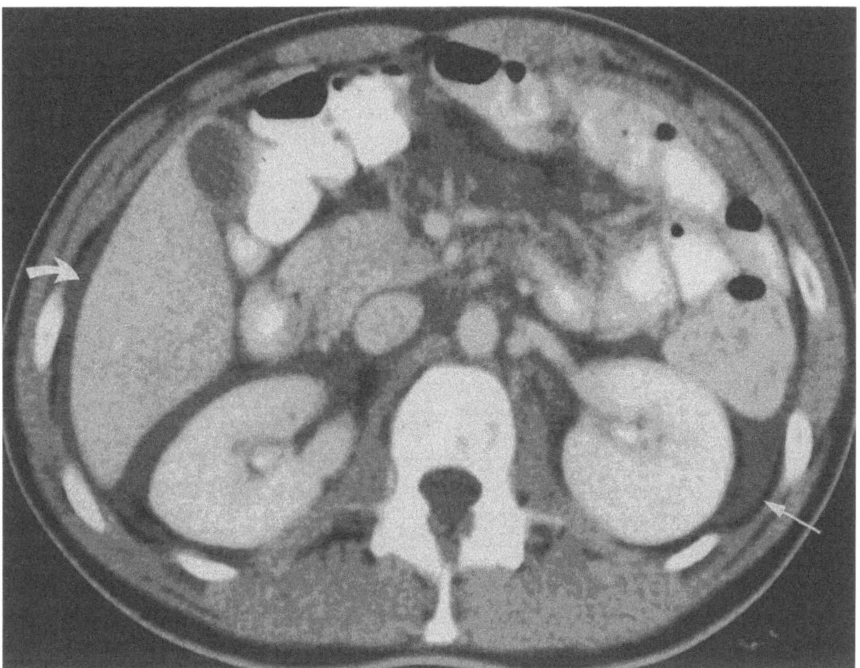

Fig. 9.4 b. Interstitial pancreatitis. Scan obtained through the head of the pancreas again demonstrates normal enhancement. There is considerable infiltration of fat with inflammatory exudate in the mesentery extending anteriorly to the transverse colon. Ascites is seen (*curved arrow*). There is also fluid within the left paracolic gutter (*straight arrow*)

Table 9.4. CT grading of acute pancreatitis according to Balthazar et al. [13, 14], slightly modified

Staging	Score
A. Normal pancreas	0
B. Focal or diffuse enlargement of the pancreas, including contour irregularities, nonhomogeneous attenuation of the gland, dilatation of pancreatic duct, foci of small fluid collections within the gland	1
C. Same as B plus involvement of peripancreatic fat	2
D. Same as B and C plus single, ill-defined fluid collection	3
E. Same as B and C plus ≥ 2 ill-defined fluid collections and/or intra-/peripancreatic gas	4
Necrosis (%)	
0	0
< 33	2
33– < 50	4
≥ 50	6
Maximum	10

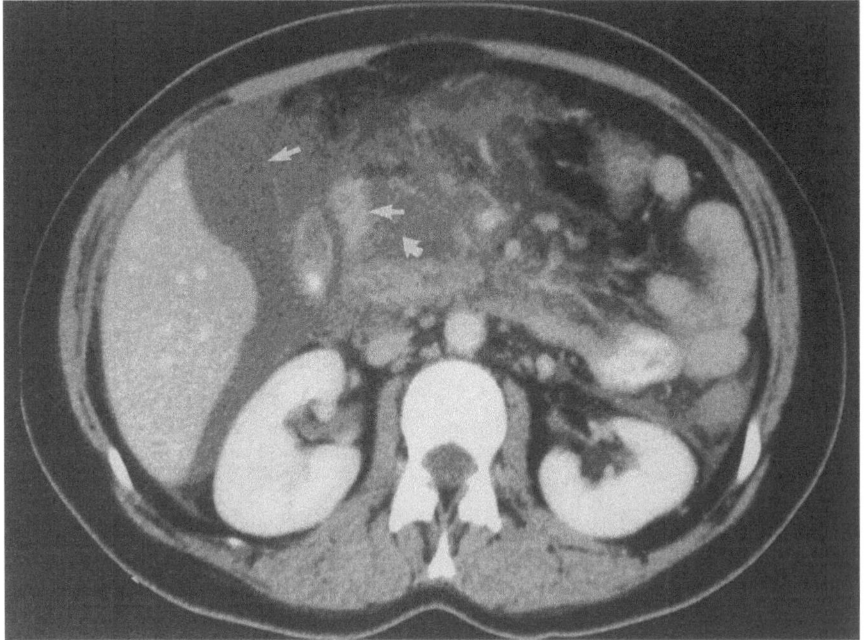

Fig. 9.5 a. Sterile necrosis of the pancreas. Dynamic contrast-enhanced CT scan performed on a 26-year-old woman on the 3rd day of gallstone pancreatitis reveals only a small portion of enhancing pancreatic parenchyma in the lateral aspect of the head of the pancreas (*horizontal arrow*). Adjacent to this, there is a large area of the head of the pancreas that does not enhance, consistent with necrosis and/or fluid (*curved arrow*). In addition, there are severe inflammatory changes extending to the anterior abdominal wall. Fluid is seen to track along the liver and surround the gallbladder (*oblique arrow*). There is a small amount of ascites around the liver. This appearance conforms to Balthazar-Ranson grade E pancreatitis with a severity score of at least 8 (see text)

enlargement of the pancreas; grade C by pancreatic gland abnormalities associated with mild peripancreatic inflammation (an appearance that is sometimes termed *stranding* to indicate a somewhat subtle disturbance of peripancreatic tissue that gives a fuzzy appearance to the silhouette of the pancreas); grade D, fluid collection in a single location (this collection invariably takes place within the anterior pararenal space and is frequently associated with enlargement of the pancreas); grade E, two or more fluid collections nearby the pancreas or gas within the pancreas or within peripancreatic inflammation (Figs. 9.5 a, b, 9.7 a–e). Fluid collections usually occur in the anterior pararenal space and in some other location such as the lesser sac or the posterior pararenal space. Gas, if present, invariably indicates the presence of infection (Fig. 9.8). However, most pancreatic infections occur in the absence of gas on CT scan [7, 76, 106, 117].

Patients with grade E pancreatitis have the most severe form of the disease [13, 14]. At least one-half of patients with grade E pancreatitis have necrotizing rather than interstitial pancreatitis. Most patients with pancreatic infection have CT evidence of grade E pancreatitis [14].

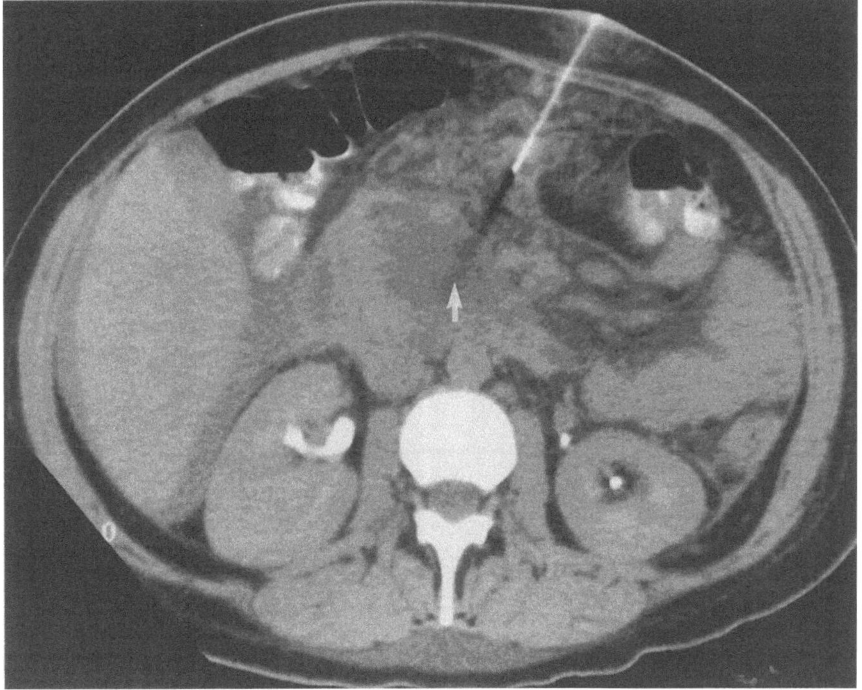

Fig. 9.5 b. Sterile necrosis of the pancreas. Because of persistent leukocytosis and temperature, guided percutaneous aspiration was performed on the 9th day of illness. The needle has been advanced under CT guidance avoiding the colon. It was then advanced further into the area of nonenhancement in the body of the pancreas (*arrow*). Gram stain and culture were negative, and the patient was managed medically

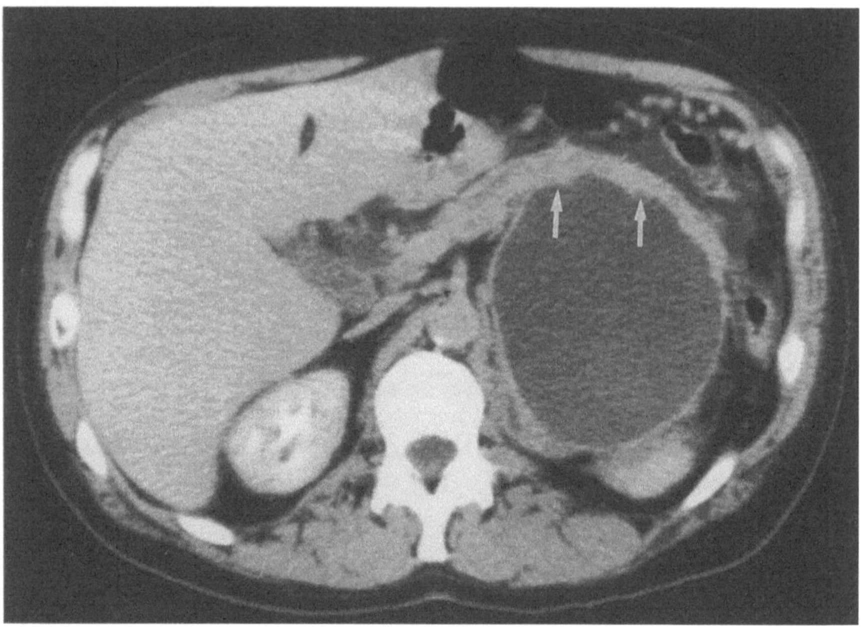

Fig. 9.6. Pseudocyst in tail of the pancreas. Dynamic contrast-enhanced CT scan shows a large homogenous low-attenuation mass posterior to the body and tail of the pancreas, which is displaced anteriorly (*arrows*). The mass is enclosed by a thin uniform capsule. The appearance is consistent with a pseudocyst. This patient had recovered from an episode of pancreatitis 2 months earlier. Because of persistence of symptoms, the patient underwent a distal pancreatectomy and splenectomy

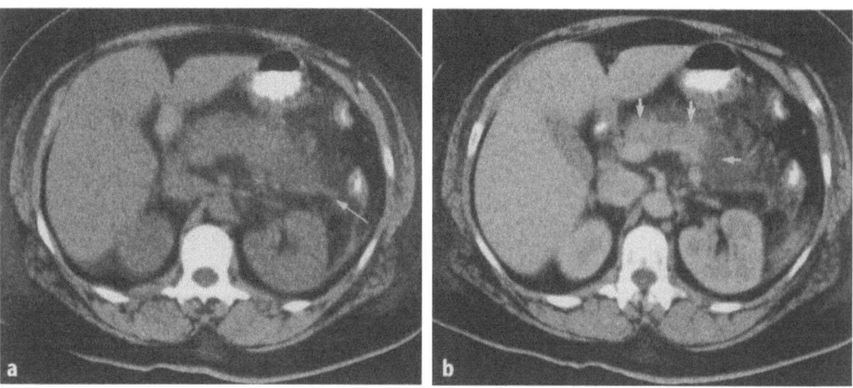

Fig. 9.7 a, b. Necrotizing pancreatitis. **a** Unenhanced CT scan on the 6th day of hospitalization of a 39-year-old woman with gallstone pancreatitis shows generalized enlargement of the pancreas with peripancreatic inflammatory changes extending into the left anterior pararenal space (*arrow*). This appearance would conform to a Balthazar-Ranson grade C pancreatitis. **b** Dynamic contrast-enhanced CT scan taken at the same level on the same day reveals uniform enhancement of the body of the pancreas (*vertical arrows*). However, there is total lack of enhancement of the distal body of the pancreas indicative of pancreatic necrosis (*horizontal arrow*). This appearance conforms to a Balthazar-Ranson severity index of 4 (2 points for grade C and 2 points for necrosis of one-third of the pancreas)

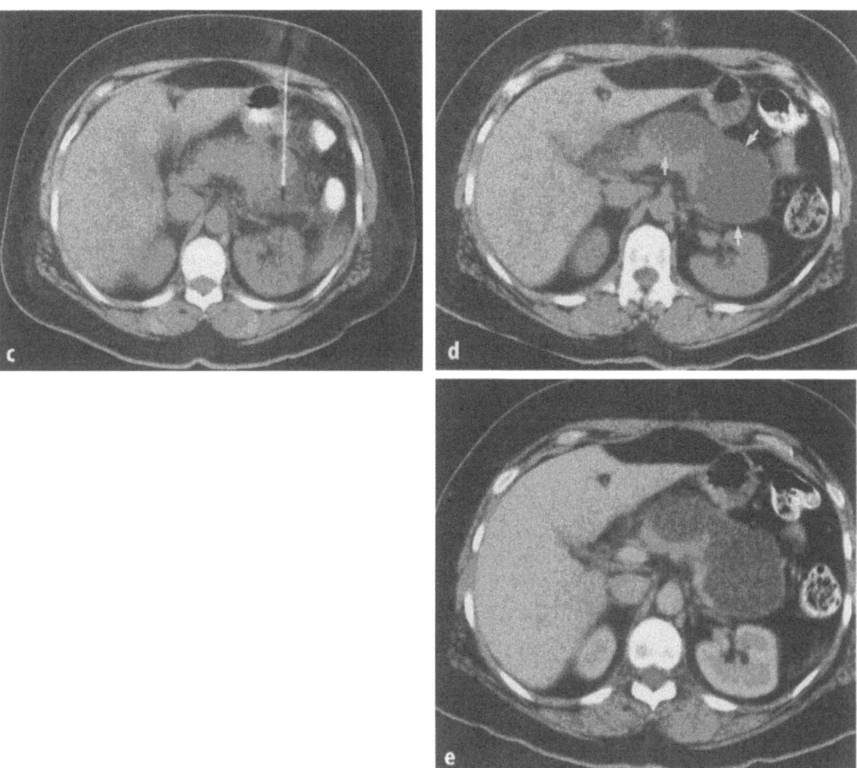

Fig. 9.7 c–e. Necrotizing pancreatitis. **c** Because of persistent leukocytosis and fever, guided percutaneous aspiration was performed 3 days later in a search for pancreatic infection. The needle was advanced between stomach and colon into the area of low attenuation replacing the tail of the pancreas. Gram stain and culture were negative, and the patient was maintained on medical therapy. **d** One month later, unenhanced CT scan reveals persistent enlargement of the pancreas. Even without intravenous contrast, there appears to be a large area of low attenuation replacing pancreatic parenchyma in the body and tail of the pancreas (*arrows*). **e** Dynamic contrast-enhanced CT scan at the same level on the same day reveals normally enhanced residual pancreatic tissue of the body of the pancreas. The body and tail of the pancreas are replaced by a 7 × 10 × 6 cm bilobed low-attenuation mass. The contents of this large mass probably represent a combination of necrosis and fluid. The peripancreatic inflammatory changes have resolved. The patient was asymptomatic and was able to eat without pain

A second grading system combines the A–E grading system of an unenhanced CT scan with a quantification of the amount of pancreatic necrosis (Table 9.4) [12, 14]. In this system, grade A is assigned 0 points; grade B, 1 point; C, 2 points; D, 3 points; and E, 4 points. To this total, an additional 2, 4, or 6 points are added depending on whether the amount of necrosis is estimated to be 30% or less, 30%–50%, or > 50%. Thus, a patient with a grade E pancreatitis is first awarded 4 points. Should dynamic contrast-enhanced CT scan reveal 30%–50% necrosis, an additional 4 points are added for a total score of 8. The higher the CT severity index, the worse the prognosis (Figs. 9.5, 9.7) [12, 14].

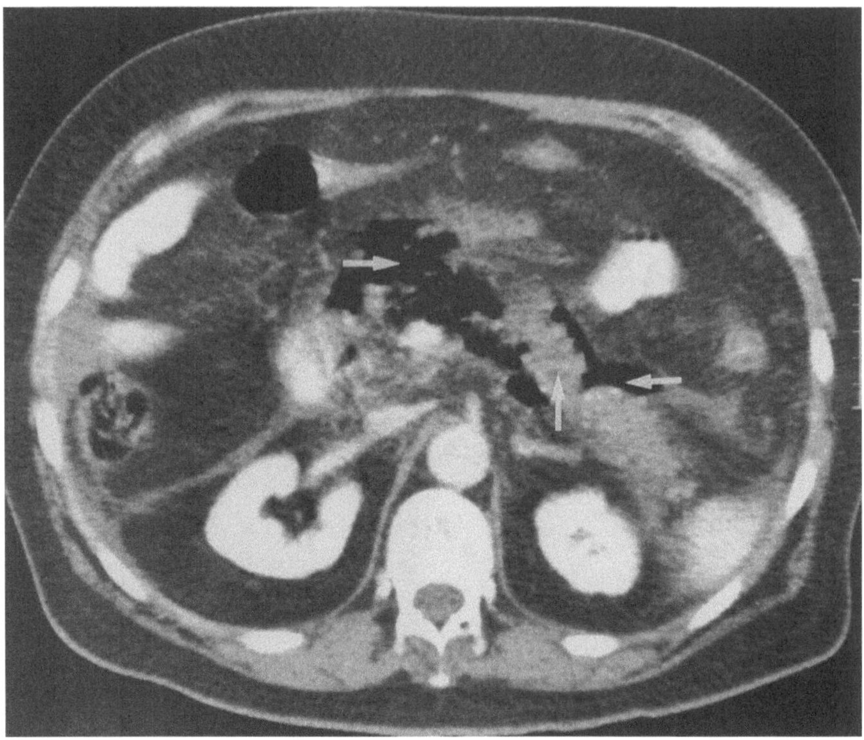

Fig. 9.8. Infected necrosis. Dynamic contrast-enhanced CT scan reveals a considerable amount of peripancreatic air (*horizontal arrows*). There is diminished and heterogenous enhancement within the visualized portions of the pancreas (*vertical arrow*). There are diffuse inflammatory changes extending to the anterior abdominal wall. This patient had entered another hospital only 3 days earlier with idiopathic pancreatitis. Following this CT scan, he was taken immediately for surgical debridement of infected pancreatic necrosis caused by a Gram-negative bacillus. He made an uneventful recovery

The term *infected pseudocyst* was deleted at the Atlanta symposium, and a recommendation was made that a pseudocyst that becomes secondarily infected should be termed an abscess. The term *phlegmon* was also deleted because authors have used this term indiscriminately for a wide variety of entities including interstitial pancreatitis, necrotizing pancreatitis, sterile necrosis, infected necrosis, and even a palpable abdominal mass. If a clinician elects to use the term phlegmon, the proper meaning is that the pancreas is considerably enlarged and that there is reason to be concerned. Unless dynamic contrast-enhanced CT scan is utilized, it is not possible to know whether the patient has interstitial or necrotizing pancreatitis. If necrotizing pancreatitis, it is not possible to know whether the patient has sterile or infected necrosis.

9.3.7
Magnetic Resonance Imaging

Information regarding the value of magnetic resonance imaging (MRI) in acute pancreatitis is fragmentary. Preliminary evidence would suggest that MRI provides essentially the same information as CT scan. The role of MRI in acute pancreatitis remains to be established.

9.3.8
Endoscopic Retrograde Cholangiopancreatography

ERCP is not required to establish a diagnosis of acute pancreatitis. In both interstitial pancreatitis and pancreatitis associated with only minimal necrosis, the main pancreatic duct is invariably normal [7, 146]. However, when there is significant pancreatic necrosis, the main pancreatic duct is normal in only one-half of cases [7]; the duct in the remainder of the cases is either blocked [7], or disrupted [146]. Since these findings are not likely to help in the decision regarding the care of the patient, ERCP is not recommended in acute pancreatitis except for its role in finding and removing common bile duct stones among patients with severe gallstone pancreatitis [68, 145].

9.4
Synopsis of Diagnostic Procedures and Grading of Severity

9.4.1
Introduction

At the Atlanta symposium, an effort was made to standardize terminology and to provide an updated clinically relevant classification system of acute pancreatitis [19, 39]. A multidisciplinary group extracted the best ideas from previous symposia and integrated these with newer concepts and new technology to develop a classification system that would have broad applicability. The importance of this symposium was several-fold. First, it was important that specialists caring for patients with pancreatitis agree on basic terminology so as to be able to communicate more effectively with one another. Second, the new classification system was important to improve the quality of clinical research. By obtaining a broad consensus pertaining to terminology and the characterization of the severity of illness, clinical research in the future would place all patients within the same broad framework such that collaborative studies could be performed and data could be interpreted properly.

In accordance with the results of the symposium, mild acute pancreatitis was defined as an illness that was associated with minimal organ dysfunction and an uneventful recovery. Severe acute pancreatitis was defined as an illness that was associated with organ failure and/or local complications, particularly necrosis, pseudocyst, and abscess [19, 39]. Essentially all deaths would take place among patients with severe acute pancreatitis.

Furthermore, it was acknowledged that severe acute pancreatitis could be anticipated early in the course of acute pancreatitis by the presence of unfavorable early predictors of severity [19]. The importance of these predictors would be to help the clinician gauge the severity of pancreatitis as early as possible and provide optimal care in the belief that early aggressive care could decrease morbidity and mortality. Two scoring systems that were mentioned in the Atlanta symposium were Ranson's scores and APACHE-II (Acute Physiology and Chronic Health Evaluation) points. Additional early predictors of severity include clinical scoring systems, peritoneal lavage, serum tests (including interleukin-6 [IL-6], C-reactive protein [CRP], polymorphonuclear [PMN] elastase, and phospholipase A_2), and urinary trypsinogen activation peptides [3, 18, 177].

9.4.2
Early Prognostic Signs

9.4.2.1
Ranson's Signs

In 1974, Ranson and his colleagues culled a large number of potential findings and identified 11 with prognostic significance (Table 9.5) [156, 157]. Of the 11, 5 are measured at the time of admission, 4 of which indicate to some extent the intensity of the local inflammatory process. The 6 that are measured within the initial 48 h of admission reflect for the most part the deleterious effects of third-space losses and systemic

Table 9.5. Early objective prognostic signs used to estimate the risk of death or major complications for acute pancreatitis according to Ranson et al. [156, 157]. (Prognostic signs for biliary acute pancreatitis do not include arterial pO_2.)

	Acute pancreatitis	
	Alcohol-induced	Biliary
On admission or diagnosis		
• Age	>55 years	>70 years
• White blood cell count	>16 000/mm³	>18 000/mm³
• Blood glucose	>200 mg/dl	>220 mg/dl
• Serum lactate dehydrogenase	>350 U/l	>400 U/l
• Serum glutamic oxaloacetic transaminase	>250 U/l	>250 U/l
During initial 48 h		
• Hematocrit decrease	>10%	>10%
• Blood urea nitrogen increase	>5 mg/dl	>2 mg/dl
• Serum calcium level	<8 mg/dl	<8 mg/dl
• Arterial pO_2	<60 mm Hg	
• Base deficit	>4 mEq/l	>5 mEq/l
• Estimated fluid sequestration	>6 l	>4 l

complications. Third-space losses are indicated by a decrease in the hematocrit >10 percentage points (reflecting the beneficial effect of fluid resuscitation in overcoming hemoconcentration caused by third-space losses), a serum calcium <8 mg% (marking the loss of unionized calcium from the circulation associated with the loss of serum albumin), and an estimated fluid sequestration of >6 l. Fluid sequestration in effect represents the differential between the amount of fluids administered intravenously minus obvious fluid losses (urine and nasogastric aspiration). The remaining signs that are measured during the initial 48 h include evidence of renal failure (an increase of blood urea nitrogen >5 mg/dl), respiratory failure (pO_2 <60 mm Hg), and cardiovascular instability (base deficit >4 mEq/l) indicating metabolic acidosis.

Ranson's prognostic signs have proven to be helpful in assessing the severity of acute pancreatitis. In one series, patients with mild pancreatitis had a mean Ranson of 1.6, severe pancreatitis 2.4, and lethal pancreatitis 5.6 [81]. In additional series, when there have been ≤ 2 positive Ranson's signs, mortality has been between 0%–5% [70, 156]; when 3–5, approximately 10% [13, 52]; ≥ 6, 60% or higher [124]. In addition to a higher mortality, patients with ≥ 6 Ranson's signs have had a higher incidence of systemic complications [52], a higher incidence of necrosis [99], and a higher incidence of infected necrosis [13, 14].

Clearly, measurement of Ranson's signs is helpful in alerting the clinician to a likelihood of a severe form of acute pancreatitis. Nonetheless, there are several important limitations. First, all 11 signs should be measured to achieve the best prediction of severity. The reason for this is the fact that individual signs may be positive in only 10%–20% of all patients with acute pancreatitis [157]. Second, a full 48 h of observation may be required before it can be concluded whether some of the signs are positive or negative. In particular, measurement of fluid sequestration requires a full 48 h. While the remaining 5 signs that are measured during the initial 48 h can be recorded as positive as soon as they occur, they may not become positive much earlier than 48 h. Accordingly, if a Ranson's score of ≥ 3 is not available to the clinician until approximately 48 h of hospitalization, the clinician may fail to maximize therapy within the first several hours.

A third limitation is that Ranson's signs are most helpful when there are either ≤ 2 positive signs (reflecting mild disease) or ≥ 6 (reflecting very serious disease), but are less helpful when there are 3–5 positive signs (with an associated mortality of approximately 10%). While the presence of ≥ 6 Ranson's signs indicates a high mortality, there are very few patients who achieve this score, and the majority of deaths in acute pancreatitis occur among patients who have 3–5 positive Ranson's signs. It would be most helpful to have additional information that would distinguish which patients with 3–5 positive signs are at high risk of a complication or a fatal outcome.

Fourth, it should be remembered that Ranson's prognostic signs have been validated as a predictor of severity only within the initial 48 h of hospitalization and should not be measured beyond this time frame. Furthermore, data have not yet been generated that would determine whether measurement of Ranson's signs is as valid when there has been a delay in hospitalization (and consequent delay in measurement of the signs) compared to when patients are admitted within 12–24 h of onset of symptoms.

Finally, when Ranson's signs have been correlated with severity of pancreatitis (bearing in mind that the definition of severity is not always the same), it would appear that not all patients with severe pancreatitis have high Ranson's signs and that a significant number of patients with high Ranson's signs do not have severe disease. For example, overall sensitivity has been reported as only 57%–85%, specificity 68%–85%, positive predictive value slightly less than 50%, and negative predictive value approximately 90% [69, 183, 197]. Hence, a good use of Ranson's signs may be to exclude severe disease [134].

9.4.2.2
Imrie's Signs

Several somewhat simplified prognostic scores have originated from Glasgow, Scotland. One representative scoring system originated from Imrie and his colleagues, who measured 9 as compared to the original 11 signs (Table 9.6) [57, 69]. Other systems from Glasgow eliminated age as a criterion. In general, Imrie's scores correlate well with Ranson's [125, 134] and also require a full 48 h for assessment. Overall, the accuracy of Imrie's signs in recognizing the presence of severe pancreatitis is similar to Ranson's [57].

9.4.2.3
Other Prognostic Systems

Bank and his colleagues evaluated broad categories of risk factors including cardiac, pulmonary, renal, metabolic, hematologic, neurologic, and hemorrhagic complications [15] (see Table 12.3). Mortality in their series was 56% if ≥ 1 criterion was positive. This system appeared to correlate well with the presence of ≥ 6 positive Ranson's signs. There are several drawbacks to this system. First, a 48-h interval is required for measurement of criteria. Second, some of the criteria in the categories are the very complications that a clinician would like to predict and thereby to prevent (such as shock and adult respiratory distress syndrome [ARDS]). Agarwal and Pitchumoni [2] developed 4 categories of signs, including cardiac, pulmonary, renal, and metabolic derangement (see Table 12.4). The presence of ≥ 1 criterion identified patients who developed complications. These criteria also require 48 h of observation.

Table 9.6. Imrie's prognostic scores [32]

- Age >55 years
- White blood cell count $>15 \times 10^9/l$
- Arterial pO$_2$ <60 mm Hg
- Plasma glucose >10 mmol/l (no diabetic history)
- Blood urea >16 mmol/l (no response to intravenous fluids)
- Serum calcium <2 mmol/l
- Serum albumin <32 g/l
- Serum lactate dehydrogenase >600 U/l
- Serum transaminases (serum glutamate-oxalacetate transaminase [SGOT] and serum glutamate pyruvic transaminase [SGPT]) >100 U/l

9.4.2.4
Peritoneal Lavage

Prognostic criteria have been developed based on the characteristics of ascitic fluid obtained percutaneously. With the recovery of any volume of peritoneal fluid with a dark color or the recovery of >20 ml of free intraperitoneal fluid of any color, mortality was approximately 33% [138]. While this technique can be utilized at any time following admission, it is invasive and has not been utilized widely [138]. The sensitivity in various series has been of the order of 36%–72%, with specificity $>90\%$ [134].

9.4.2.5
Clinical Scoring Systems

Clinical scoring systems utilizing information available at the bedside have been generated and compared with Ranson's, Imrie's, and other scoring systems. A clinical scoring system has certain benefits, including the fact that it is inexpensive, available on the first day of admission and easy to administer. Overall, on admission, clinical scoring systems have been insensitive ($<40\%$) [49, 197] but highly specific [197]. After 48 h, clinical assessment has been comparable to Ranson's and Imrie's scoring systems. As indicated earlier, information that is available after 48 h may be too late to overcome systemic complications.

There is a variety of observations that can be made at the bedside that should sensitize the clinician to corrective action. The first is evidence of hypovolemia. This can be manifested by hemoconcentration (with the hematocrit >50 percentage points), oliguria (with urine output <30 mL), hypotension (with systolic blood pressure <90 mm Hg), and tachycardia (with pulse >120 beats/min). Another is early evidence of hypoxemia with pO_2 on blood gas determination ≤ 60 mm Hg. A third is disorientation and even frank coma. Individual danger signals such as these should result in prompt corrective action (see Sect. 11.1.3).

9.4.2.6
APACHE-II Scores

The APACHE-II grading system awards points of severity on the basis of a quantitative measure of degree of abnormality of 12 physiologic variables, age, and chronic health status (Table 9.7). In several studies, measurement of APACHE-II scores on admission and at 48 h have helped identify patients who are at high risk of fatal outcome [52, 57, 109, 197]. In general, patients with APACHE-II scores ≤ 9 within the first 48 h have survived, whereas those with scores of ≥ 13 have a high likelihood of a fatal outcome. In one study, for example, the mortality was 4% among patients with APACHE-II ≤ 9, 16% with values 11–15, and 33% with values 16–20 [52]. Overall, on admission, sensitivity of APACHE-II has varied between 34%–70%, specificity 76%–98%. At 48 h, sensitivity may still be below 50%, whereas specificity is close to 100% [197]. Accordingly, on admission, this system lacks sensitivity, and at 48 h appears to be no better than other scoring systems [134].

Table 9.7. APACHE-II severity of disease classification system (see also Table 12.5) [111]

Physiologic variable	+4	+3	+2	+1	0	+1	+2	+3	+4
Temperature – rectal (°C)	$\geq 41°$	39°–40.9°	—	38.5°–38.9°	36°–38.4°	34°–35.9°	32°–33.9°	30°–31.9°	$\leq 29.9°$
Mean arterial pressure (mm Hg)	≥ 160	130–159	110–129	—	70–109	—	50–69	—	≤ 49
Heart rate (ventricular response)	≥ 180	140–179	110–139	—	70–109	—	55–69	40–54	≤ 39
Respiratory rate (nonventilated or ventilated)	≥ 50	35–49	—	25–34	12–24	10–11	6–9	—	≤ 5
Oxygenation: A-aDO$_2$ or pO$_2$ (mm Hg)									
a. FIO$_2$ ≥ 0.5 record A-aDO$_2$	≥ 500	350–499	200–349	—	< 200	—	—	—	—
b. FIO$_2$ < 0.5 record only pO$_2$	—	—	—	—	pO$_2$ >70	pO$_2$ 61–70	—	pO$_2$ 55–60	pO$_2$ <55
Arterial pH	≥ 7.7	7.6–7.69	—	7.5–7.59	7.33–7.49	—	7.25–7.32	7.15–7.24	< 7.15
Serum sodium (mmol/l)	≥ 180	160–179	155–159	150–154	130–149	—	120–129	111–119	<110
Serum potassium (mmol/l)	≥ 7	6–6.9	—	5.5–5.9	3.5–5.4	3–3.4	2.5–2.9	—	< 2.5
Serum creatinine (mg/100 ml) (double point score for acute renal failure)	> 3.5	2–3.4	1.5–1.9	—	0.6–1.4	—	< 0.6	—	—
Hematocrit (%)	≥ 60	—	50–59.9	46–49.9	30–45.9	—	20–29.9	—	< 20
White blood count (total/mm^3) (in 1000 s)	≥ 40	—	20–39.9	15–19.9	3–14.9	—	1–2.9	—	< 1
Glasgow coma score (GCS): Score – 15 minus actual GCS	—	—	—	—	—	—	—	—	—
A Total acute physiology score (APS): Sum of the 12 individual variable points	—	—	—	—	—	—	—	—	—
Serum HCO$_2$ (venous-mmol/l) (not preferred, use if no ABGs)	≥ 52	41–51.9	—	32–40.9	22–31.9	—	18–21.9	15–17.9	< 15

B   Age Points
Assign points to age as follows:

Age (yrs)	Points
≤ 44	0
45–54	2
55–64	3
65–74	5
≥ 75	6

C   Chronic Health Points
If the patient has a history of severe organ system insufficiency or is immuno-compromised, assign points as follows:

A-aDO$_2$ = alveolar-arterial difference for oxygen
FIO$_2$ = fraction of inspired oxygen

a. For nonoperative or emergency postoperative patients – 5 points   *or*
b. For elective postoperative patients – 2 points

Definitions   Organ insufficiency or immuno-compromised state must have been evident prior to this hospital admission and conforms to the following criteria:

Liver   Biopsy-proven cirrhosis and documented portal hypertension, episodes of past upper gastrointestinal bleeding attributed to portal hypertension; or prior episodes of hepatic failure/encephalopathy/coma.

Cardiovascular   NY Heart Association Class IV.

Respiratory   Chronic restrictive, obstructive, or vascular diseases resulting in severe exercise restriction, i.e., unable to climb stairs or perform household duties; or documented chronic hypoxia, hypercapnia, secondary polycythemia, severe pulmonary hypertension (>40 mm Hg), or respirator dependence.

Renal   Recurring chronic dialysis.

Immuno-compromised   The patient has received therapy that suppresses resistance to infection (e.g. immuno-suppression, chemotherapy, radiation, long-term or recent high-dose steroids) or has a disease that is sufficiently advanced to suppress resistance to infection (e.g. leukemia, lymphoma, AIDS).

APACHE-II Score
Sum of A + B + C

A   APS points _________
B   Age points _________
C   Chronic Health points _________
Total APACHE-II Score _________

9.4.2.7
Serum Markers

Measurement of serum amylase is not helpful in distinguishing mild from severe pancreatitis [91, 127, 148, 157].

CRP is an acute phase reactant that is produced by the liver. Evidence thus far indicates that its levels are higher in severe than mild pancreatitis and are usually higher in necrotizing than interstitial pancreatitis [44, 58, 91, 127, 184, 189, 196]. The peak concentration of CRP occurs at 36–48 h. Its sensitivity is somewhat better than other scoring systems, but specificity, positive predictive value, and negative predictive value are similar to other scoring systems. Because its peak activity is well beyond the time of admission, measurement of CRP is not recommended on admission.

IL-6 is an acute phase reactant cytokine that is produced by a variety of cells. IL-6 induces the synthesis of CRP in the liver. Its peak activity is between 24 and 36 h [91]. It would appear that its value is similar to other scoring systems [134].

PMN-elastase has also been shown to be higher in severe than in mild pancreatitis [26, 58, 81] and higher in necrotizing than interstitial pancreatitis [184]. Sensitivity and specificity of PMN-elastase on admission is very high, comparable to IL-6, and somewhat better than other scoring systems and individual tests [134].

9.4.2.8
Urine Tests

Trypsinogen activation peptide (TAP) is the amino terminus peptide released from the activation of trypsinogen by trypsin. In acute pancreatitis, it is released from the acinar cell and appears in plasma, peritoneum, and urine. In two recent studies, measurement of urinary TAP among patients who presented within 48 h of onset of symptoms distinguished mild from severe pancreatitis [82, 91]. Accordingly, measurement of urinary TAP appears to be very accurate in identifying patients with severe disease within the first 48 h of onset of symptoms.

9.4.2.9
Obesity

Several reports have called attention to obesity as a prognostic factor in acute pancreatitis. In two earlier reports, obese patients had a higher incidence of respiratory failure than nonobese patients [122, 154]. In a more recent report, patients with severe acute pancreatitis had a higher body mass index (BMI) and were obese when compared to those with mild disease [77]. In a fourth report, among patients with severe sterile necrosis, patients who died had a higher BMI and were obese as compared to those that lived [109]. Additional information will be required to substantiate the importance of obesity as an early prognostic sign.

9.4.2.10
Chest X-ray

In two reports, patients showing pleural effusion on either contrast-enhanced CT scan within 72 h after admission [115] or on chest X-ray obtained within the initial 6 days of hospitalization [83] had more severe disease than those who did not experience pleural effusions. Recently, also the presence of pulmonary infiltrates on chest X-ray was shown to be a prognostic factor [116]. Additional studies will be required to substantiate these results.

9.4.2.11
Summary

There are a variety of scoring systems that provide early prognostic information. A major weakness of some systems is that the data is not complete until 48 h (Ranson's and Imrie's scoring systems) and others is that the peak response is delayed (IL-6 and CRP). Some that are available on admission (clinical assessment and APACHE-II) have low sensitivity and positive predictive value. Tests that are promising on admission but are not yet generally available include serum PMN-elastase and urinary TAP.

Nonetheless, measurement of early prognostic signs has some value in clinical assessment of patients. Measurement also may help in assuring comparability of patients in clinical trials. The clinician should keep in mind that good clinical judgment may be very helpful in recognizing patients with a high probability of severe pancreatitis and the need for transfer to a specialized unit for aggressive fluid resuscitation and general care.

9.4.3
Organ Failure

The definition of organ failure has varied considerably in reports of acute pancreatitis. Accordingly, at the Atlanta symposium, it was important to define organ failure in specific terms. The major components of organ failure that were agreed to were, as follows: shock was defined as systolic blood pressure <90 mm Hg; pulmonary insufficiency was defined as pO_2 ≤ 60 mm Hg; renal failure was defined as creatinine level >2 mg/dl after rehydration; and gastrointestinal bleeding as more than 500 ml/24 h.

Mortality is determined largely by the presence of organ system failure. As many as 10%–28% of cases of acute pancreatitis are complicated by organ system failure [49, 52, 57, 58, 69, 82, 183]. In the absence of organ failure, mortality is very low; in the presence of organ system failure, mortality is reported to be 10%–62% [49, 52, 57, 58, 81, 82, 99, 127, 131, 133, 151, 164, 183, 197]. This wide variation in mortality probably has several explanations. One may be the variation in definition of organ system failure among papers published prior to the Atlanta symposium. Another might be the patient population itself (that is, mortality in a surgical department that specializes in the care of acute pancreatitis may attract the sickest patients and have a high mortality).

9.4.4
Local Complications

Local complications include pancreatic necrosis, pancreatic pseudocyst, and pancreatic abscess. Whereas the mortality of interstitial pancreatitis is only 1%–2%, mortality in necrotizing pancreatitis is considerably higher. In one study, mortality was 33% in infected necrosis compared to 10% in sterile necrosis [163]. Other reports have also pointed out the favorable prognosis in interstitial pancreatitis and the higher mortality in necrotizing pancreatitis [14, 189].

Overall, mortality associated with infected necrosis of the pancreas is higher than that of a pancreatic abscess [31, 72].

9.4.5
Mortality

On the basis of recent reports, mortality in acute pancreatitis is 3%–17% with a median of 8% [2, 14, 15, 25, 43, 49, 52, 57, 58, 69, 70, 81, 82, 97, 117, 126, 127, 131, 133, 136, 138, 156, 157, 165, 183, 189, 197, 200]. Several additional reports have also noted that of all hospitalized patients with acute pancreatitis, the diagnosis was made for the first time at autopsy in 12%–42% [43, 123, 136, 199, 200]. Hence, the overall mortality of acute pancreatitis is even higher than 8%.

Throughout the years, it has been recognized that some patients die within the first 7–10 days of organ failure and comorbid conditions, whereas others die somewhat later, frequently secondary to pancreatic infection. More recently, clinicians have gained the impression that they are more successful in overcoming the early manifestations of organ failure and that the majority of deaths occur late as a result of complications of pancreatic necrosis [109]. Indeed, it has been stated that 80% of all deaths in acute pancreatitis are as a result of late pancreatic infection [40, 41]. A careful review of published reports over the past several years indicate that a considerable number of deaths continue to take place within the first 14 days [123, 131, 136, 160, 165, 200]. It may be that reports noting a preponderance of late deaths originate from surgical services which specialize in the treatment of pancreatic necrosis and care for a large number of patients referred after 7–10 days from other hospitals. It is also possible that reports that mention early deaths include patients admitted to medical services who do not come under surgical scrutiny.

Late deaths are invariably related to the presence of pancreatic necrosis [109, 159, 163]. Whereas the mortality of interstitial pancreatitis is close to zero, patients with necrotizing pancreatitis have a considerable mortality [14, 109, 159, 163, 189]. In several series, the mortality has been reported as 10%–12% in sterile necrosis and approximately 30% in infected necrosis [159, 163]. When pancreatic necrosis has been associated with significant organ system failure, the mortality of both sterile and infected necrosis is even higher [20, 109, 163]. Indeed, there is some evidence that the mortality of sterile necrosis may be equivalent to infected necrosis [20, 159]. It is possible that patients with severe organ system failure have a high (and possibly equally high) mortality in both sterile and infected necrosis.

There are factors other than unfavorable early prognostic signs, organ failure and local complications such as necrosis that influence mortality. One such factor is coma on admission. In one study [43], one-third of the patients who entered comatose expired. Another is age. While the influence of age remains somewhat controversial, a number of reports have pointed out that older patients with acute pancreatitis are more likely to expire [25, 70, 136, 200], and that comorbid disease may play an important role in deaths in the older population [70, 200]. Indeed, several scoring systems of early prognostic signs include age as a risk factor of severity in acute pancreatitis [156, 157]. Another important factor appears to be the absence of prior episodes of acute pancreatitis. In a number of reports, it has been pointed out that patients are much more likely to have serious pancreatitis or a fatal outcome during their initial episode [43, 123, 157, 200].

Another factor is etiology. In general, the mortality of gallstone pancreatitis is comparable to that of alcoholic pancreatitis [25, 52, 81, 136] and usually in the order of 5% or lower [25, 52, 136]. Mortality appears to be somewhat higher in other etiologies including idiopathic and postoperative pancreatitis [25, 136]. In several series, the mortality of ERCP-induced pancreatitis has been higher than of the alcohol- and biliary induced form of the disease [25, 136]. This information originated from hospitals that specialize in acute pancreatitis and included patients with ERCP-induced pancreatitis who were referred from other hospitals.

References

1. Adler G, Hupp T, Kern HF (1979) Course and spontaneous regression of acute pancreatitis in the rat. Virchows Arch [Pathol Anat] 382:31–47
2. Agarwal N, Pitchumoni CS (1986) Simplified prognostic criteria in acute pancreatitis. Pancreas 1:69–73
3. Agarwal N, Pitchumoni CS (1991) Assessment of severity in acute pancreatitis. Am J Gastroenterol 86:1385–1391
4. Agarwal N, Pitchumoni CS, Sivaprasad AV (1990) Evaluating tests for acute pancreatitis. Am J Gastroenterol 85:356–366
5. Allam BF, Imrie CW (1977) Serum ionized calcium in acute pancreatitis. Br J Surg 64:665–668
6. Amouyal P, Amouyal G, Lévy P, Tuzet S, Palazzo L, Vilgrain V, Gayet B, Belghiti J, Fékété F, Bernades P (1994) Diagnosis of choledocholithiasis by endoscopic ultrasonography. Gastroenterology 106:1062–1067
7. Angelini G, Cavallini G, Pederzoli P, Bovo P, Bassi C, Di Francesco V, Frulloni L, Sgarbi D, Talamini G, Castagnini A (1993) Long-term outcome of acute pancreatitis: a prospective study with 118 patients. Digestion 54:143–147
8. Apple F, Benson P, Preese L, Eastep S, Bilodeau L, Heiler G (1991) Lipase and pancreatic amylase activities in tissues and in patients with hyperamylasemia. Am J Clin Pathol 96:610–614
9. Avioli LV, Birge SJ, Scott S, Shieber W (1969) Role of the thyroid gland during glucagon-induced hypocalcemia in the dog. Am J Physiol 216:939–945
10. Balthazar EJ, Chako AC (1990) Computed tomography of pancreatic masses. Am J Gastroenterol 85:343–349
11. Balthazar EJ, Freeny PC (1994) Contrast-enhanced computed tomography in acute pancreatitis: is it beneficial or harmful? Gastroenterology 106:259–262
12. Balthazar EJ, Freeny PC, vanSonnenberg E (1994) Imaging and intervention in acute pancreatitis. Radiology 193:297–306
13. Balthazar EJ, Ranson JHC, Naidich DP, Megibow AJ, Caccavale R, Cooper MM (1985) Acute pancreatitis: prognostic value of CT. Radiology 156:767–772

14. Balthazar EJ, Robinson DL, Megibow AJ, Ranson JHC (1990) Acute pancreatitis: value of CT in establishing prognosis. Radiology 174:331–336
15. Bank S, Wise L, Gersten M (1983) Risk factors in acute pancreatitis. Am J Gastroenterol 78: 637–640
16. Banks PA (1979) Pancreatitis. Plenum Medical Book Comp., New York–London
17. Banks PA (1986) Acute pancreatitis: clinical presentation. In: Go VLW, DiMagno EP, Gardner JD, Lebenthal E, Reber HA, Scheele GA (eds) The Exocrine Pancreas: Biology, Pathobiology, and Diseases. Raven Press, New York, pp 475–479
18. Banks PA (1991) Predictors of severity in acute pancreatitis. Pancreas 6, Suppl. 1:S7–S12
19. Banks PA (1994) A new classification system for acute pancreatitis. Am J Gastroenterol 89: 151–152
20. Banks PA, Gerzof SG, Langevin RE, Silverman SG, Sica GT, Hughes MD (1995) CT-guided aspiration of suspected pancreatic infection. Bacteriology and clinical outcome. Int J Pancreatol 18: 265–270
21. Banks PA, Gerzof SG, Sullivan JG (1988) Central cavitary necrosis: differentiation from pancreatic pseudocyst on CT scan. Pancreas 3:83–88
22. Banks PA, Sidi S, Gelman ML, Lee K-H, Warshaw AL (1979) Amylase-creatinine clearance ratios and serum amylase isoenzymes in moderate renal insufficiency. J Clin Gastroenterol 1:331–335
23. Baron M, Paltiel H, Lander P (1984) Aseptic necrosis of the talus and calcaneal insufficiency fractures in a patient with pancreatitis, subcutaneous fat necrosis, and arthritis. Arthritis Rheumatism 27:1309–1313
24. Barrows D, Berk JE, Fridhandler L (1972) Macroamylasemia – Survey of prevalence in a mixed population. N Engl J Med 286:1352
25. Beaux ACde, Palmer KR, Carter DC (1995) Factors influencing morbidity and mortality in acute pancreatitis; an analysis of 279 cases. Gut 37:121–126
26. Bergenfeldt M, Berling R, Ohlsson K (1994) Levels of leukocyte proteases in plasma and peritoneal exudate in severe, acute pancreatitis. Scand J Gastroenterol 29:371–375
27. Berk JE (1995) Macroamylasemia. In: Haubrich WS, Schaffner F, Berk JE (eds) Bockus Gastroenterology, vol. 4, 5th edn. W.B. Saunders Comp., Philadelphia-London-Toronto etc, pp 2851–2860
28. Berk JE, Kizu H, Wilding P, Searcy RL (1967) Macroamylasemia: a newly recognized cause for elevated serum amylase activity. N Engl J Med 277:941–946
29. Berman B, Conteas C, Smith B, Leong S, Hornbeck III L (1987) Fatal pancreatitis presenting with subcutaneous fat necrosis. Evidence that lipase and amylase alone do not induce lipocyte necrosis. J Am Acad Dermatol 17:359–364
30. Berry AR, Taylor TV, Davies GC (1982) Diagnostic tests and prognostic indicators in acute pancreatitis. J R Coll Surg Edinb 27:345–352
31. Bittner R, Block S, Büchler M, Beger HG (1987) Pancreatic abscess and infected pancreatic necrosis. Different local septic complications in acute pancreatitis. Dig Dis Sci 32:1082–1087
32. Blamey SL, Imrie CW, O'Neill J, Gilmour WH, Carter DC (1984) Prognostic factors in acute pancreatitis. Gut 25:1340–1346
33. Blamey SL, Osborne DH, Gilmour WH, O'Neill J, Carter DC, Imrie CW (1983) The early identification of patients with gallstone associated pancreatitis using clinical and biochemical factors only. Ann Surg 198:574–578
34. Block S, Maier W, Bittner R, Büchler M, Malfertheiner P, Beger HG (1986) Identification of pancreas necrosis in severe acute pancreatitis: imaging procedures versus clinical staging. Gut 27: 1035–1042
35. Bode C, Riederer J, Brauner B, Bode JC (1990) Macrolipasemia: a rare cause of persistently elevated serum lipase. Am J Gastroenterol 85:412–416
36. Borgström A, Bohe M (1989) Severe acute pancreatitis and normal serum amylase activity due to pancreatic isoamylase deficiency. Dig Dis Sci 34:644–646
37. Bowen M, Cooper EH, McMahon MJ (1983) The diagnosis of acute pancreatitis: enhanced sensitivity from an ELISA assay of lipase. Biomed Pharmacother 37:395–398
38. Boyle CEL, Fraser CG (1985) Macroamylasaemia: how common is it? Br Med J 291:1389
39. Bradley III EL (1993) A clinically based classification system for acute pancreatitis. Summary of the International Symposium on Acute Pancreatitis, Atlanta, Ga, September 11 through 13, 1992. Arch Surg 128:586–590

40. Bradley III EL (1994) Necrosectomy in acute pancreatitis. J HBP Surg 2:152–154
41. Bradley III EL, Murphy F, Ferguson C (1989) Prediction of pancreatic necrosis by dynamic pancreatography. Ann Surg 210:495–504
42. Bretzke G, Bretzke K (1987) Beitrag zur Retinopathie bei akuter Pankreatitis. Z Gesamte Inn Med 42:369–370
43. Buggy BP, Nostrant TT (1983) Lethal pancreatitis. Am J Gastroenterol 78:810–814
44. Büchler M, Malfertheiner P, Schoetensack C, Uhl W, Beger HG (1986) Sensitivity of antiproteases, complement factors and C-reactive protein in detecting pancreatic necrosis. Results of a prospective clinical study. Int J Pancreatol 1:227–235
45. Cannon JR, Pitha JV, Everett MA (1979) Subcutaneous fat necrosis in pancreatitis. J Cutan Pathol 6:501–506
46. Casey JE, Porter KA, Langevin RE, Banks PA (1993) Clinical features and natural history of central cavitary necrosis. Pancreas 8:141–145
47. Clavien P-A, Robert J, Meyer P, Borst F, Hauser H, Herrmann F, Dunand V, Rohner A (1989) Acute pancreatitis and normoamylasemia. Not an uncommon combination. Ann Surg 210: 614–620
48. Condon JR, Ives D, Knight MJ, Day J (1975) The aetiology of hypocalcaemia in acute pancreatitis. Br J Surg 62:115–118
49. Corfield AP, Cooper MJ, Williamson RCN, Mayer AD, McMahon MJ, Dickson AP, Shearer MG, Imrie CW (1985) Prediction of severity in acute pancreatitis: prospective comparison of three prognostic indices. Lancet 2:403–407
50. Croton RS, Warren RA, Stott A, Roberts NB (1981) Ionized calcium in acute pancreatitis and its relationships with total calcium and serum lipase. Br J Surg 68:241–244
51. Dati F, Habenstein K (1983) Teststreifen für den schnellen Nachweis der α-Amylase im Urin. Eine kooperative Studie. Dtsch Med Wochenschr 108:1308–1311
52. Demmy TL, Burch JM, Feliciano DV, Mattox KL, Jordan GL Jr (1988) Comparison of multiple-parameter prognostic systems in acute pancreatitis. Am J Surg 156:492–496
53. Dennison AR, Royle GT (1984) Acute pancreatitis – presentation as a discoloured lump in the groin. Postgrad Med J 60:374–375
54. Dhawan SS, Jimenez-Acosta F, Poppiti RJ Jr, Barkin JS (1990) Subcutaneous fat necrosis associated with pancreatitis: histochemical and electron microscopic findings. Am J Gastroenterol 85: 1025–1028
55. Dickson AP, Imrie CW (1984) The incidence and prognosis of body wall ecchymosis in acute pancreatitis. Surg Gynecol Obstet 159:343–347
56. Dickson AP, O'Neill J, Imrie CW (1984) Hyperlipidaemia, alcohol abuse and acute pancreatitis. Br J Surg 71:685–688
57. Domínguez-Muñoz JE, Carballo F, García MJ, de Diego JM, Campos R, Yangüela J, de la Morena J (1993) Evaluation of the clinical usefulness of APACHE II and SAPS systems in the initial prognostic classification of acute pancreatitis: a multicenter study. Pancreas 8:682–686
58. Domínguez-Muñoz JE, Carballo F, García MJ, de Diego JM, Gea F, Yangüela J, de la Morena J (1993) Monitoring of serum proteinase-antiproteinase balance and systemic inflammatory response in prognostic evaluation of acute pancreatitis. Results of a prospective multicenter study. Dig Dis Sci 38:507–513
59. Donhauser JL, Bigelow NH (1958) Atypical symptom-sign complex of acute pancreatitis. Am J Surg 96:61–65
60. Dooner HP, Aliaga C (1965) Painless acute necrotic pancreatitis. Arch Intern Med 116:828–831
61. Dunne MJ, Shenkin A, Imrie CW (1979) Misleading hyponatraemia in acute pancreatitis with hyperlipaemia. Lancet 1:211
62. Dürr HK, Bode C, Krupinski R, Bode JC (1978) A comparison between naturally occurring macroamylasaemia and macroamylasaemia induced by hydroxyethyl-starch. Eur J Clin Invest 8: 189–191
63. Dürr HK, Bode JC, Lankisch PG, Koop H (1977) Amylase-creatinine clearance ratio in pancreatitis. N Engl J Med 296:635
64. Eckfeldt JH, Kolars JC, Elson MK, Shafer RB, Levitt MD (1985) Serum tests for pancreatitis in patients with abdominal pain. Arch Pathol Lab Med 109:316–319

65. Edmondson HA, Fields IA (1942) Relation of calcium and lipids to acute pancreatic necrosis. Report of fifteen cases, in one of which fat embolism occurred. Arch Intern Med 69:177–190
66. Elman R, Arneson N, Graham EA (1929) Value of blood amylase estimations in the diagnosis of pancreatic disease. A clinical study. Arch Surg 19:943–967
67. Falk A, Gustafsson L, Gamklou R (1984) Silent pancreatitis. Report of 4 cases of acute pancreatitis with atypical symptomatology. Acta Chir Scand 150:341–342
68. Fan S-T, Lai ECS, Mok FPT, Lo C-M, Zheng S-S, Wong J (1993) Early treatment of acute biliary pancreatitis by endoscopic papillotomy. N Engl J Med 328:228–232
69. Fan S-T, Lai ECS, Mok FPT, Lo C-M, Zheng S-S, Wong J (1993) Prediction of the severity of acute pancreatitis. Am J Surg 166:262–269
70. Fan ST, Choi TK, Lai CS, Wong J (1988) Influence of age on the mortality from acute pancreatitis. Br J Surg 75:463–466
71. Farrar WH, Calkins WG (1978) Sensitivity of the amylase-creatinine clearance ratio in acute pancreatitis. Arch Intern Med 138:958–962
72. Fedorak IJ, Ko TC, Djuricin G, McMahon M, Thompson K, Prinz RA (1992) Secondary pancreatic infections: are they distinct clinical entities? Surgery 112:824–831
73. Flaggl E, Heer M, Hany A, Branda L (1988) Visusverlust als Komplikation der akuten Pankreatitis. Schweiz Med Wochenschr 118:722–725
74. Flamion B, Delhaye M, Horanyi Z, Delange A, Demanet H, Quenon M, Van Melsen A, Cremer M, Delcourt A (1987) Comparison of elastase-1 with amylase, lipase, and trypsin-like immunoreactivity in the diagnosis of acute pancreatitis. Am J Gastroenterol 82:532–535
75. Foitzik T, Bassi DG, Schmidt J, Lewandrowski KB, Fernandez-del Castillo C, Rattner DW, Warshaw AL (1994) Intravenous contrast medium accentuates the severity of acute necrotizing pancreatitis in the rat. Gastroenterology 106:207–214
76. Freeny PC (1993) Incremental dynamic bolus computed tomography of acute pancreatitis. Int J Pancreatol 13:147–158
77. Funnell IC, Bornman PC, Weakley SP, Terblanche J, Marks IN (1993) Obesity: an important prognostic factor in acute pancreatitis. Br J Surg 80:484–486
78. Garden OJ, Dominiczak MH, Shenkin A, Carter DC (1985) The diagnosis of acute pancreatitis in the presence of hyperlipaemia. Scot Med J 30:235–236
79. Gibbons CP (1984) Pancreatitis and inguinal swelling. Postgrad Med J 60:711
80. Good LI, Long WB (1977) Prognostic significance of hypertension in acute pancreatitis. Gastroenterology 72:1064 (abstr)
81. Gross V, Schölmerich J, Leser H-G, Salm R, Lausen M, Rückauer K, Schöffel U, Lay L, Heinisch A, Farthmann EH, Gerok W (1990) Granulocyte elastase in assessment of severity of acute pancreatitis. Comparison with acute-phase proteins, C-reactive protein, α_1-antitrypsin, and protease inhibitor α_2-macroglobulin. Dig Dis Sci 35:97–105
82. Gudgeon AM, Heath DI, Hurley P, Jehanli A, Patel G, Wilson C, Shenkin A, Austen BM, Imrie CW, Hermon-Taylor J (1990) Trypsinogen activation peptides assay in the early prediction of severity of acute pancreatitis. Lancet 335:4–8
83. Gumaste V, Singh V, Dave P (1992) Significance of pleural effusion in patients with acute pancreatitis. Am J Gastroenterol 87:871–874
84. Gumaste VV (1994) Diagnostic tests for acute pancreatitis. Gastroenterologist 2:119–130
85. Gumaste VV, Dave PB, Weissman D, Messer J (1991) Lipase/amylase ratio. A new index that distinguishes acute episodes of alcoholic from nonalcoholic acute pancreatitis. Gastroenterology 101:1361–1366
86. Gumaste VV, Roditis N, Mehta D, Dave PB (1993) Serum lipase levels in nonpancreatic abdominal pain versus acute pancreatitis. Am J Gastroenterol 88:2051–2055
87. Gwozdz GP, Steinberg WM, Werner M, Henry JP, Pauley C (1990) Comparative evaluation of the diagnosis of acute pancreatitis based on serum and urine enzyme assays. Clin Chim Acta 187:243–254
88. Haffter D, Meyer N, Scholer A, Gyr K (1983) Der diagnostische Wert der Bestimmung von Serumamylase und Serumlipase bei Verdacht auf akuten Schub einer akuten oder chronischen Pankreatitis. Schweiz Med Wochenschr 113:184–188
89. Haffter D, Reichlin B, Gyr K (1981) Der Quotient aus Amylaseclearance und Kreatininclearance in der Diagnose der akuten Pankreatitis. Schweiz Med Wochenschr 111:806–808

90. Hathaway JA, Kitt D, Wingate B (1983) A comparison of currently used serum lipase and amylase procedures in the serial detection of enzyme elevations in acute pancreatitis. Clin Chim Acta 133:327–330

91. Heath DI, Cruickshank A, Gudgeon AM, Jehanli A, Shenkin A, Imrie CW (1995) The relationship between pancreatic enzyme release and activation and the acute-phase protein response in patients with acute pancreatitis. Pancreas 10:347–353

92. Heer M, Pei P, Streuli R, Bühler H, Ammann R (1983) Pankreatitis-Diagnostik am Krankenbett mittels Urinamylase-Test-Tape. Schweiz Med Wochenschr 113:1950–1952

93. Helfat A, Berk JE, Fridhandler L (1974) The prevalence of macroamylasemia. Further study. Am J Gastroenterol 62:54–58

94. Heresbach D, Boutroux D, Bretagne J-F, Raoul J-L, Siproudhis L, Lebert P, Nicol M, Gosselin M (1994) L'identification des pancréatites aiguës biliaires et alcooliques par le dosage précore des enzymes pancréatiques est-elle possible? Gastroenterol Clin Biol 18:135–140

95. Hiatt JR, Calabria RP, Passaro E Jr, Wilson SE (1987) The amylase profile: a discriminant in biliary and pancreatic disease. Am J Surg 154:490–492

96. Higgins E, Ive FA (1990) Subcutaneous fat necrosis in pancreatic disease. Br J Surg 77:532–533

97. Ho HS, Frey CF (1995) Gastrointestinal and pancreatic complications associated with severe pancreatitis. Arch Surg 130:817–823

98. Hoffbrand BI (1975) Haemorrhagic discoloration of the penis in acute pancreatitis. Lancet 2:1049–1050

99. Howard TJ, Wiebke EA, Mogavero G, Kopecky K, Baer JC, Sherman S, Hawes RH, Lehman GA, Goulet RJ, Madura JA (1995) Classification and treatment of local septic complications in acute pancreatitis. Am J Surg 170:44–50

100. Imrie CW, Beastall GH, Allam BF, O'Neill J, Benjamin IS, McKay AJ (1978) Parathyroid hormone and calcium homeostasis in acute pancreatitis. Br J Surg 65:717–720

101. Imrie CW, Benjamin IS, Ferguson JC, McKay AJ, Mackenzie I, O'Neill J, Blumgart LH (1978) A single-centre double-blind trial of Trasylol therapy in primary acute pancreatitis. Br J Surg 65:337–341

102. Imrie CW, King J, Henderson AR (1972) Macroamylasemia – Survey of prevalence in a mixed population. N Engl J Med 287:931

103. Isgar B, Blunt J, Wolinski AP (1994) Pancreatitis presenting with unilateral scrotal pain and swelling. Br J Surg 81:101

104. Jaakkola M, Sillanaukee P, Löf K, Koivula T, Nordback I (1994) Blood tests for detection of alcoholic cause of acute pancreatitis. Lancet 343:1328–1329

105. Jipp P, Mayer H, Reinold H-M, Schrader K-E (1985) Akute Pankreatitis und ischämische Netzhautveränderungen. Med Klin 80:363–366

106. Johnson CD, Stephens DH, Sarr MG (1991) CT of acute pancreatitis: correlation between lack of contrast enhancement and pancreatic necrosis. Am J Roentgenol 156:93–95

107. Jones PA (1985) Survival after profound hypocalcaemia with tetany complicating severe haemorrhagic acute pancreatitis. Postgrad Med J 61:43–45

108. Kaiser AM, Grady T, Gerdes D, Saluja M, Steer ML (1995) Intravenous contrast medium does not increase the severity of acute necrotizing pancreatitis in the opossum. Dig Dis Sci 40:1547–1553

109. Karimgani I, Porter KA, Langevin RE, Banks PA (1992) Prognostic factors in sterile pancreatic necrosis. Gastroenterology 103:1636–1640

110. Klöppel G, Maillet B (1993) Pathology of acute and chronic pancreatitis. Pancreas 8:659–670

111. Knaus WA, Draper EA, Wagner DP, Zimmerman JE (1985) APACHE II: a severity of disease classification system. Critical Care Med 13:818–829

112. Kolars JC, Ellis CJ, Levitt MD (1984) Comparison of serum amylase, pancreatic isoamylase and lipase in patients with hyperamylasemia. Dig Dis Sci 29:289–293

113. Koop H (1984) Serum levels of pancreatic enzymes and their clinical significance. Clin Gastroenterol 13:739–761

114. Lankisch PG, Buschmann-Kaspari H, Otto J, Schröder K, Koop H (1990) Correlation of pancreatic enzyme levels with the patient's recovery from acute edematous pancreatitis. Klin Wochenschr 68:565–569

115. Lankisch PG, Dröge M, Becher R (1994) Pleural effusions: a new negative prognostic parameter for acute pancreatitis. Am J Gastroenterol 89:1849–1851
116. Lankisch PG, Dröge M, Becher R (1996) Pulmonary infiltrations. Sign of severe acute pancreatitis. Int J Pancreatol 19:113–115
117. Lankisch PG, Haseloff M, Becher R (1994) No parallel between the biochemical course of acute pancreatitis and morphologic findings. Pancreas 9:240–243
118. Lankisch PG, Koop H, Otto J, Oberdieck U, Winckler K, Wolfrum DI (1977) Specificity of increased amylase to creatinine clearance ratio in acute pancreatitis. Digestion 16:160–164
119. Lankisch PG, Mahlke R, Graf D, Becher R, Riesner K (1995) Painless acute pancreatitis mimicking pancreatic carcinoma. Pancreas 10:413–414
120. Lankisch PG, Müller C-H, Niederstadt H, Brand A (1990) Painless acute pancreatitis subsequent to anticholinesterase insecticide (parathion) intoxication. Am J Gastroenterol 85:872–875
121. Lankisch PG, Petersen M (1994) Lipase/amylase ratio: not helpful in the early etiological differentiation of acute pancreatitis. Z Gastroenterol 32:8–11
122. Lankisch PG, Schirren CA (1990) Increased body weight as a prognostic parameter for complications in the course of acute pancreatitis. Pancreas 5:626–629
123. Lankisch PG, Schirren CA, Kunze E (1991) Undetected fatal acute pancreatitis: why is the disease so frequently overlooked? Am J Gastroenterol 86:322–326
124. Larvin M, Chalmers AG, McMahon MJ (1990) Dynamic contrast enhanced computed tomography: a precise technique for identifying and localising pancreatic necrosis. Br Med J 300: 1425–1428
125. Larvin M, McMahon MJ (1989) APACHE-II score for assessment and monitoring acute pancreatitis. Lancet 2:201–205
126. Leese T, Shaw D (1988) Comparison of three Glasgow multifactor prognostic scoring systems in acute pancreatitis. Br J Surg 75:460–462
127. Leese T, Shaw D, Holliday M (1988) Prognostic markers in acute pancreatitis: can pancreatic necrosis be predicted? Ann R C Surg Engl 70:227–232
128. Lesser PB, Warshaw AL (1975) Diagnosis of pancreatitis masked by hyperlipemia. Ann Intern Med 82:795–798
129. Levitt MD, Eckfeldt JH (1993) Diagnosis of acute pancreatitis. In: Go VLW, DiMagno EP, Gardner JD, Lebenthal E, Reber HA, Scheele GA (eds) The Pancreas: Biology, Pathobiology, and Disease, 2nd edn. Raven Press, New York, pp 613–635
130. Love L, Meyers MA, Churchill RJ, Reynes CJ, Moncada R, Gibson D (1981) Computed tomography of extraperitoneal spaces. Am J Roentgenol 136:781–789
131. Lucarotti ME, Virjee J, Alderson D (1993) Patient selection and timing of dynamic computed tomography in acute pancreatitis. Br J Surg 80:1393–1395
132. Lucas PF, Owen TK (1962) Subcutaneous fat necrosis, "polyarthritis", and pancreatic disease. Gut 3:146–148
133. Luiten EJT, Hop WCJ, Lange JF, Bruining HA (1995) Controlled clinical trial of selective decontamination for the treatment of severe acute pancreatitis. Ann Surg 222:57–65
134. Malfertheiner P, Domínguez-Muñoz JE (1993) Prognostic factors in acute pancreatitis. Int J Pancreatol 14:1–8
135. Manji N, Hulyalkar AR, Keroack MA, Vekshtein VI, Kirshenbaum JM, Sugarman DI, Chopra S (1988) Cutaneous pseudo abscesses: an unusual presentation of severe pancreatitis. Am J Gastroenterol 83:177–179
136. Mann DV, Hershman MJ, Hittinger R, Glazer G (1994) Multicentre audit of death from acute pancreatitis. Br J Surg 81:890–893
137. Mayer H (1985) Zur Pathogenese der Retinopathie bei akuter Pankreatitis. Klin Monatsbl Augenheilkd 187:293–295
138. McMahon MJ, Playforth MJ, Pickford IR (1980) A comparative study of methods for the prediction of severity of attacks of acute pancreatitis. Br J Surg 67:22–25
139. McMahon MJ, Playforth MJ, Rashid SA, Cooper EH (1982) The amylase-to-creatinine clearance ratio – a non-specific response to acute illness? Br J Surg 69:29–32
140. Mishler JM, Dürr GH-K (1980) Macroamylasemia induced by hydroxyethyl starch – confirmation by gel filtration analysis of serum and urine. Am J Clin Pathol 74:387–391

141. Mitchell CE (1964) Relapsing pancreatitis with recurrent pericardial and pleural effusions. A case report and review of the literature. Ann Intern Med 60:1047–1053
142. Morand P, Lanfranchi J, Curelli J-P (1977) Péricardites aiguës et pancréatites. Coeur Med Interne 16:19–28
143. Murata A, Ogawa M, Fujimoto K, Kitahara T, Kosaki G (1982) Changes in serum immunoreactive pancreatic elastase 1 in acute pancreatitis. Hepatogastroenterology 29:278–280
144. Neher M, Kümmerle F (1978) Gastrointestinale Komplikationen bei akuter Pankreatitis. Dtsch Med Wochenschr 103:1400–1404
145. Neoptolemos JP, Carr-Locke DL, London NJ, Bailey IA, James D, Fossard DP (1988) Controlled trial of urgent endoscopic retrograde cholangiopancreatography and endoscopic sphincterotomy versus conservative treatment for acute pancreatitis due to gallstones. Lancet 2:979–983
146. Neoptolemos JP, London NJM, Carr-Locke DL (1993) Assessment of main pancreatic duct integrity by endoscopic retrograde pancreatography in patients with acute pancreatitis. Br J Surg 80:94–99
147. Nord HJ, Weis HJ, Cölle H (1973) Untersuchungen zum Stoffwechsel der Serumamylase. Verh Dtsch Ges Inn Med 79:868–870
148. Nordestgaard AG, Wilson SE, Williams RA (1988) Correlation of serum amylase levels with pancreatic pathology and pancreatitis etiology. Pancreas 3:159–162
149. Paloyan D, Simonowitz D (1976) Diagnostic considerations in acute alcoholic and gallstone pancreatitis. Am J Surg 132:329–331
150. Paxton JR, Payne JH (1948) Acute pancreatitis. A statistical review of 307 established cases of acute pancreatitis. Surg Gynecol Obstet 86:69–75
151. Pederzoli P, Bassi C, Vesentini S, Campedelli A (1993) A randomized multicenter clinical trial of antibiotic prophylaxis of septic complications in acute necrotizing pancreatitis with imipenem. Surg Gynecol Obstet 176:480–483
152. Phillips RM Jr, Sulser RE, Songcharoen S (1980) Inflammatory arthritis and subcutaneous fat necrosis associated with acute and chronic pancreatitis. Arthritis Rheumatism 23:355–360
153. Pieper-Bigelow C, Strocchi A, Levitt MD (1990) Where does serum amylase come from and where does it go? Gastroenterol Clin North Am 19:793–810
154. Porter KA, Banks PA (1991) Obesity as a predictor of severity in acute pancreatitis. Int J Pancreatol 10:247–252
155. Potts DE, Mass MF, Iseman MD (1975) Syndrome of pancreatic disease, subcutaneous fat necrosis and polyserositis. Case report and review of literature. Am J Med 58:417–423
156. Ranson JHC (1982) Etiological and prognostic factors in human acute pancreatitis: a review. Am J Gastroenterol 77:633–638
157. Ranson JHC, Rifkind KM, Roses DF, Fink SD, Eng K, Spencer FC (1974) Prognostic signs and the role of operative management in acute pancreatitis. Surg Gynecol Obstet 139:69–81
158. Ranson JHC, Rifkind KM, Turner JW (1976) Prognostic signs and nonoperative peritoneal lavage in acute pancreatitis. Surg Gynecol Obstet 143:209–219
159. Rattner DW, Legermate DA, Lee MJ, Mueller PR, Warshaw AL (1992) Early surgical débridement of symptomatic pancreatic necrosis is beneficial irrespective of infection. Am J Surg 163:105–110
160. Renner IG, Savage III WT, Pantoja JL, Renner VJ (1985) Death due to acute pancreatitis. A retrospective analysis of 405 autopsy cases. Dig Dis Sci 30:1005–1018
161. Robertson GM Jr, Moore EW, Switz DM, Sizemore GW, Estep HL (1976) Inadequate parathyroid response in acute pancreatitis. N Engl J Med 294:512–516
162. Robison JC, Gitlin N, Morrelli HF, Mann LJ (1982) Factitious hyperamylasuria. A trap in the diagnosis of pancreatitis. N Engl J Med 305:1211–1212
163. Roscher R, Beger HG (1987) Bacterial infection of pancreatic necrosis. In: Beger HG, Büchler M (eds) Acute Pancreatitis. Springer, Berlin-Heidelberg, pp 314–317
164. Rotman N, Chevret S, Pezet D, Mathieu D, Trovero C, Cherqui D, Chastang C, Fagniez P-L, The French Association for Surgical Research (1994) Prognostic value of early computed tomographic scans in severe acute pancreatitis. J Am Coll Surg 179:538–544
165. Sainio V, Kemppainen E, Puolakkainen P, Taavitsainen M, Kivisaari L, Valtonen V, Haapiainen R, Schröder T, Kivilaakso E (1995) Early antibiotic treatment in acute necrotising pancreatitis. Lancet 346:663–667
166. Salt II WB, Schenker S (1976) Amylase – its clinical significance: a review of the literature. Medicine 55:269–289

167. Scholhamer CF Jr, Spiro HM (1979) The first attack of acute pancreatitis: a clinical study. J Clin Gastroenterol 1:325–329
168. Schräpler P, Popp G, Putzka A (1974) Ätiologische, klinische, therapeutische und prophylaktische Aspekte der akuten Pankreatitis. Eine statistisch-kasuistische Studie. Wehrmed Monatsschr H. 7:205–212
169. Schrier RW, Melmon KL, Fenster LF (1965) Subcutaneous nodular fat necrosis in pancreatitis. Arch Intern Med 116:832–836
170. Schuster MM, Iber FL (1965) Psychosis with pancreatitis. A frequent occurrence infrequently recognized. Arch Intern Med 116:228–233
171. Semlacher EA, Chan-Yan C (1993) Acute pancreatitis presenting with visual disturbance. Am J Gastroenterol 88:756–759
172. Shewring DJ, Naerger HG, Steer HW (1991) Rare intrathoracic complications in acute pancreatitis. Thorax 46:399–400
173. Snady-McCoy L, Morse PH (1985) Retinopathy associated with acute pancreatitis. Am J Ophthalmol 100:246–251
174. Solomon R, Werner C, Mann D, D'Elia J, Silva P (1994) Effects of saline, mannitol, and furosemide on acute decreases in renal function induced by radiocontrast agents. N Engl J Med 331:1416–1420
175. Song H, Tietz NW, Tan C (1970) Usefulness of serum lipase, esterase, and amylase estimation in the diagnosis of pancreatitis – a comparison. Clin Chem 16:264–268
176. Stein W, Bohner J, Bahlinger M (1987) Macro lipase – a new member of the family of immunoglobulin-linked enzymes. J Clin Chem Clin Biochem 25:837–843
177. Steinberg WM (1990) Predictors of severity of acute pancreatitis. Gastroenterol Clin North Am 19:849–861
178. Steinberg WM, Goldstein SS, Davis ND, Shamma'a J, Anderson K (1985) Diagnostic assays in acute pancreatitis. A study of sensitivity and specificity. Ann Intern Med 102:576–580
179. Tenner SM, Steinberg W (1992) The admission serum lipase:amylase ratio differentiates alcoholic from nonalcoholic acute pancreatitis. Am J Gastroenterol 87:1755–1758
180. Thomson HJ, Obekpa PO, Smith AN, Brydon WG (1987) Diagnosis of acute pancreatitis: a proposed sequence of biochemical investigations. Scand J Gastroenterol 22:719–724
181. Toffler AH, Spiro HM (1962) Shock or coma as the predominant manifestation of painless acute pancreatitis. Ann Intern Med 57:655–659
182. Toskes PP (1990) Hyperlipidemic pancreatitis. Gastroenterol Clin North Am 19:783–791
183. Tran DD, Cuesta MA (1992) Evaluation of severity in patients with acute pancreatitis. Am J Gastroenterol 87:604–608
184. Uhl W, Büchler M, Malfertheiner P, Martini M, Beger HG (1991) PMN-elastase in comparison with CRP, antiproteases, and LDH as indicators of necrosis in human acute pancreatitis. Pancreas 6:253–259
185. Variyam EP, Shah A (1987) Pericardial effusion and left ventricular function in patients with acute alcoholic pancreatitis. Arch Intern Med 147:923–925
186. Ventrucci M, Gullo L, Daniele C, Bartolucci C, Priori P, Platé L, Bonora G, Labò G (1983) Comparative study of serum pancreatic isoamylase, lipase, and trypsin-like immunoreactivity in pancreatic disease. Digestion 28:114–121
187. Ventrucci M, Pezzilli R, Gullo L, Platé L, Sprovieri G, Barbara L (1989) Role of serum pancreatic enzyme assays in diagnosis of pancreatic disease. Dig Dis Sci 34:39–45
188. Ventrucci M, Pezzilli R, Naldoni P, Platé L, Baldoni F, Gullo L, Barbara L (1987) Serum pancreatic enzyme behavior during the course of acute pancreatitis. Pancreas 2:506–509
189. Vesentini S, Bassi C, Talamini G, Cavallini G, Campedelli A, Pederzoli P (1993) Prospective comparison of C-reactive protein level, Ranson score and contrast-enhanced computed tomography in the prediction of septic complications of acute pancreatitis. Br J Surg 80:755–757
190. Wapnick S, Evans MI, Hadas N, Grosberg SJ (1980) Limitation of amylase creatinine clearance ratio as a diagnostic test for postoperative pancreatitis. Surg Gynecol Obstet 150:694–698
191. Warshaw AL, Bellini CA, Lesser PB (1975) Inhibition of serum and urine amylase activity in pancreatitis with hyperlipemia. Ann Surg 182:72–75
192. Warshaw AL, Fuller AF Jr (1975) Specificity of increased renal clearance of amylase in diagnosis of acute pancreatitis. N Engl J Med 292:325–328

193. Weir GC, Lesser PB, Drop LJ, Fischer JE, Warshaw AL (1975) The hypocalcemia of acute pancreatitis. Ann Intern Med 83:185–189
194. Wells AD, McDonnell PJ, Burnand KG (1990) Purtscher's retinopathy in acute pancreatitis. Br J Surg 77:820
195. Wilding P, Cooke WT, Nicholson GI (1964) Globulin-bound amylase. A cause of persistently elevated levels in serum. Ann Intern Med 60:1053–1059
196. Wilson C, Heads A, Shenkin A, Imrie CW (1989) C-reactive protein, antiproteases and complement factors as objective markers of severity in acute pancreatitis. Br J Surg 76:177–181
197. Wilson C, Heath DI, Imrie CW (1990) Prediction of outcome in acute pancreatitis: a comparative study of APACHE II, clinical assessment and multiple factor scoring systems. Br J Surg 77:1260–1264
198. Wilson C, Imrie CW (1986) Amylase and gut infarction. Br J Surg 73:219–221
199. Wilson C, Imrie CW (1988) Deaths from acute pancreatitis: why do we miss the diagnosis so frequently? Int J Pancreatol 3:273–282
200. Wilson C, Imrie CW, Carter DC (1988) Fatal acute pancreatitis. Gut 29:782–788
201. Wilson HA, Askari AD, Neiderhiser DH, Johnson AM, Andrews BS, Hoskins LC (1983) Pancreatitis with arthropathy and subcutaneous fat necrosis. Evidence for the pathogenicity of lipolytic enzymes. Arthritis Rheumatism 26:121–126
202. Winslet M, Hall C, London NJM, Neoptolemos JP (1992) Relation of diagnostic serum amylase levels to aetiology and severity of acute pancreatitis. Gut 33:982–986
203. Wohlgemuth J (1910) Beitrag zur funktionellen Diagnostik des Pankreas. Berl Klin Wochenschr 47:92–95
204. Zastrow R (1978) Death due to pancreas necrosis. Clinical and pathological anatomic findings. Tijdschr Gastroenterol 21:217–232

10 Acute Pancreatitis: Complications

10.1
Local Complications

Local complications are those that involve the pancreas or peripancreatic area. Local complications include acute fluid collections, pancreatic necrosis, acute pseudocyst, and pancreatic abscess (Table 10.1).

Table 10.1. Local complications of acute pancreatitis

- Acute fluid collections
- Pancreatic necrosis
- Acute pseudocyst
- Pancreatic abscess

The Atlanta symposium held in 1992 reviewed and updated definitions of these local complications [22]. The following information represents a synthesis of the conclusions of this symposium correlated with other important information pertaining to these entities.

10.1.1
Acute Fluid Collection

Acute fluid collections are collections of enzyme-rich pancreatic juice [6, 22, 43]. They occur early in approximately 30%–50% of cases of acute pancreatitis and resolve spontaneously in the majority. On computed tomography (CT) scan, an acute fluid collection appears as low attenuation, poorly marginated collections of fluid with no recognized capsule (Fig. 10.1 a, b). Most acute fluid collections develop at the periphery of the gland in the anterior pararenal space. From this location, a fluid collection may extend to the posterior pararenal space, the lesser sac, the peritoneal cavity, and even the mediastinum. Occasionally, fluid collections are intrapancreatic and appear as one or more very small areas of low attenuation.

A fluid collection that persists eventually becomes encapsulated and after 4–6 weeks is properly termed a pseudocyst.

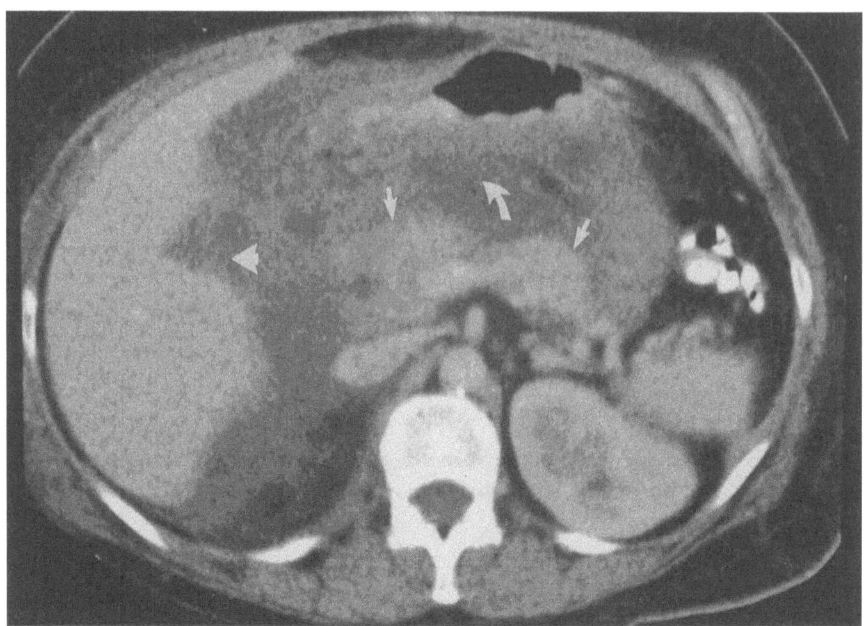

Fig. 10.1 a. Interstitial pancreatitis. Dynamic contrast-enhanced CT scan performed on a 53-year-old woman with pancreatitis secondary to hypertriglyceridemia reveals somewhat diminished and heterogenous enhancement of the pancreas (*oblique arrows*). The pancreatic margins are ill-defined. There is extensive peripancreatic fluid extending into the lesser sac (*curved arrow*) and into the porta hepatis (*arrowhead*). This appearance is consistent with severe interstitial pancreatitis with a severity score of 4 (4 points for grade E and 0 points for necrosis)

10.1.2
Pancreatic Necrosis

According to the Atlanta symposium, pancreatic necrosis is best defined as a process characterized by diffuse or focal areas of nonviable pancreatic parenchyma, usually associated with peripancreatic fat necrosis as well [22]. The determination whether a patient has interstitial or necrotizing pancreatitis can be made by dynamic contrast-enhanced CT scan [6, 8, 19, 25, 43, 85] (Fig. 10.1 a, b; see also Sect. 9.3 and Figs. 9.4, 9.5, 9.7, 9.8).

The clinician has several methods of determining on contrast-enhanced CT scan whether there are areas of necrosis. First, a well marginated zone of nonenhanced pancreatic parenchyma can readily be distinguished by visual inspection from surrounding well-perfused, uniformly enhancing parenchyma. Second, the clinician can make a visual comparison of pancreatic and splenic densities, which normally are similar. The liver should not be used for this comparison because if it contains a substantial amount of fat, the overall density of this organ is reduced. Third, the clinician can ask the radiologist to put a cursor over areas of suspected necrosis and determine the density of tissue in Hounsfield units. In general, the density of normal pancreatic paren-

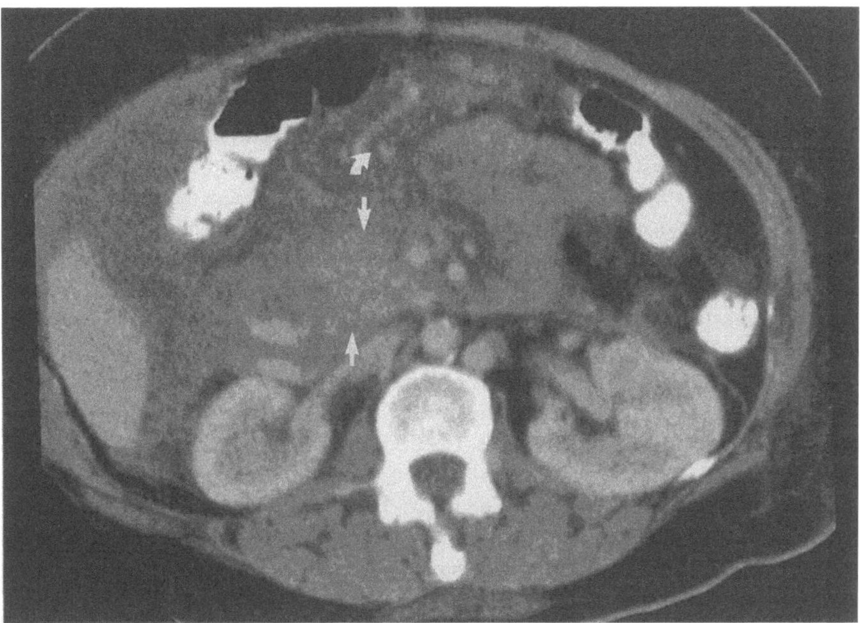

Fig. 10.1 b. Interstitial pancreatitis. At a lower level, the head of the pancreas is ill-defined and demonstrates diminished and heterogenous enhancement (*vertical arrows*). The peripancreatic inflammatory changes are again well seen extending into the mesentery (*curved arrow*) and into the right paracolic and subhepatic locations. Follow-up CT scans revealed no evidence of pancreatic necrosis. The patient made an uneventful recovery

chyma in the absence of intravenous contrast is approximately 40–50 Hounsfield units [8, 25, 43]. Following dynamic contrast-enhanced CT scan, normal pancreatic parenchyma enhances to at least 80–90 Hounsfield units [25, 43]. If the Hounsfield units fall short of this number, pancreatic necrosis should be strongly suspected. If the density fails to exceed 50 Hounsfield units, pancreatic necrosis is assured.

A very important question is whether findings that are termed pancreatic necrosis on CT scan can be verified. Thus far, several reports in man have confirmed by reasonable quantitative means that the amount of necrosis visualized by CT scan can be verified at surgery or autopsy [19, 25, 68, 85]. In addition, in the opossum, the amount of necrosis visualized by CT scan has been confirmed by pathologic examination [125].

In most cases of pancreatic necrosis, there is at least some peripancreatic necrosis; in some cases, peripancreatic necrosis is considerable and occurs with little if any pancreatic necrosis (see Fig. 7.2). Unfortunately, the CT characteristics of peripancreatic inflammation cannot distinguish between fat necrosis and fluid [6, 68, 85].

Studies thus far have strongly suggested that pancreatic necrosis may take place as early as the first 48–72 h of illness [63]. Accordingly, efforts to prevent or minimize pancreatic necrosis must be made within the first 48 h of illness.

Overall, almost all patients with interstitial pancreatitis can be expected to survive. However, overall mortality in necrotizing pancreatitis is at least 10% in the absence of associated pancreatic infection (termed *sterile necrosis*), and approximately 33% when there is associated pancreatic infection (a process termed *infected necrosis*) [120, 122]. Accordingly, in terms of prognosis, there is a high priority in determining whether a patient has interstitial or necrotizing pancreatitis.

An important question is the timing of the initial CT scan in acute pancreatitis. If the diagnosis of acute pancreatitis is in doubt, CT scan should be performed as early as possible in an effort to exclude alternative diagnoses such as a perforated duodenal ulcer. If the diagnosis of acute pancreatitis is secure, CT scan should be obtained if there is evidence of organ failure and/or marked clinical deterioration of the patient. Under these circumstances, the clinician needs to know whether the patient has necrotizing pancreatitis, and if so, whether the patient has infected necrosis of the pancreas. It is not clear that this information is mandatory during the first 3–5 days of hospitalization. First, even if the patient has necrotizing pancreatitis, clinical efforts during the first several days are directed to overcoming organ failure whether the patient has interstitial or necrotizing pancreatitis. The finding by CT scan at a very early stage that the patient has necrotizing pancreatitis does not impact on the resuscitative efforts that are being made. Second, while pancreatic infection takes place during the first 2 weeks in the majority of cases of necrotizing pancreatitis [9, 45], it is not likely to take place during the first several days. Accordingly, guided percutaneous aspiration for the purposes of discovering the presence of pancreatic infection usually does not take place until after the first 5 days. The necessity of a contrast-enhanced CT on admission of a patient with acute pancreatitis is not finally established. It is our policy to perform this investigation within 72 h after admission if there is need for further proof of the diagnosis or earlier recognition of pancreatic necrosis [143].

This policy is supported by the finding that early administration of imipenem among patients with pancreatic necrosis reduces the incidence of pancreatic infection [113]. Thus, it may be important to detect pancreatic necrosis as soon as possible. In a prospective study on more than 200 patients, the result of an initial contrast-enhanced CT on admission was significantly correlated with parameters of severity in the course of the disease. None of the patients with a normal CT on admission deteriorated, whereas 9% of patients with slight to moderate changes showed severe abnormalities on follow-up CTs [143]. Further studies are of interest.

Once pancreatic necrosis is determined on the basis of dynamic contrast-enhanced CT scan, the clinician is faced with a likelihood that the illness will be more severe than if CT scan demonstrated interstitial pancreatitis. First, 34%–70% of patients with necrotizing pancreatitis have evidence of multiorgan failure [113, 122]. Second, Ranson's scores are usually less than 2 in interstitial pancreatitis and between 3–5 in necrotizing pancreatitis [7, 8, 15, 28, 113, 154]. The interplay between early prognostic scores and pancreatic necrosis help alert the clinician as to the severity of illness and the likelihood of a fatal outcome, as follows (for grading scores see Tables 9.4–9.6): with a CT grade of E and a low Ranson's score of 1–3, there are essentially no deaths; with a CT grade of E and a Ranson's score of 5–8, mortality in one series was 44% [7]; with a CT grade of D or E and an Imrie score of ≥ 3, mortality in one series was 30%–55% [93].

Mortality in necrotizing pancreatitis has also been correlated with the extent of pancreatic necrosis. In some series [15, 122, 123, 154], but not in others [8, 70], patients with very extensive pancreatic necrosis had a higher mortality than those with < 30% necrosis. A major concern in pancreatic necrosis is the development of secondary pancreatic infection. Some reports have indicated that pancreatic infection is much more likely to take place when there is > 50% pancreatic necrosis than when there are lesser amounts of necrosis [15, 113, 154], but there are other series in which the majority of patients with almost complete pancreatic necrosis had a very low incidence of infection (Fig. 10.2 a, b) [31]. The overall incidence of secondary pancreatic infection associated with necrotizing pancreatitis in reported series is between 20% and 60% [9, 14, 15, 42, 91, 113, 122, 123]. Whereas the incidence of infection in earlier reports was in general ≥ 40%, it is lower in more recent reports [9, 113]. While the explanation for this apparent decline in infection associated with necrotizing pancreatitis is not clear, one factor might be the use of potent antibiotics that either prevent the development of pancreatic infection or possibly even might treat it successfully before it becomes clinically apparent.

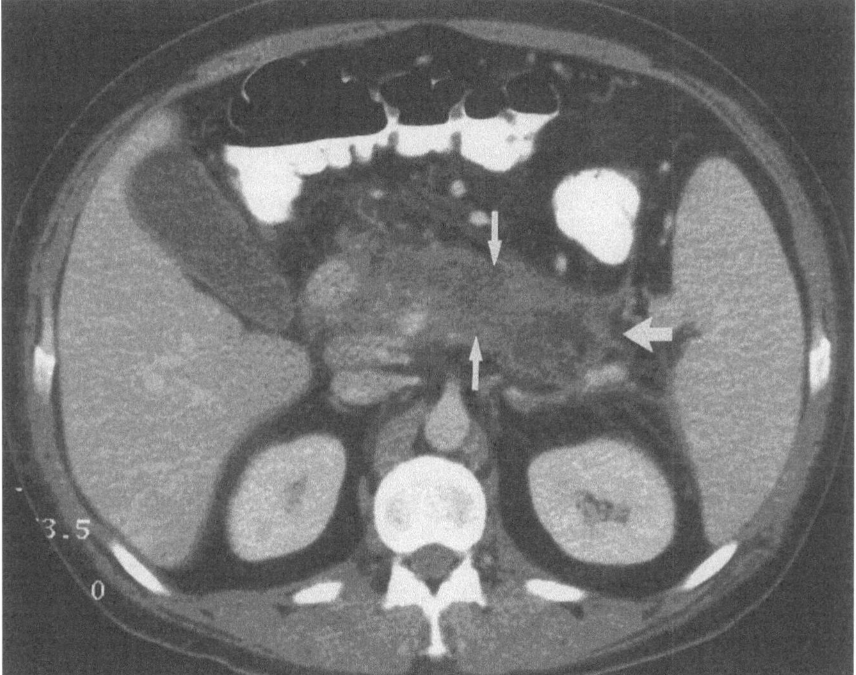

Fig. 10.2 a. Necrotizing pancreatitis with splenic vein thrombosis. Dynamic contrast-enhanced CT scan in a 36-year-old man recovering from his first episode of alcoholic pancreatitis reveals considerable necrosis of the body and tail of the pancreas (*vertical arrows*). There is a residual inflammatory response in the peripancreatic area (*horizontal arrow*). He made an uneventful recovery and was maintained on insulin for diabetes and on pancreatic enzymes for steatorrhea associated with extensive pancreatic necrosis

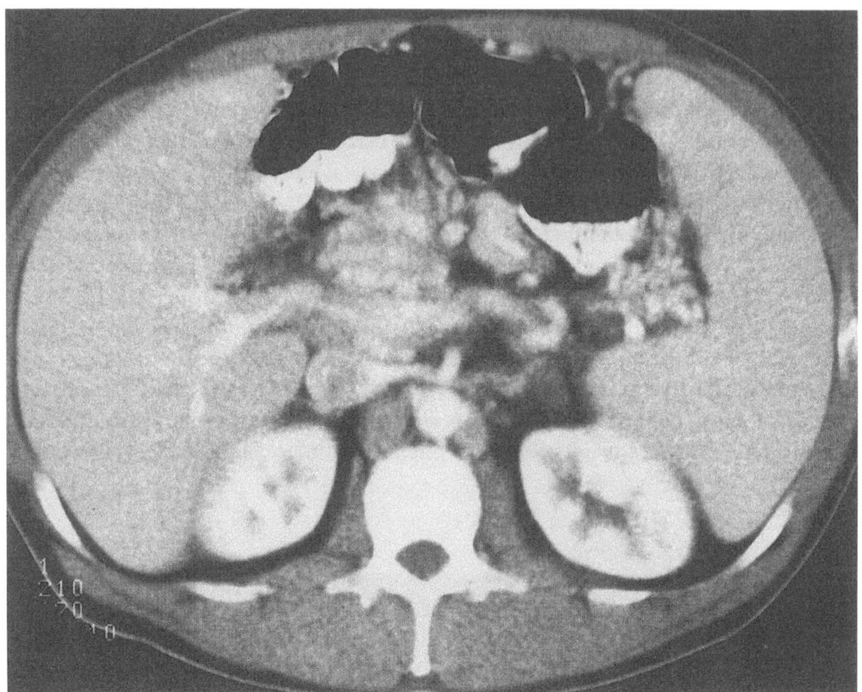

Fig. 10.2 b. Necrotizing pancreatitis with splenic vein thrombosis. One year later, dynamic contrast-enhanced CT scan demonstrates nonvisualization of the body and tail of the pancreas at this level and at other levels, indicating total necrosis and resorption of this tissue. More inferiorly, a normally enhancing head of the pancreas is visualized. The spleen is enlarged, and collateral vessels are seen in the splenic hilum

For many years, it has been thought that mortality in infected necrosis was higher than that of sterile necrosis [15, 23, 68, 122]. However, some reports [9, 120] have suggested that the mortality of infected necrosis is not greater than that of sterile necrosis. Indeed, there is evidence that sterile necrosis associated with severe organ dysfunction is a very serious illness with a high mortality [70]. Higher mortality in infected necrosis and sterile necrosis appears to be associated with severe organ dysfunction [70, 122]. Death in infected necrosis has also been correlated with the presence of 3 or more organisms, widespread extravasation of pancreatic exudate including intraperitoneal spread, deterioration of renal function, and the need for surgical reexploration [44].

In summary, pancreatic necrosis can be diagnosed on dynamic contrast-enhanced CT scan. In the absence of organ failure, mortality is usually very low. When there is organ failure, there is an increased mortality in both infected necrosis and sterile necrosis. When there is severe organ dysfunction, it is not clear that infected necrosis has a higher mortality than sterile necrosis.

10.1.3
Acute Pseudocyst

At the Atlanta symposium, a *pseudocyst* was defined as a collection of pancreatic juice enclosed by a wall of fibrous or granulation tissue [6, 22, 43] (see Fig. 9.6). A pseudocyst can arise as a result of acute pancreatitis, pancreatic trauma, or chronic pancreatitis, and can be distinguished from an acute fluid collection by the presence of a well-defined wall composed of fibrous or granulation tissue. A pseudocyst usually contains a high concentration of pancreatic enzymes and variable amounts of particulate material. The majority is sterile. Experience has shown that the formation of a well-defined wall takes 4 or more weeks from the onset of acute pancreatitis. Hence, a fluid collection with a duration of less than 4 weeks should be assumed to lack a well-defined wall and should be termed an acute fluid collection. On occasion, within this time frame, dynamic contrast-enhanced CT scan may suggest that the capsule is sufficiently thick to be suitable for a surgical anastomosis. However, there have been no formal studies that have correlated *wall thickness* following dynamic contrast-enhanced CT scan with maturity of the wall [6].

Most pseudocysts are located in the peripancreatic area, but some occur in other sites in the abdomen, within the mediastinum [10, 75], and in the pelvis [46]. Complications of a pancreatic pseudocyst include infection, occlusion of the splenic vein with secondary development of varices, arterial pseudoaneurysm formation, acute hemorrhage, invasion into spleen or liver [77, 157], perforation into the gastrointestinal tract, and obstruction of the common bile duct, stomach, or other areas in the gastrointestinal tract [6]. A diagnosis of pancreatic infection can be made by CT guided percutaneous aspiration with bacteriological sampling for Gram stain and culture [9, 45]. The presence of intracyst bleeding can be noted by the presence of high attenuation material within the cyst on CT scan. Arterial pseudoaneurysm formation is usually well seen by dynamic contrast-enhanced CT scan and if need by arteriography. The remaining complications are also well seen by CT scan.

The differential diagnosis of a cystic structure within the pancreas may be difficult. It includes pancreatic pseudocysts, cystic neoplasm [51, 89, 155, 159, 160], hematoma, hydatid cyst [98], von Hippel-Lindau syndrome [145], urinoma [141], metastatic tumor, and true cyst [142]. Cystic neoplasms include serous cystadenomas, mucinous cystadenomas, mucinous cystadenocarcinoma [90], and rarely cystic islet-cell tumors [160].

Cystic conditions other than pseudocyst and cystic neoplasm are quite rare. Unless there is epidemiologic evidence in favor of a hydatid cyst or features suggestive of von Hippel-Lindau syndrome such as renal cysts, retinal angiomas, and hemangioblastomas of the central nervous system, the differential diagnosis usually involves only pseudocyst or cystic neoplasm. A cystic neoplasm should be suspected in an individual who has not suffered a recent episode of acute pancreatitis and does not have evidence indicative of chronic pancreatitis, such as characteristic abnormalities on CT scan or ERCP.

Most cystic neoplasms are discovered because an ultrasound or CT scan is performed for symptoms totally unrelated to a pancreatic process or for very mild symptoms associated with the neoplasm (Fig. 10.3).

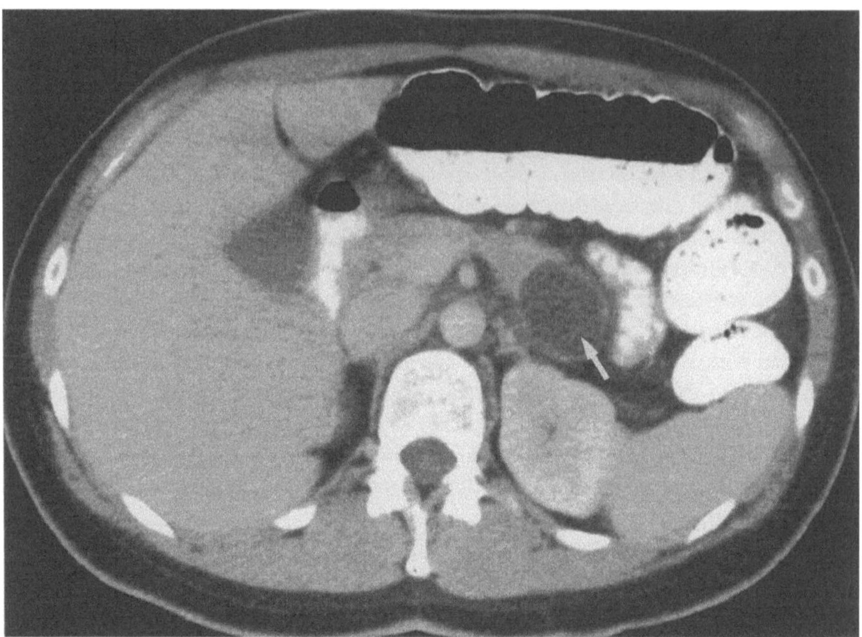

Fig. 10.3. Cystic neoplasm. Dynamic contrast-enhanced CT scan in a 30-year-old woman with mild recurrent left upper quadrant pain reveals a low-attenuation mass in the tail of the pancreas (*arrow*). She had been told several years earlier on the basis of an abdominal ultrasound that she had a cyst in her pancreas. The differential diagnosis included cystic neoplasm and pseudocyst of the pancreas. In the absence of a previous episode of acute pancreatitis, evidence of chronic pancreatitis, or evidence of another process such as hydatid cyst or hematoma, cystic neoplasm should be the first diagnosis. Distal pancreatectomy and splenectomy were performed. This proved to be a mucinous cystadenoma of the pancreas

The appearance on CT scan does not reliably distinguish among pseudocyst, serous cystadenoma, mucinous cystadenoma, and cystadenocarcinoma [155]. The presence of septations is helpful in distinguishing pseudocyst from neoplasm but not for distinguishing serous from mucinous tumors. When there are multiple small loculations, serous cystadenoma is strongly suggested. However, small loculations have been noted in only 50% of serous cystadenoma [155]. The presence of a central scar or *sunburst* calcification is highly suggestive of serous cystadenomas but are rarely seen [155].

ERCP is usually not essential in the preoperative evaluation of a suspected pancreatic cystic neoplasm unless there is some clinical or radiologic evidence that the patient may have chronic pancreatitis and that the cystic structure could be a pseudocyst. In chronic pancreatitis, there should be characteristic ductal abnormalities of this condition, and contrast may flow into the pseudocyst. In the case of cystic neoplasm, the pancreatic duct should be entirely normal, and only on rare occasions can the cystic neoplasm be filled with contrast. If a cystic neoplasm is strongly suspected and there is obstruction to the flow of contrast in the main pancreatic duct, this finding may indicate that the cystic neoplasm is malignant [155].

If a suspected cystic neoplasm is producing symptoms, it should be resected. First, at the time of surgery, it is not possible for a surgeon even with multiple biopsies of the wall of the cyst to provide sufficient histologic material for the pathologist to be confident that a lesion is a pseudocyst rather than a cystic neoplasm. The reason is that a considerable amount of the epithelium of a cystic neoplasm may be denuded simulating a pseudocyst. A thorough histologic inspection of the lining of the entire cystic structure by the pathologist is required to exclude a cystic neoplasm. If the surgeon were to perform a cystenterostomy in the mistaken belief that the lesion is a pseudcyst rather than a cystic neoplasm, an opportunity for cure of a malignant cystic neoplasm would be lost. There are many examples of individuals with malignant cystic neoplasms treated in this fashion who, during the next several years, were then found to have incurable metastatic disease [160].

If a suspected cystic neoplasm is producing no symptoms, the choices are to perform a resection or to maintain medical surveillance. In general, cystic neoplasms have been resected among patients who are considered to be good surgical candidates because there have been no preoperative techniques that have determined with certainty that a cystic neoplasm is benign. Medical surveillance would be reasonable if the clinician could distinguish between serous cystadenoma (which is almost always benign) and mucinous cystic neoplasm (which may or may not be benign). Recently, it has been suggested that aspiration for mucin content, cytology, amylase, and a variety of tumor markers is helpful in distinguishing serous cystadenomas and pseudocysts from mucinous cystadenomas and mucinous cystadenocarcinomas [51, 89]. A carcino-embryonic antigen (CEA) of < 5 has been shown to be strong evidence that a tumor is not mucinous. Cytology is usually positive in mucinous cystic neoplasms. Amylase is invariably high in pseudocysts, low in serous cystadenomas, and variable in mucinous neoplasms. Additional studies involving aspiration of cyst fluid will be required to confirm these findings. Since it is not possible by any preoperative test to distinguish mucinous cystadenoma from mucinous cystadenocarcinoma (it may also be difficult for the pathologist as well), mucinous tumors should be resected.

10.1.4
Pancreatic Abscess

Pancreatic abscess was defined at the Atlanta symposium as a circumscribed intraabdominal collection of pus following an episode of acute pancreatitis or pancreatic trauma [22]. An abscess is usually close to the pancreas and contains little, if any, pancreatic necrosis. General experience has been that pancreatic abscesses occur later than infected necrosis, frequently 4 weeks or more following the onset of pancreatitis [18]. The substrate of a pancreatic abscess may take two forms. The first is an area of limited necrosis with secondary liquefaction and eventual infection. The second is infection of a pancreatic pseudocyst. In general, mortality of a pancreatic abscess is less than that of infected necrosis [18, 40].

10.2
Systemic and Other Extrapancreatic Complications

Although local, intrapancreatic complications of acute pancreatitis may present a difficult clinical problem, extrapancreatic complications of the disease (Table 10.2) may be equally important since many of them occur in an early stage and may seriously influence the course of the disease [79].

10.2.1
Shock

Experimental evidence underscores the significance of shock. Hemorrhagic shock in rats converts edematous pancreatitis to hemorrhagic [74].

Shock is one of the most serious complications of acute pancreatitis. Data on its frequency vary considerably from study to study (1%–60%) and depend on whether or not milder forms of the disease are included [38].

Shock is assumed to be due to leakage of pancreatic exudate into the interstitial, retroperitoneal, and peritoneal spaces which may severely reduce intravascular volume and lead to systemic hypotension. There is some experimental evidence that toxic substances liberated in acute pancreatitis contribute to shock and to its high mortality [4, 82]. Prognosis of shock is poor. Jacobs et al. [66] reported a mortality rate of 29% and 39% when patients with acute pancreatitis had a systolic blood pressure of 100 and 90 mm Hg on admission, respectively. In patients with fatal acute pancreatitis, refractory hypotension or respiratory failure were the lethal mechanisms in 20% of the cases [27]. In another series, shock requiring intensive resuscitative measures was observed in 25 (6.4%) of 389 patients, 22 (88%) of whom died. This mortality rate was significantly higher than for patients never in shock [127].

Shock may be associated with coagulation disorders. The exact frequency of these disorders is not known, but they are obviously more frequent in cases with a poor prognosis [105, 117].

Furthermore, postmortem examinations in patients dying after oligemic shock showed the importance of the presence of acute renal tubular necrosis. When acute renal tubular necrosis was present, there was a 50% incidence of major pancreatic inju-

Table 10.2. Extrapancreatic complications of acute pancreatitis

- Shock
- Renal insufficiency
- Respiratory insufficiency
- Cardiac complications
- Common bile duct obstruction
- Gastrointestinal bleeding
- Stenosis of an adjacent hollow organ (duodenum, colon, ureter)
- Ileus of the small intestine
- Fat necrosis
- Pancreatic encephalopathy
- Cutaneous manifestations
- Ophthalmological changes

ry but only a 9% incidence in its absence. Similarly, among patients dying after non-oligemic shock, 12% of those without acute renal tubular necrosis had major pancreatic injury compared to 35% of patients with this complication. Pancreatic ischemia due to hypoperfusion was considered to be a critical factor which could cause a progression from interstitial to necrotizing pancreatitis also in man [158].

Finally, it should be mentioned that it may be difficult to diagnose acute pancreatitis in the presence of shock, because shock may be the predominant manifestation of painless acute pancreatitis [150].

10.2.2
Renal Insufficiency

Evidence of renal insufficiency in acute pancreatitis differs considerably in the literature since there is no generally accepted definition for this complication. Minor abnormalities, such as protein, red and white cells in the urine, have been found in up to 50% of the cases [36]. In a personal series of 602 patients we found that serum creatinine levels within the first 48 h after admission of the patient were slightly elevated (1.1–2.0 mg/dl) in 24% of the patients and were >2.0 mg/dl in another 8.5%. A dialysis procedure was necessary in 7% of the cases because of acute renal failure [78]. In severe necrotizing pancreatitis, the incidence of elevated serum creatinine (>1.4 mg/dl) was reported to be as high as 29.8% [15]. Similarly to Jacobs [66], we found that an elevated serum creatinine within 48 h after admission is significantly associated with an increase in mortality [78].

Acute renal failure may be due to hypovolemia and hypotension [88]. However, renal failure has also been found in the absence of demonstrable hypotension [47]. Transient systemic hypertension has been reported to occur during acute pancreatitis [126], and in another study, all patients with acute pancreatitis had hypertension during the acute phase of the disease. The occurrence of renal failure in this series was considered to be due to a release of vasopressin in the circulation to increase the total peripheral resistance (causing systemic hypertension) and renal vascular resistance (causing a decrease in renal plasma flow and glomerular filtration) [162]. In this context, it is of interest that in 17% of patients with malignant hypertension, acute pancreatitis occurred, and all of these had renal failure [11].

10.2.3
Respiratory Insufficiency

Pleural effusions have long been recognized as secondary occurrences in acute pancreatitis, usually due to transdiaphragmatic lymphatic blockage and, less often, to pancreaticopleural fistulas. For the most part, they are left-sided or bilateral, and the amylase level in the pleural effusion is much higher than the corresponding serum amylase level. In a recent comparison of the occurrence of pleural effusions with the findings of contrast-enhanced CT, it was shown that pleural effusions occur in 50% of the patients and are significantly associated with more severe morphological changes of the pancreas including necrosis [80]. In patients with pleural effusions, pancreatic pseudocysts occur more frequently and the mortality rate is higher than in patients without these complications [80]. Furthermore, pulmonary infiltrates are also frequent in acute pancreatitis. They may occur in 18%–25% [62, 81]. If pulmonary infiltrates and severe hypoxemia occur together, mortality rate may be as high as 56% [62]. In a study comparing the occurrence of pulmonary infiltrates with morphological changes seen on contrast-enhanced CT, it was found that patients with pulmonary infiltrates have significantly more severe pancreatic changes and necrosis and develop more frequently a pancreatic pseudocyst and have a higher mortality [81]. Thus, pleural effusions and pulmonary infiltrates are important prognostic factors in acute pancreatitis.

The list of thoracic complications in acute pancreatitis also includes pancreatic pseudocysts with mediastinal extension and enzymatic mediastinitis which occur in 0.3%–0.4% of the patients [55].

Only a few decades ago, patients with severe necrotizing pancreatitis usually died from shock and renal failure. Improved intensive therapy now enable many patients to survive these early complications. It was only after this early mortality rate was lowered that the danger of subsequent development of acute respiratory failure became apparent [21, 79]. Data on its frequency vary considerably from study to study, due to the variable severity of acute pancreatitis and the equally variable evaluation of respiratory insufficiency. Marked respiratory insufficiency has been reported in one series in 22% of the cases, and 60% of these died from uncontrollable hypoxemia [144]. In a personal series of 204 patients with acute pancreatitis in whom blood gas analysis was performed within 48 h after admission, 63% had an arterial pO_2 <70 mm Hg, and in 30%, a pO_2 <60 mm Hg was measured [78]. In another series, respiratory insufficiency defined as an arterial pO_2 below 75 mm Hg within 48 h after admission was observed in 58% [118]. The same authors reported in a further study incidences for respiratory insufficiency of 69% (pO_2 <76 mm Hg), 52% (pO_2 <71 mm Hg), and 38% (pO_2 <66 mm Hg) [119].

A decrease of arterial pO_2 is associated with increased mortality. In two studies from Imrie and coworkers [59, 106], patients in whom arterial pO_2 levels fell below 70 mm Hg had a mortality rate of 3% [106] and 5.9% [59], whereas this rate increased to 14.3% and 13.2% when the arterial pO_2 was <60 mm Hg.

Septic complications in acute pancreatitis were the major cause for death in 80% of the cases in one series; refractory hypotension or respiratory failure were the cause for death in the remaining 20% [27]. Between 8.55% and 12.5% of the patients require artificial ventilation during the course of the disease [66, 78] and mortality may be as high as 75% in these cases [66].

The pathogenesis of acute respiratory failure is still yet unclear [107]. The following possibilities are under discussion: hypoventilation due to painful abdominal distension and/or pleural effusion; high output respiratory failure due to generalized inflammation of the abdomen; release of enzymes and biogenic amines such as histamine, trypsin, phospholipase A, triglycerides [71, 72, 156].

In a postmortem study we found with increasing progression of the disease from its onset until death due to necrotizing pancreatitis, interstitial edema, stickiness of granulocytes, thrombus formation, hyaline membranes, and proliferation of pneumocytes, and finally, interstitial fibrosis – all histological findings which are also seen in the so-called shock lung of other causes (Figs. 10.4–10.6) [84]. An adult respiratory distress syndrome (ARDS) model may be helpful in understanding the underlying pathogenetic mechanism and in improving the prognosis of the disease.

Internal pancreatic fistulas are well-known complications of acute pancreatitis. In very rare cases, these may reach the bronchial tree [56].

10.2.4
Cardiac Complications

Several decades ago, experimental and clinical studies showed electrocardiographic changes simulating myocardial infarction [13, 115]. In some cases recently reported, ECG changes were so pronounced that acute myocardial infarction was assumed and thrombolytic therapy started [29]. A prospective study showed electrocardiographic changes, mostly inversion of T-waves and displacement of ST segment in 51% of patients with acute pancreatitis [112].

The etiology of cardiac complications in acute pancreatitis is unclear. Vagal reflexes associated with acute pancreatitis either acting directly on the myocardium, or indirectly altering coronary blood flow, or through the increased secretion of pancreatic protolytic enzymes, are possibilities. Electrolyte abnormalities such as hypokalemia, hypocalcemia, and hyponatremia are common in acute pancreatitis and can modify the repolarization phase on the ECG [29].

Pericarditis and significant pericardial effusions may occur and result in cardiac tamponade [101, 102, 165]. Ventricular function studies have demonstrated primary

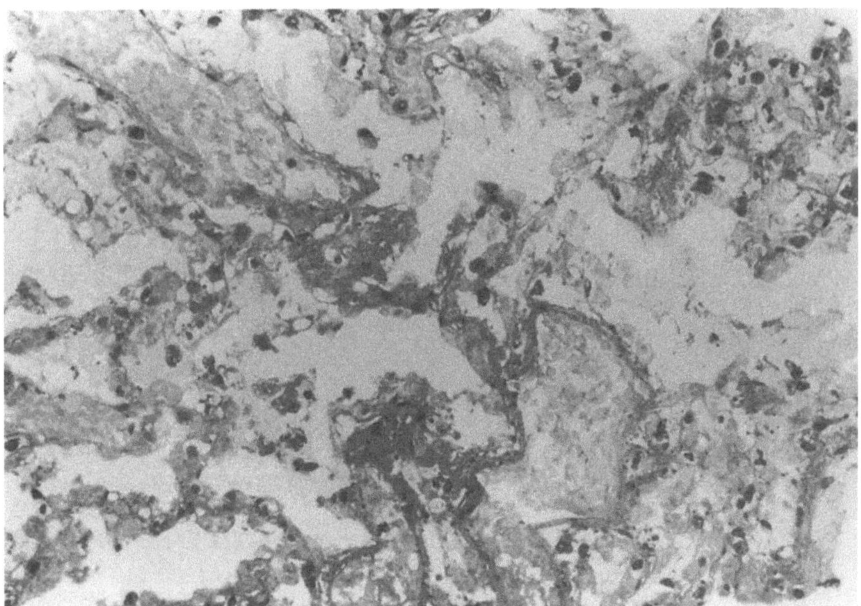

Fig. 10.4. Lung tissue in the early phase with interstitial and intraalveolar edema 4 days after the onset of the disease. Semithin section, Giemsa, × 225. (From [84] with permission)

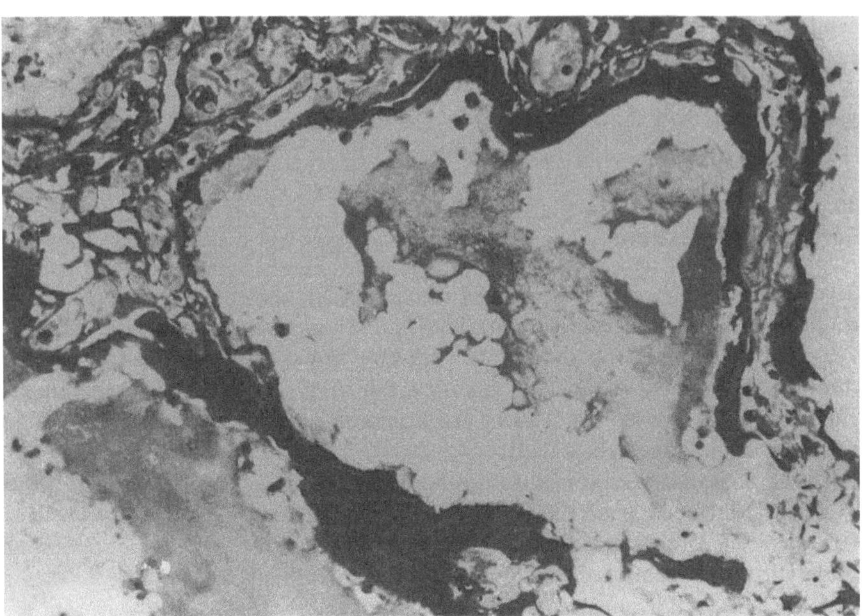

Fig. 10.5. Lung tissue in the late phase with hyaline membranes coating the alveolar ducts 10 days after the onset of the disease. Semithin section, Giemsa, × 225. (From [84] with permission)

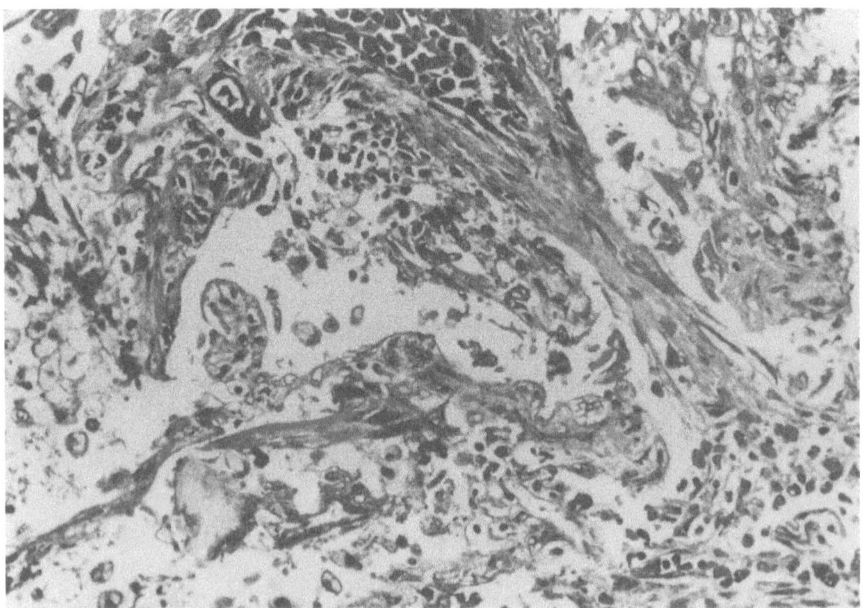

Fig. 10.6. Lung tissue in the final phase with interstitial fibrosis 18 days after the onset of the disease. Semithin section, Goldner's trichrome, × 225. (From [84] with permission)

myocardial depression [64, 86]. More recently, echocardiographic studies have shown pericardial effusion in 47% of alcoholics with acute pancreatitis [152] and in 17% of patients with acute pancreatitis of all etiologies [97], thus indicating a very high frequency of this extrapancreatic complication. Left ventricular function was unimpaired [152].

10.2.5
Common Bile Duct Obstruction

In acute pancreatitis, jaundice may occur in 39% of the patients. This is due to a stenosis of the common bile duct induced by edematous swelling of the head of the pancreas in mild acute pancreatitis and due to necrosis of the head of the pancreas in the severe form of the disease [109].

The treatment depends on the course of the disease. In less severe forms of pancreatitis, common bile duct obstruction will return to normal, with spontaneous resolution of the acute inflammation of the gland. In severe cases, common bile duct obstruction may persist and may be complicated by jaundice, fever, and sepsis. In these cases, a biliodigestive anastomosis or even a Whipple's operation may be necessary.

If common bile duct obstruction is due to a gallstone, endoscopic sphincterotomy is indicated.

10.2.6
Gastrointestinal Bleeding

Gastrointestinal bleeding is a rare event in acute pancreatitis with an incidence of 2%–4% [20, 60, 135]. Its incidence is much higher in necrotizing (11.3%) than in edematous (1.5%) pancreatitis [108]. The etiology of gastrointestinal bleeding in acute pancreatitis is unknown, but there is probably a direct relation to the effect of alcohol. Intestinal bleeding occurs more often in alcoholics than in nonalcoholics [20]. Local factors for gastrointestinal bleeding are alcoholic gastritis, Mallory-Weiss syndrome, active gastric or duodenal ulcer, intrapancreatic bleeding (Fig. 10.7 a, b), segmental hypertension with esophageal varices, and visceral vessel erosions. Bleeding from erosions of vessels in pancreatic pseudocysts or from gastroduodenal or pancreaticoduodenal pseudoaneurysm occurs more frequently in chronic than in acute pancreatitis (see Sect. 18.3.4). Mortality rate is high: 2 out of 4 [60] and 7 out of 10 patients died [135]. Gastrointestinal bleeding can be diagnosed by upper gastrointestinal endoscopy and/or CT; angiography is rarely necessary.

10.2.7
Stenosis of an Adjacent Hollow Organ (Duodenum, Colon, Ureter)

10.2.7.1
Stenosis of the Duodenum

Duodenal obstruction subsequent to acute pancreatitis is a rare event. Until 1981, this complication has been described in only 4 patients [24]. In one study, idiopathic duo-

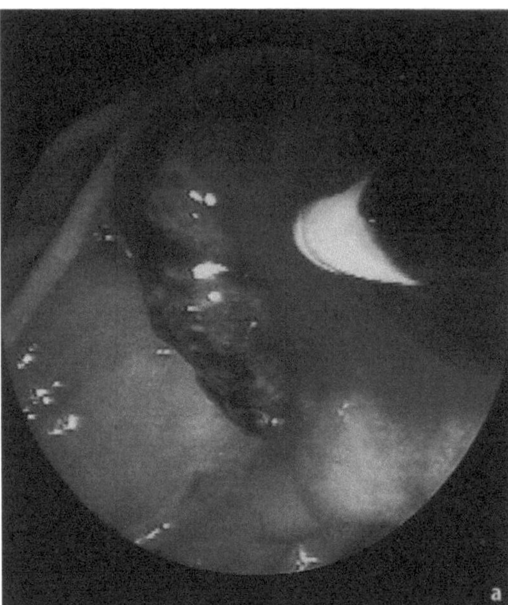

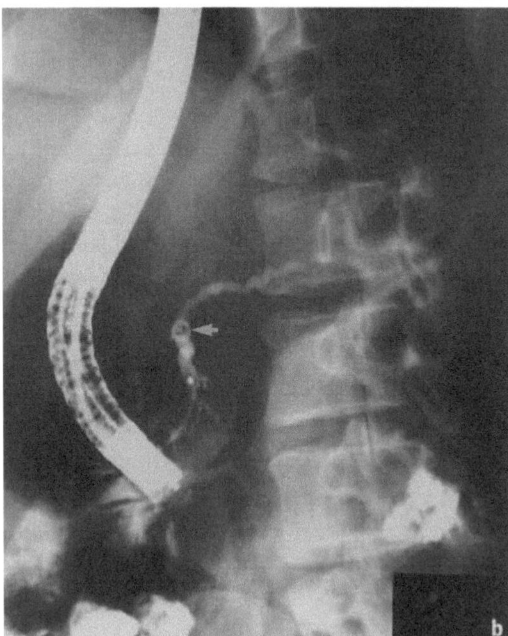

Fig. 10.7 a, b. Hemisuccus pancreaticus. **a** Endoscopic view of the duodenum with catheter inserted into the ampulla of Vater in a 48-year-old woman with recurrent idiopathic pancreatitis and recurrent episodes of gastrointestinal bleeding. There is clot adherent to the ampullary region and fresh blood issuing forth from the ampulla. **b** ERCP reveals slight dilatation of the pancreatic duct and an intraluminal filling defect consistent with a blood clot (*arrow*). She underwent Whipple operation and was found to have adenocarcinoma of the pancreas. This is an unusual cause of hemisuccus pancreaticus. A more common cause is bleeding from a pseudoaneurysm

denal obstruction was observed in 9 (1%) of 878 patients. The complication resolved completely within 3 weeks in 4 patients who had moderately severe pancreatitis. In the remaining 5, a surgical bypass operation was necessary. It seems likely that these were patients with chronic pancreatitis involving the head of the pancreas [24]. In a second study, 65 patients with edematous, 37 patients with necrotizing pancreatitis and 78 patients in whom pancreatic abscesses were diagnosed after the acute attack, were reported. None of the first, but 2 and 8 patients (10/115 patients = 9%) of the second and third group had duodenal stenosis [108].

10.2.7.2
Stenosis of the Colon

Lesions of the colon in acute pancreatitis include necrosis [129], partial or complete stenosis and fistulas [83], and even an incarceration of a transverse colon within a ventral hernia following the development of a severe ileus [146]. Colonic necrosis is probably due to ischemia, whereas stenosis of the colon may follow either ischemia or fibrosis of the pancreas. Data on the incidence of this complication vary considerably, depending on whether they were collected in a medical, or a surgical, or a mixed medical/surgical series of patients and whether or not patients with acute attacks of chronic pancreatitis were included. In a combined retrospective and prospective study, partial or complete chronic stenosis was present in 14% of the patients and a review of the literature at that time showed that the splenic flexure was mostly involved (Fig. 10.8) [1, 83]. In another series, 7 of 115 patients with acute hemorrhagic and septic pancreatitis showed colonic stenosis, whereas this complication was not found in the edematous form of the disease. Four (18%) of 22 patients with acute pancreatitis showed changes of the chronic pattern on plain X-ray of the abdomen, but only 1 developed a stenosis at the splenic flexure. Finally, 5 (26%) of 19 patients with pancreatic necrosis had a concomitant necrosis of the colon too [121].

Colonic stenosis may occur during an acute attack or several weeks later [83, 148]. Clinically, many patients had occult or evident gastrointestinal bleeding [149], or obstipation [137]. Colonic stenosis may be suspected from plain abdominal X-ray performed during the diagnosis of acute pancreatitis [137] or during the diagnosis of a colonic ileus when acute pancreatitis is not suspected [94]. Colonic ileus may take a stormy course right from the beginning in the form of cecal perforation [140], or occur postoperatively in severe acute pancreatitis [129]. Spontaneous resolution is possible; however, in a number of cases, surgical procedures are necessary [83, 124].

Pancreaticocolonic fistula, a rare complication, may occur with almost no symptoms, but the majority of cases are associated with severe necrotizing or septic complications [3, 147].

10.2.7.3
Stenosis of the Ureter

Ureteral obstruction due to acute pancreatitis is rare. Until 1994, 18 cases had been reported, but only 10 had urological signs or symptoms. The most common of them were flank pain on the affected side and fever. Pancreatitis may be acute or chronic, and ureteral obstruction may occur either during the acute attack or up to 7 months later, in this case due to a pancreatic pseudocyst [110]. In another series, 6 (5%) of 124

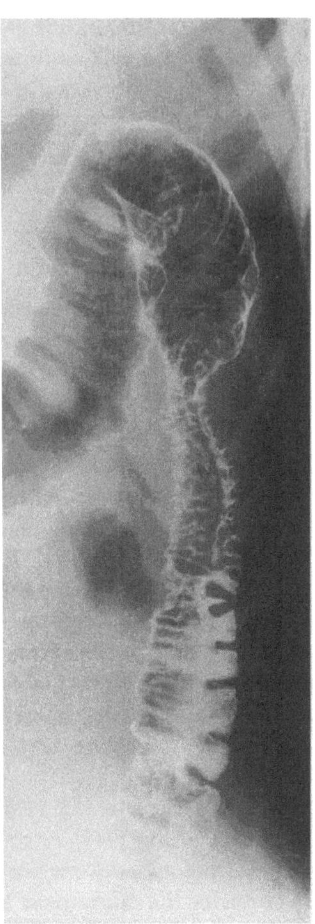

Fig. 10.8. Subtotal colonic stenosis below the splenic flexure (double-contrast barium enema investigation). (From [83] with permission)

patients with acute pancreatitis, or acute exacerbation of chronic pancreatitis, showed mild to moderate right hydronephrosis and proximal hydroureter. Follow-up examinations in available patients showed an improvement of obstruction with the resolution of pancreatitis [103]. However, a fatal outcome has been described in a patient with involvement of both ureters [46, 54, 69].

10.2.8
Ileus of the Small Intestine

Paralytic ileus due to peritonitis, electrolyte imbalance, toxic substances or *extravasation* of pancreatic exudation through the mesentery of the small intestine may occur in up to 50% of the patients [108]. Its frequency is higher in necrotizing (95%) than in edematous (25%) pancreatitis [108]. The prognosis is usually good.

More than 2 decades ago, when prognostic scores had not been developed and imaging procedures such as ultrasound and CT were not available, the best clinical index of severity or of improvement of acute pancreatitis was believed to be provided by the duration of the ileus. An ileus vanishes after 2 or 3 days in the majority of patients. The longer it lasts, the higher is the severity of the disease [151].

Another very rare involvement of the small intestine in acute pancreatitis, small intestinal infarction, was described in 3 patients, 2 of whom died [33, 49].

10.2.9
Fat Necrosis

Fat necrosis in acute pancreatitis has been of scientific interest for more than a century. It is well known that fat necrosis does not only occur within or surrounding the pancreas but everywhere in the body and may be associated with a fatal outcome [5, 76, 111]. It is assumed to be due to lipase-induced release of fatty acids and glycerol from triglycerides and the subsequent combination of free fatty acids with calcium-forming calcium soaps. In animal experiments and in postmortem studies of humans, pancreatitis was shown to start with fat necrosis around and within the pancreas. In a second step, acinar cell necrosis as well as vascular destruction and thrombosis arose in the immediate neighborhood of the fat necrosis [130, 131]. It may occur in a wide variety of tissues including retroperitoneal tissue, peritoneal tissue including the mesentery, mediastinum, pleura, pericardium, subcutaneous tissue, bones, and joints.

There are no data on its frequency in acute pancreatitis so that it is not known whether or not it has any influence on the prognosis of the disease.

Sometimes, the most striking feature is the large extent of extraperitoneal necrosis despite the comparatively normal residual pancreas [95].

Among the localizations of fat necrosis in acute pancreatitis, subcutaneous and intraosseous manifestations with or without involvement of joints have attracted particular interest.

Subcutaneous fat necrosis in acute pancreatitis may look like erythema nodosum [30, 52], but may occasionally resemble cutaneous pseudoabscesses [96]. Subcutaneous fat necrosis may be associated with a number of other complications of acute pancreatitis [132]. However, fat necrosis may be the initial manifestation of the disease in patients without abdominal pain, and the course of the disease in these cases may be even fatal [17, 30]. Occasionally, subcutaneous fat necrosis may occur after paracentesis of the anterior abdominal wall, probably secondary to leakage of pancreatic enzymes [87]. Recent intracellular staining of adipocytes with a monoclonal antibody to pancreatic lipase in a lesion of subcutaneous pancreatic fat necrosis has confirmed the role of pancreatic lipase in the pathogenesis of this complication. In 5 out of 8 cases of subcutaneous fat necrosis, acute pancreatitis was fatal [17, 30, 52, 87, 96, 132]. In patients who survived this complication, subcutaneous fat necrosis resolved within 4 weeks to 1 year [52].

Subcutaneous fat necrosis and an involvement of joints with the appearance of inflammatory arthritis have been described in a few patients. Most of the cases were fatal [92, 114, 116, 164]. In a patient who survived this complication, surgical removal of a giant pancreatic pseudocyst resulted in remission of the inflammatory process in the joints as well as within the subcutaneous tissue [166].

Several case reports have also dealt with intraosseous fat necrosis. In a postmortem study, 7 (10.4%) of 67 patients with necrotizing pancreatitis had fat necrosis in the bone marrow. This was obviously associated with wide-spread abdominal fat necrosis and especially with extraabdominal fat necrosis. None of the patients with acute necrotizing pancreatitis but without fat necrosis, or with only focal fat necrosis, showed any involvement of the bone marrow [128].

Bone lesions, both in acute and chronic pancreatitis, have been described for more than 30 years [2, 57, 58]. More recently, they have been found to occur with both cutaneous and arthritis syndromes in acute pancreatitis (for review see [12]).

Diagnosis was mostly made by X-ray. Magnetic resonance imaging (MRI) is now recommended for the detection of intraosseous fat necrosis [50]. Osteolytic lesions may occur 3–4 weeks after the onset of pancreatitis and even after discharge of the patient. Osteolytic lesions may resolve spontaneously, but at least in one case, total pancreatectomy was held necessary to relieve all symptoms and to heal destroyed bones [104].

10.2.10
Pancreatic Encephalopathy

Psychosis in acute pancreatitis has been described as a frequent extrapancreatic complication [133]. The incidence of pancreatic encephalopathy is between 4% and 19% [34]. However, it remains unclear whether these transient hallucinations in alcoholics are due to the withdrawal of alcohol, to the use of atropine at that time for inhibition of pancreatic secretion, or to the disease itself (see Sect. 9.1.2).

In one study [27], one-third of the patients who entered comatous expired. In a prospective study, nonspecific electroencephalographic changes were found in 35% of patients with acute pancreatitis. There was a significant increase in lipase in the cerebrospinal fluid of these patients. Encephalopathy had no obvious effect on the course of the disease [39]. Further studies are required.

10.2.11
Cutaneous Manifestations

In severe acute pancreatitis, cyanosis may be apparent on the face and extremities. In the event of retroperitoneal hemorrhage, there may be dissection of blood causing ecchymosis in the flanks (Grey-Turner's sign) (see Fig. 9.1) or in the umbilicus (Cullen's sign), both signs having been described many decades ago [35, 48].

CT examinations have shown that Grey-Turner sign is produced by spread of an inflammatory process from the anterior pararenal space to between the two leaves of the posterior renal fascia and subsequently to the lateral edge of the quadratus lumborum muscle. Communication may be established to the posterior pararenal space and to the structures of the flank wall. The lumbar triangle, a site of anatomic weakness on the flank wall, may serve as a structural predisposition.

Cullen's sign was shown to be secondary to the tracking of inflammatory exudate to the anterior abdominal wall from the inflamed gastrohepatic ligament and across the falciform ligament. Another more direct pathway may be extension from inflammatory changes of the small mesentery or greater omentum to the round ligament, and then to properitoneal fat deep to the umbilicus [100].

Both signs are infrequent (Grey-Turner's sign 0.8%, Cullen's sign 1.1%) [66]. When they occur, they are associated with a poor prognosis. In one study, 23 of 770 patients developed one or both of these skin signs and 8 (35%) of the 23 patients died (see Table 9.1) [37]. However, both skin signs should be considered with caution since they may be not specific [32] and even self-infliction has been reported [163].

Finally, a case of thrombophlebitis migrans in association with acute relapsing pancreatitis has been described [153].

10.2.12
Ophthalmological Changes

Episodes of sudden blindness, with retinal changes, most closely corresponding to Purtscher's retinopathy, have been described in case reports during the last decades [26, 41, 61, 65, 67, 73, 99, 134, 136, 138, 139, 161]. The frequency of this extrapancreatic complication is unknown. It may be overlooked because it is overshadowed by other overwhelming systemic complications.

The pathogenesis of retinopathy is also unknown. Fat embolism of retinal arteries may produce ischemic infarctions in the retina [41, 99]. However, these fat embolisms are too small to produce an occlusion of the central retinal artery [139]. Embolism of posterior retinal vessels by complement-induced leukoaggregates in fibrin clots has also been described [16, 53, 65, 73, 136].

The prognosis is poor. Visual field defects may disappear [134], but severe ophthalmological changes may persist [61, 65].

References

1. Abcarian H, Eftaiha M, Kraft AR, Nyhus LM (1979) Colonic complications of acute pancreatitis. Arch Surg 114:995–1001
2. Achord JL, Gerle RD (1966) Bone lesions in pancreatitis. Am J Dig Dis 11:453–460
3. Alsumait AR, Jabbari M, Goresky CA (1978) Pancreaticocolonic fistula: a complication of pancreatitis. Can Med Assoc J 119:715–719
4. Amundsen E, Ofstad E, Hagen P-O (1968) Experimental acute pancreatitis in dogs. I. Hypotensive effect induced by pancreatic exudate. Scand J Gastroenterol 3:659–664
5. Balser W (1882) Ueber Fettnekrose, eine zuweilen tödtliche Krankheit des Menschen. Arch Pathol Anat 90:520–535
6. Balthazar EJ, Freeny PC, vanSonnenberg E (1994) Imaging and intervention in acute pancreatitis. Radiology 193:297–306
7. Balthazar EJ, Ranson JHC, Naidich DP, Megibow AJ, Caccavale R, Cooper MM (1985) Acute pancreatitis: prognostic value of CT. Radiology 156:767–772
8. Balthazar EJ, Robinson DL, Megibow AJ, Ranson JHC (1990) Acute pancreatitis: value of CT in establishing prognosis. Radiology 174:331–336

9. Banks PA, Gerzof SG, Langevin RE, Silverman SG, Sica GT, Hughes MD (1995) CT-guided aspiration of suspected pancreatic infection. Bacteriology and clinical outcome. Int J Pancreatol 18: 265–270

10. Banks PA, McLellan PA, Gerzof SG, Splaine EF, Lintz RM, Brown ND (1984) Mediastinal pancreatic pseudocyst. Dig Dis Sci 29:664–668

11. Barcenas CG, Gonzalez-Molina M, Hull AR (1978) Association between acute pancreatitis and malignant hypertension with renal failure. Arch Intern Med 138:1254–1256

12. Baron M, Paltiel H, Lander P (1984) Aseptic necrosis of the talus and calcaneal insufficiency fractures in a patient with pancreatitis, subcutaneous fat necrosis, and arthritis. Arthritis Rheumatism 27:1309–1313

13. Bauerlein TC, Stobbe LHO (1954) Acute pancreatitis simulating myocardial infarction with characteristic electrocardiographic changes. Gastroenterology 27:861–864

14. Beaux ACde, Palmer KR, Carter DC (1995) Factors influencing morbidity and mortality in acute pancreatitis; an analysis of 279 cases. Gut 37:121–126

15. Beger HG, Bittner R, Block S, Büchler M (1986) Bacterial contamination of pancreatic necrosis. A prospective clinical study. Gastroenterology 91:433–438

16. Behrens-Baumann W, Scheurer G, Schroer H (1992) Pathogenesis of Purtscher's retinopathy. An experimental study. Graefe's Arch Clin Exp Ophthalmol 230:286–291

17. Berman B, Conteas C, Smith B, Leong S, Hornbeck III L (1987) Fatal pancreatitis presenting with subcutaneous fat necrosis. Evidence that lipase and amylase alone do not induce lipocyte necrosis. J Am Acad Dermatol 17:359–364

18. Bittner R, Block S, Büchler M, Beger HG (1987) Pancreatic abscess and infected pancreatic necrosis. Different local septic complications in acute pancreatitis. Dig Dis Sci 32:1082–1087

19. Block S, Maier W, Bittner R, Büchler M, Malfertheiner P, Beger HG (1986) Identification of pancreas necrosis in severe acute pancreatitis: imaging procedures versus clinical staging. Gut 27: 1035–1042

20. Bonebrake RG, Watson P, Lanspa SJ (1992) Upper gastrointestinal bleeding in acute pancreatitis. J Clin Gastroenterol 14:274–275

21. Boumghar M, Cavin R (1978) Respiratorische Komplikationen bei schwerer akuter Pankreatitis. Schweiz Rundschau Med 67:1394–1401

22. Bradley III EL (1993) A clinically based classification system for acute pancreatitis. Summary of the International Symposium on Acute Pancreatitis, Atlanta, Ga, September 11 through 13, 1992. Arch Surg 128:586–590

23. Bradley III EL, Allen K (1991) A prospective longitudinal study of observation versus surgical intervention in the management of necrotizing pancreatitis. Am J Surg 161:19–25

24. Bradley III EL, Clements JL Jr (1981) Idiopathic duodenal obstruction. An unappreciated complication of pancreatitis. Ann Surg 193:638–648

25. Bradley III EL, Murphy F, Ferguson C (1989) Prediction of pancreatic necrosis by dynamic pancreatography. Ann Surg 210:495–504

26. Bretzke G, Bretzke K (1987) Beitrag zur Retinopathie bei akuter Pankreatitis. Z Gesamte Inn Med 42:369–370

27. Buggy BP, Nostrant TT (1983) Lethal pancreatitis. Am J Gastroenterol 78:810–814

28. Büchler M, Malfertheiner P, Schädlich H, Nevalainen TJ, Friess H, Beger HG (1989) Role of phospholipase A2 in human acute pancreatitis. Gastroenterology 97:1521–1526

29. Cafri C, Basok A, Katz A, Abuful A, Gilutz H, Battler A (1995) Thrombolytic therapy in acute pancreatitis presenting as acute myocardial infarction. Int J Cardiol 49:279–281

30. Cannon JR, Pitha JV, Everett MA (1979) Subcutaneous fat necrosis in pancreatitis. J Cutan Pathol 6:501–506

31. Casey JE, Porter KA, Langevin RE, Banks PA (1993) Clinical features and natural history of central cavitary necrosis. Pancreas 8:141–145

32. Chung MA, Oung C, Szilagyi A (1992) Cullen's sign: it doesn't always mean hemorrhagic pancreatitis. Am J Gastroenterol 87:1026–1028

33. Collins JJ Jr, Peterson LM, Wilson RE (1968) Small intestinal infarction as a complication of pancreatitis. Ann Surg 167:433–436

34. Colmant HJ, Noltenius H (1977) Pankreatische Enzephalopathie. Med Klin 72:2146–2154

35. Cullen TS (1918) A new sign in ruptured extrauterine pregnancy. Am J Obstet Gynecol 78:457

36. Dabels J, Diwok K, Gülzow M (1966) Nierenschädigung bei akuten Pankreaserkrankungen. Dtsch Z Verdau Stoffwechselkr 26:229–241
37. Dickson AP, Imrie CW (1984) The incidence and prognosis of body wall ecchymosis in acute pancreatitis. Surg Gynecol Obstet 159:343–347
38. Dürr H-K (1979) Acute pancreatitis. In: Howat HT, Sarles H (eds) The Exocrine Pancreas. W.B. Saunders Comp., London-Philadelphia-Toronto, pp 352–401
39. Estrada RV, Moreno J, Martinez E, Hernandez MC, Gilsanz G, Gilsanz V (1979) Pancreatic encephalopathy. Acta Neurol Scand 59:135–139
40. Fedorak IJ, Ko TC, Djuricin G, McMahon M, Thompson K, Prinz RA (1992) Secondary pancreatic infections: are they distinct clinical entities? Surgery 112:824–831
41. Flaggl E, Heer M, Hany A, Branda L (1988) Visusverlust als Komplikation der akuten Pankreatitis. Schweiz Med Wochenschr 118:722–725
42. Foitzik T, Bassi DG, Schmidt J, Lewandrowski KB, Fernandez-del Castillo C, Rattner DW, Warshaw AL (1994) Intravenous contrast medium accentuates the severity of acute necrotizing pancreatitis in the rat. Gastroenterology 106:207–214
43. Freeny PC (1993) Incremental dynamic bolus computed tomography of acute pancreatitis. Int J Pancreatol 13:147–158
44. Gerkin TM, Eckhauser FE, Raper SE, Mulholland MW, Knol JA, Schork MA (1995) Are traditional prognostic criteria useful in pancreatic abscess? Pancreas 10:331–337
45. Gerzof SG, Banks PA, Robbins AH, Johnson WC, Spechler SJ, Wetzner SM, Snider JM, Langevin RE, Jay ME (1987) Early diagnosis of pancreatic infection by computed tomography-guided aspiration. Gastroenterology 93:1315–1320
46. Gibson GE, Tiernan E, Cronin CC, Ferriss JB (1993) Reversible bilateral ureteric obstruction due to a pancreatic pseudocyst. Gut 34:1267–1268
47. Goldstein DA, Llach F, Massry SG (1976) Acute renal failure in patients with acute pancreatitis. Arch Intern Med 136:1363–1365
48. Grey Turner G (1920) Local discoloration of the abdominal wall as a sign of acute pancreatitis. Br J Surg 7:394–395
49. Griffiths RW, Brown PW Jr (1970) Jejunal infarction as a complication of pancreatitis. Gastroenterology 58:709–712
50. Haller J, Greenway G, Resnick D, Kindynis P, Kang HS (1989) Intraosseous fat necrosis associated with acute pancreatitis: MR imaging. Radiology 173:193–195
51. Hammel P, Levy P, Voitot H, Levy M, Vilgrain V, Zins M, Flejou J-F, Molas G, Ruszniewski P, Bernades P (1995) Preoperative cyst fluid analysis is useful for the differential diagnosis of cystic lesions of the pancreas. Gastroenterology 108:1230–1235
52. Higgins E, Ive FA (1990) Subcutaneous fat necrosis in pancreatic disease. Br J Surg 77:532–533
53. Holló G, Popik G (1992) Is retinopathy in pancreatitis caused by leukocyte emboli? Acta Ophthalmol 70:820–823
54. Höfler H (1978) Symmetrische hämorrhagische Infarcierung der Ureteren als Komplikation der akuten Pankreatitis. Virchows Arch [Pathol Anat] 379:151–156
55. Iacono C, Procacci C, Frigo F, Bergamo Andreis IA, Cesaro G, Caia S, Bassi C, Pederzoli P, Serio G, Dagradi A (1989) Thoracic complications of pancreatitis. Pancreas 4:228–236
56. Iglehart JD, Mansback C, Postlethwait R, Roberts L Jr, Ruth W (1986) Pancreaticobronchial fistula. Case report and review of the literature. Gastroenterology 90:759–763
57. Immelman E, Krige H, Bank S (1963) Radiological changes in bone due to intramedullary fat necrosis in pancreatitis. Clin Radiol 14:273–275
58. Immelman EJ, Bank S, Krige H, Marks IN (1964) Roentgenologic and clinical features of intramedullary fat necrosis in bones in acute and chronic pancreatitis. Am J Med 36:96–105
59. Imrie CW, Ferguson JC, Murphy D, Blumgart LH (1977) Arterial hypoxia in acute pancreatitis. Br J Surg 64:185–188
60. Imrie CW, Whyte AS (1975) A prospective study of acute pancreatitis. Br J Surg 62:490–494
61. Inkeles DM, Walsh JB, Matz R (1976) Purtscher's retinopathy in acute pancreatitis. Am J Med Sci 272:335–338
62. Interiano B, Stuard ID, Hyde RW (1972) Acute respiratory distress syndrome in pancreatitis. Ann Intern Med 77:923–926

63. Isenmann R, Büchler M, Uhl W, Malfertheiner P, Martini M, Beger HG (1993) Pancreatic necrosis: an early finding in severe acute pancreatitis. Pancreas 8:358–361
64. Ito K, Ramirez-Schon G, Shah PM, Agarwal N, Delguercio LRM, Reynolds BM (1981) Myocardial function in acute pancreatitis. Ann Surg 194:85–88
65. Jacob HS, Goldstein IM, Shapiro I, Craddock PR, Hammerschmidt DE, Weissmann G (1981) Sudden blindness in acute pancreatitis. Possible role of complement-induced retinal leukoembolization. Arch Intern Med 141:134–136
66. Jacobs ML, Daggett WM, Civetta JM, Vasu MA, Lawson DW, Warshaw AL, Nardi GL, Bartlett MK (1977) Acute pancreatitis: analysis of factors influencing survival. Ann Surg 185:43–51
67. Jipp P, Mayer H, Reinold H-M, Schrader K-E (1985) Akute Pankreatitis und ischämische Netzhautveränderungen. Med Klin 80:363–366
68. Johnson CD, Stephens DH, Sarr MG (1991) CT of acute pancreatitis: correlation between lack of contrast enhancement and pancreatic necrosis. Am J Roentgenol 156:93–95
69. Justich E, Höfler H, Fink W, Kratochvil K (1978) Nekrose beider Ureteren nach Pankreatitis. Fortschr Röntgenstr 128:636–637
70. Karimgani I, Porter KA, Langevin RE, Banks PA (1992) Prognostic factors in sterile pancreatic necrosis. Gastroenterology 103:1636–1640
71. Kimura T, Toung JK, Margolis S, Bell WR, Cameron JL (1980) Respiratory failure in acute pancreatitis: the role of free fatty acids. Surgery 87:509–513
72. Kimura T, Toung JK, Margolis S, Permutt S, Cameron JL (1979) Respiratory failure in acute pancreatitis. A possible role for triglycerides. Ann Surg 189:509–514
73. Kincaid MC, Green WR, Knox DL, Mohler C (1982) A clinicopathological case report of retinopathy of pancreatitis. Br J Ophthalmol 66:219–226
74. Kyogoku T, Manabe T, Tobe T (1992) Role of ischemia in acute pancreatitis. Hemorrhagic shock converts edematous pancreatitis to hemorrhagic pancreatitis in rats. Dig Dis Sci 37:1409–1417
75. Landreneau RJ, Johnson JA, Keenan RJ, Thompson WM, Megison S, Ferson PF (1994) "Spontaneous" mediastinal pancreatic pseudocyst fistulization to the esophagus. Ann Thorac Surg 57:208–210
76. Langerhans R (1890) Ueber multiple Fettgewebsnekrose. Arch Pathol Anat 122:252–270
77. Lankisch PG (1990) The spleen in inflammatory pancreatic disease. Gastroenterology 98:509–516
78. Lankisch PG, Burchard-Reckert S, Petersen M, Lehnick D, Schirren CA, Köhler H, Stöckmann F, Peiper HJ, Creutzfeldt W (1996) Morbidity and mortality in 602 patients with acute pancreatitis seen between the years 1980–1994. Z Gastroenterol 34:371–377
79. Lankisch PG, Buschmann H (1984) Extrapancreatic complications of acute pancreatitis. In: Banks PA, Bianchi Porro G (eds) Acute Pancreatitis. Advances in pathogenesis, diagnosis and treatment. Masson Italia, Milano, pp 49–56
80. Lankisch PG, Dröge M, Becher R (1994) Pleural effusions: a new negative prognostic parameter for acute pancreatitis. Am J Gastroenterol 89:1849–1851
81. Lankisch PG, Dröge M, Becher R (1996) Pulmonary infiltrations. Sign of severe acute pancreatitis. Int J Pancreatol 19:113–115
82. Lankisch PG, Koop H, Winckler K, Schmidt H (1979) Continuous peritoneal dialysis as treatment of acute experimental pancreatitis in the rat. II. Analysis of its beneficial effect. Dig Dis Sci 24:117–122
83. Lankisch PG, Lopez E, Winckler K, Schuster R (1976) Kolonstenosen nach Pankreatitis. Schweiz Med Wochenschr 106:1243–1247
84. Lankisch PG, Rahlf G, Koop H (1983) Pulmonary complications in fatal acute hemorrhagic pancreatitis. Dig Dis Sci 28:111–116
85. Larvin M, Chalmers AG, McMahon MJ (1990) Dynamic contrast enhanced computed tomography: a precise technique for identifying and localising pancreatic necrosis. Br Med J 300:1425–1428
86. Lee WK, Frasca M, Lee C, Haider B, Regan TJ (1981) Depression of myocardial function during acute pancreatitis. Circ Shock 8:369–374
87. Levine N, Lazarus GS (1976) Subcutaneous fat necrosis after paracentesis. Report of a case in a patient with acute pancreatitis. Arch Dermatol 112:993–994
88. Levy M, Geller R, Hymovitch S (1986) Renal failure in dogs with experimental acute pancreatitis: role of hypovolemia. Am J Physiol 251:F969–F977

89. Lewandrowski K, Lee J, Southern J, Centeno B, Warshaw A (1995) Cyst fluid analysis in the differential diagnosis of pancreatic cysts: a new approach to the preoperative assessment of pancreatic cystic lesions. Am J Roentgenol 164:815–819

90. Lewandrowski KB, Southern JF, Pins MR, Compton CC, Warshaw AL (1993) Cyst fluid analysis in the differential diagnosis of pancreatic cysts. A comparison of pseudocysts, serous cystadenomas, mucinous cystic neoplasms, and mucinous cystadenocarcinoma. Ann Surg 217:41–47

91. Lucarotti ME, Virjee J, Alderson D (1993) Patient selection and timing of dynamic computed tomography in acute pancreatitis. Br J Surg 80:1393–1395

92. Lucas PF, Owen TK (1962) Subcutaneous fat necrosis, "polyarthritis", and pancreatic disease. Gut 3:146–148

93. Luiten EJT, Hop WCJ, Lange JF, Bruining HA (1995) Controlled clinical trial of selective decontamination for the treatment of severe acute pancreatitis. Ann Surg 222:57–65

94. Macerollo P, Segal I, Epstein B, Essop R, Elisseos C (1983) Total obstruction of the ascending colon complicating acute pancreatitis. Am J Gastroenterol 78:28–30

95. Maclean N (1977) The role of the surviving pancreas in late fatalities of acute pancreatitis. Br J Surg 64:345–346

96. Manji N, Hulyalkar AR, Keroack MA, Vekshtein VI, Kirshenbaum JM, Sugarman DI, Chopra S (1988) Cutaneous pseudo abscesses: an unusual presentation of severe pancreatitis. Am J Gastroenterol 83:177–179

97. Maringhini A, Ciambra M, Patti R, Randazzo MA, Dardanoni G, Mancuso L, Termini A, Pagliaro LP (1996) Ascites, pleural, and pericardial effusions in acute pancreatitis. A prospective study of incidence, natural history, and prognostic role. Dig Dis Sci 41:848–852

98. Mathai V, Banerjee Jesudason SR, Muthusami JC, Kuruvilla R, Idikula J, Sada P (1994) Chronic pancreatitis caused by intraductal hydatic cysts of the pancreas. Br J Surg 81:1029

99. Mayer H (1985) Zur Pathogenese der Retinopathie bei akuter Pankreatitis. Klin Monatsbl Augenheilkd 187:293–295

100. Meyers MA, Feldberg MAM, Oliphant M (1989) Grey Turner's sign and Cullen's sign in acute pancreatitis. Gastrointest Radiol 14:31–37

101. Mitchell CE (1964) Relapsing pancreatitis with recurrent pericardial and pleural effusions. A case report and review of the literature. Ann Intern Med 60:1047–1053

102. Morand P, Lanfranchi J, Curelli J-P (1977) Péricardites aiguës et pancréatites. Coeur Med Interne 16:19–28

103. Morehouse HT, Thornhill BA, Alterman DD (1985) Right ureteral obstruction associated with pancreatitis. Urol Radiol 7:150–152

104. Morgan JE, Robbins AH, Matsumoto G, Nabseth D (1976) Total pancreatectomy for recurrent medullary fat necrosis. Arch Surg 111:1394–1398

105. Murphy D, Imrie CW, Davidson JF (1977) Haematological abnormalities in acute pancreatitis. A prospective study. Postgrad Med J 53:310–314

106. Murphy D, Imrie CW, Pack A, Davidson JF, Blumgart LH (1976) The mechanism of acute respiratory insufficiency in acute pancreatitis. Br J Surg 63:669 (abstr)

107. Murphy D, Pack AI, Imrie CW (1980) The mechanism of arterial hypoxia occurring in acute pancreatitis. Quart J Med 49:151–163

108. Neher M, Kümmerle F (1978) Gastrointestinale Komplikationen bei akuter Pankreatitis. Dtsch Med Wochenschr 103:1400–1404

109. Neher M, Mangold G, Kümmerle F (1977) Ursachen und Behandlung des Ikterus bei entzündlichen Pankreaserkrankungen. Dtsch Med Wochenschr 102:644–647

110. Newman RM, Provet JA, Ranson JHC (1994) Clinically significant ureteral obstruction caused by inflammatory complications of severe pancreatitis. Surgery 115:656–660

111. Opie (1901) The relation of cholelithiasis to disease of the pancreas and to fat-necrosis. Bull Johns Hopkins Hosp 12:19–21

112. Oteyza CP, Rebollar JL, Chantres MT, Estella J (1979) Alteraciones electrocardiográficas en la pancreatitis aguda. Rev Clin Esp 152:287–290

113. Pederzoli P, Bassi C, Vesentini S, Campedelli A (1993) A randomized multicenter clinical trial of antibiotic prophylaxis of septic complications in acute necrotizing pancreatitis with imipenem. Surg Gynecol Obstet 176:480–483

114. Phillips RM Jr, Sulser RE, Songcharoen S (1980) Inflammatory arthritis and subcutaneous fat necrosis associated with acute and chronic pancreatitis. Arthritis Rheumatism 23:355–360
115. Pollock AV, Bertrand CA (1956) Electrocardiographic changes in acute pancreatitis. Surgery 40:951–960
116. Potts DE, Mass MF, Iseman MD (1975) Syndrome of pancreatic disease, subcutaneous fat necrosis and polyserositis. Case report and review of literature. Am J Med 58:417–423
117. Ranson JHC, Lackner H, Berman IR, Schinella R (1977) The relationship of coagulation factors to clinical complications of acute pancreatitis. Surgery 81:502–511
118. Ranson JHC, Roses DF, Fink SD (1973) Early respiratory insufficiency in acute pancreatitis. Ann Surg 178:75–79
119. Ranson JHC, Turner JW, Roses DF, Rifkind KM, Spencer FC (1974) Respiratory complications in acute pancreatitis. Ann Surg 179:557–566
120. Rattner DW, Legermate DA, Lee MJ, Mueller PR, Warshaw AL (1992) Early surgical débridement of symptomatic pancreatic necrosis is beneficial irrespective of infection. Am J Surg 163:105–110
121. Ravindra KV, Sikora SS, Kumar A, Kapoor VK, Saxena R, Kaushik SP (1995) Colonic necrosis in an adverse prognostic factor in pancreatic necrosis. Br J Surg 82:109–110
122. Roscher R, Beger HG (1987) Bacterial infection of pancreatic necrosis. In: Beger HG, Büchler M (eds) Acute Pancreatitis. Springer, Berlin-Heidelberg, pp 314–317
123. Rotman N, Chevret S, Pezet D, Mathieu D, Trovero C, Cherqui D, Chastang C, Fagniez P-L, The French Association for Surgical Research (1994) Prognostic value of early computed tomographic scans in severe acute pancreatitis. J Am Coll Surg 179:538–544
124. Russell JC, Welch JP, Clark DG (1983) Colonic complications of acute pancreatitis and pancreatic abscess. Am J Surg 146:558–564
125. Rünzi M, Raptopoulos V, Saluja AK, Kaiser AM, Nishino H, Gerdes D, Steer ML (1995) Evaluation of necrotizing pancreatitis in the opossum by dynamic contrast-enhanced computed tomography: correlation between radiographic and morphologic changes. J Am Coll Surg 180:673–682
126. Sankaran S, Lucas CE, Walt AJ (1974) Transient hypertension with acute pancreatitis. Surg Gynecol Obstet 138:235–238
127. Satiani B, Stone HH (1979) Predictability of present outcome and future recurrence in acute pancreatitis. Arch Surg 114:711–716
128. Scarpelli DG (1956) Fat necrosis of bone marrow in acute pancreatitis. Am J Pathol 32:1077–1087
129. Schein M, Saadia R, Decker G (1985) Colonic necrosis in acute pancreatitis. A complication of massive retroperitoneal suppuration. Dis Col Rect 28:948–950
130. Schmidt H, Lankisch PG (1978) Fat necrosis - a cause of pancreatic parenchymal necrosis? Digestion 17:84–91
131. Schmitz-Moormann P (1981) Comparative radiological and morphological study of the human pancreas. IV. Acute necrotizing pancreatitis in man. Pathol Res Pract 171:325–335
132. Schrier RW, Melmon KL, Fenster LF (1965) Subcutaneous nodular fat necrosis in pancreatitis. Arch Intern Med 116:832–836
133. Schuster MM, Iber FL (1965) Psychosis with pancreatitis. A frequent occurrence infrequently recognized. Arch Intern Med 116:228–233
134. Semlacher EA, Chan-Yan C (1993) Acute pancreatitis presenting with visual disturbance. Am J Gastroenterol 88:756–759
135. Simma W, Brücke P (1976) Zur Diagnostik und Therapie der oberen gastrointestinalen Blutung bei der akuten Pankreatitis und deren Folgezustände. Wien Klin Wochenschr 88:592–595
136. Slater G, Goldblum SE, Tzamaloukas AH, Jones WL, Goldhahn RT (1984) Renal cortical necrosis and Purtscher's retinopathy in hemorrhagic pancreatitis. Am J Med Sci 288:37–39
137. Slavin J, Smedley FH, Cahill CJ (1990) Closed loop large bowel obstruction secondary to pancreatitis. J R Soc Med 83:530–531
138. Snady-McCoy L, Morse PH (1985) Retinopathy associated with acute pancreatitis. Am J Ophthalmol 100:246–251
139. Soledad Donoso Flores M, Narváez Rodríguez I, López Bernal I, del Mar Alcalde Rubio M, Galván Ledesma A, Pascasio Acevedo JM, Soria Monge A (1995) Retinopathy as a systemic complication of acute pancreatitis. Am J Gastroenterol 90:321–324
140. Sonnenshein MA, Bruckner B, Pitchumoni CS (1979) Cecal perforation in alcoholic pancreatitis. Am J Gastroenterol 72:556–560

141. Sorgman JA, Langevin E, Banks PA (1992) Urinoma masquerading as pancreatic pseudocyst. Int J Pancreatol 11:195–198

142. Sperti C, Pasquali C, Costantino V, Perasole A, Liessi G, Pedrazzoli S (1995) Solitary true cyst of the pancreas in adults. Report of three cases and review of the literature. Int J Pancreatol 18: 161–167

143. Struckmann K, Assmus C, Lehnick D, Becher R, Lankisch PG (1996) Has contrast-enhanced computed tomography performed on admission any prospective value for the course of acute pancreatitis: results of a prospective study. Digestion 57:267 (abstr)

144. Talvik R, Liigant A, Sissak HM, O'Konnel-Bronina N (1977) Respiratory failure in acute pancreatitis. Intensive Care Med 3:97–98

145. Tenner S, Roston A, Lichtenstein D, Sica G, Carr-Locke D, Banks PA (1995) Von Hippel-Lindau disease complicated by acute pancreatitis and Evan's syndrome. Int J Pancreatol 18:271–275

146. Tenner S, Silverman ST, Brooks D, Banks PA (1995) Strangulation of the colon complicating acute pancreatitis. Am J Gastroenterol 90:1511–1513

147. Thomas CT, Hinton PJ, Thomas E (1986) Spontaneous pancreatic duct-colon fistula. J Clin Gastroenterol 8:69–73

148. Thompson WM, Kelvin FM, Rice RP (1977) Inflammation and necrosis of the transverse colon secondary to pancreatitis. Am J Roentgenol 128:943–948

149. Thompson WM, Pizzo SV, Kelvin FM, Rice RP (1978) Necrosis of the colon secondary to pancreatitis. Am J Dig Dis 23 (Suppl.):92s–96s

150. Toffler AH, Spiro HM (1962) Shock or coma as the predominant manifestation of painless acute pancreatitis. Ann Intern Med 57:655–659

151. Trapnell J (1972) The natural history and management of acute pancreatitis. Clin Gastroenterol 1:147–166

152. Variyam EP, Shah A (1987) Pericardial effusion and left ventricular function in patients with acute alcoholic pancreatitis. Arch Intern Med 147:923–925

153. Vaughan MM, Thomas WEG (1995) Thrombophlebitis migrans in association with acute relapsing pancreatitis. Br J Surg 82:674

154. Vesentini S, Bassi C, Talamini G, Cavallini G, Campedelli A, Pederzoli P (1993) Prospective comparison of C-reactive protein level, Ranson score and contrast-enhanced computed tomography in the prediction of septic complications of acute pancreatitis. Br J Surg 80:755–757

155. Warshaw AL, Compton CC, Lewandrowski K, Cardenosa G, Mueller PR (1990) Cystic tumors of the pancreas. New clinical, radiologic, and pathologic observations in 67 patients. Ann Surg 212:432–445

156. Warshaw AL, Lesser PB, Rie M, Cullen DJ (1975) The pathogenesis of pulmonary edema in acute pancreatitis. Ann Surg 182:505–510

157. Warshaw AL, McC.Chesney T, Evans GW, McCarthy HF (1972) Intrasplenic dissection by pancreatic pseudocysts. N Engl J Med 287:72–75

158. Warshaw AL, O'Hara PJ (1978) Susceptibility of the pancreas to ischemic injury in shock. Ann Surg 188:197–201

159. Warshaw AL, Rutledge PL (1987) Cystic tumors mistaken for pancreatic pseudocysts. Ann Surg 205:393–398

160. Weissmann D, Lewandrowski K, Godine J, Centeno B, Warshaw A (1994) Pancreatic cystic islet-cell tumors. Clinical and pathologic features in two cases with cyst fluid analysis. Int J Pancreatol 15:75–79

161. Wells AD, McDonnell PJ, Burnand KG (1990) Purtscher's retinopathy in acute pancreatitis. Br J Surg 77:820

162. Werner MH, Hayes DF, Lucas CE, Rosenberg IK (1974) Renal vasoconstriction in association with acute pancreatitis. Am J Surg 127:185–190

163. Wilson C (1988) Artefactual body wall ecchymosis in acute pancreatitis. Br J Surg 75:704

164. Wilson HA, Askari AD, Neiderhiser DH, Johnson AM, Andrews BS, Hoskins LC (1983) Pancreatitis with arthropathy and subcutaneous fat necrosis. Evidence for the pathogenicity of lipolytic enzymes. Arthritis Rheumatism 26:121–126

165. Withrington R, Collins P (1980) Cardiac tamponade in acute pancreatitis. Thorax 35:959–960

166. Zimmermann-Górska I, Urbaniak M, Karwowski A (1986) Coexistence of arthritis, subcutaneous fat necrosis, and pseudocyst of pancreas. Rheumatol Int 6:45–48

11 Acute Pancreatitis: Treatment

11.1
Basic Treatment

11.1.1
Goals

Thus far, medical strategy in acute pancreatitis has relied on supportive measures, with emphasis on vigorous fluid resuscitation, careful pulmonary care, and if required, close supervision in an intensive care unit. In the future, success in reducing morbidity and mortality will depend in large measure on innovative strategies to limit systemic complications, prevent pancreatic necrosis, and prevent pancreatic infection if necrosis has taken place.

11.1.1.1
Limitation of Systemic Complications

Systemic complications include respiratory failure, hypotension, and renal failure. For many years, efforts to eliminate systemic complications have been directed primarily to eliminating inflammatory mediators, such as activated pancreatic enzymes. Three methods to accomplish this goal have included the reduction of pancreatic secretion of enzymes, inhibition of circulating inflammatory mediators, and peritoneal lavage to rinse out inflammatory mediators (Table 11.1).

Reduction of pancreatic secretion of enzymes has been accomplished with the use of nasogastric suction, H_2-blocking agents, atropine, glucagon, calcitonin, 5-fluorouracil, somatostatin, or the long-acting somatostatin analogue, octreotide. In controlled clinical trials in man, none of these measures have been proven conclusively to be effective [7, 8, 52, 68, 74, 78, 88, 92]. There have been several deficiencies in these clinical trials. First, in some trials, patients with mild pancreatitis were included. A new agent would not be expected to improve morbidity or mortality in mild pancreatitis. Second, some of the trials have not been double-blinded. As a result, a conclusion that a medication was helpful might be flawed by the possibility of inadvertent observer bias [52, 68, 74, 78].

A second method of eliminating inflammatory mediators has been their inhibition in the circulation. There are two main types of inflammatory mediators. One type consists of activated pancreatic enzymes. Thus far, randomized prospective trials using

Table 11.1. Elimination of inflammatory mediators

- Reduction of pancreatic secretion
  Nasogastric suction
  H$_2$-blocking agents
  Atropine
  Glucagon
  Calcitonin
  5-fluorouracil
  Octreotide
- Inhibition of inflammatory mediators
  Aprotinin
  Gabexate mesilate
  Indomethacin
  CaNa$_2$ EDTA
  Acetylcysteine
  Fresh frozen plasma
- Removal of toxic factors
  Peritoneal lavage
- Endoscopic sphincterotomy

antiproteases including aprotinin (Trasylol) and gabexate mesilate have also been ineffective [7, 8, 26, 76, 92]. Further, the use of fresh frozen plasma to replenish levels of naturally occurring antiproteases such as α_2-macroglobulin (and also to improve pancreatic perfusion and thereby prevent pancreatic necrosis) has been ineffective [92]. The second type of inflammatory mediators is produced by white blood cells and platelets. These inflammatory mediators include cytokines, lysosomal hydrolases, reactive oxygen species, nitric oxide, elastase, phospholipase A$_2$, and others [85]. Preliminary results with the use of a platelet-activating factor receptor antagonist to overcome systemic complications have been encouraging, and additional studies are in progress [54].

The third method of eliminating inflammatory mediators is peritoneal lavage for the purpose of removing mediators that are present in ascitic fluid. Controlled clinical trials with peritoneal lavage carried out for a period of 2–4 days have thus far been ineffective in reducing morbidity and mortality [72, 92]. In one additional study, patients who received peritoneal lavage for 7 days as compared to 2 days experienced a reduction in pancreatic sepsis and death from sepsis but no reduction in overall mortality [81].

More recently, a fourth method of eliminating inflammatory mediators has been introduced in an effort to limit systemic complications and improve the morbidity and mortality of acute pancreatitis. This method involves endoscopic retrograde cholangiopancreatography (ERCP) for the purpose of removing gallstones in the common bile duct among patients with gallstone pancreatitis. In one study, endoscopic sphincterotomy (ES) within 72 h was shown to reduce morbidity (including systemic complications) but not mortality in severe gallstone pancreatitis among elderly patients [34]. Because computed tomography (CT) scan was not available, it is not known whether ES reduced morbidity by reducing the severity of pancreatitis or possibly by relieving biliary sepsis. In a second study from Hong Kong, ES performed within 24 h among patients with both mild and severe gallstone pancreatitis reduced morbidity by eliminating biliary sepsis but also did not reduce mortality [77].

On the basis of these reports, ERCP is recommended within the first 2–3 days of hospitalization among patients with gallstone pancreatitis who are exhibiting evidence of biliary sepsis and among patients with severe gallstone pancreatitis who are exhibiting evidence of organ failure. If stones are found in the common bile duct, they should be removed endoscopically. If the organ failure was caused specifically by biliary sepsis, one would expect improvement in the natural history of pancreatitis. However, if the organ failure was related to the pancreatitis itself rather than biliary sepsis, it remains unclear at present whether the removal of gallstones under these circumstances will improve the natural history of acute pancreatitis.

11.1.1.2
Prevention of Pancreatic Necrosis

Among the many factors that contribute to pancreatic necrosis, impairment of the microcirculation of the pancreas appears to be the most important [18]. There are many factors that contribute to impairment of the microcirculation. These include hypovolemia with decreased blood flow in the pancreas, the injurious effects of inflammatory mediators on capillaries and small arteries, and venous and capillary thrombi [18]. While aggressive fluid resuscitation may be helpful in counteracting shock and renal failure, it is not clear that fluid resuscitation alone can prevent pancreatic necrosis. Hemodilution with dextran-60 is an innovative technique that may prevent pancreatic necrosis. In the experimental animal, for example, hemodilution with dextran-60 has been shown to limit the progression of pancreatic necrosis by protecting the pancreatic microcirculation and improving oxygen delivery to the pancreas [50]. Dextran-60 may have achieved this benefit either by increasing intravascular volume thereby increasing capillary oncotic pressure or by improving the rheologic characteristics of blood. In one uncontrolled study utilizing isovolemic hemodilution in 13 patients, the hematocrit was reduced within hours to a level of approximately 30%, and results were considered encouraging [67]. A controlled study will be required to determine the benefit of isovolemic hemodilution in man.

Additional techniques to prevent pancreatic necrosis have been unsuccessful [92]. In one study, the use of fresh frozen plasma did not achieve significant benefit. In another study, the intravenous infusion of prostaglandin A_2 did not provide clinical benefit. In a further study, the use of indomethacin, a prostaglandin inhibitor, did not influence the outcome among patients with mild disease. Prostaglandins may be of help in improving the microcirculation of the pancreas but as mediators of inflammation, could potentially intensify the course of acute pancreatitis.

11.1.1.3
Prevention of Pancreatic Infection

There have been many randomized controlled studies that have failed to show a benefit of antibiotics in preventing pancreatic infection [7, 92]. However, the majority of patients in these studies did not have necrotizing pancreatitis, and furthermore, the antibiotics that were utilized may not have provided effective therapeutic levels within pancreatic tissue.

The mechanism of secondary bacterial infection in necrotizing pancreatitis appears to be translocation of bacteria from the colon and most particularly the transverse colon [14]. Potential methods to prevent pancreatic infection include sterilization of the colon, prevention of translocation of bacteria, or the use of an antibiotic that is effective against enteric organisms and achieves bacteriocidal levels in pancreatic tissue. In recent studies, approximately 75% of organisms that secondarily infect the pancreas include E. coli, klebsiella, and other Gram-negative rods; staphylococcus and streptococcus species compose approximately 20% [12, 43]. The antibiotics that have the highest bacteriocidal activity against the majority of bacteria in pancreatic infection and achieve the best levels in pancreatic tissue appear to be imipenem, ofloxacin, and ciprofloxacin [24].

There have been three recent studies that have attempted to show benefit of antibiotics in the prevention of pancreatic infection [69, 79, 87]. In one randomized prospective nonblinded study, the use of imipenem among patients with necrotizing pancreatitis was associated with a reduction of pancreatic infection (from 30% in the control group to 12% in the imipenem group) [79]. However, there was no improvement in mortality. Imipenem appeared to achieve the most striking benefit in preventing infection among patients with less than 33% pancreatic necrosis. In this group, survival was as favorable among patients who developed secondary infection and underwent surgical debridement as those who did not have secondary infection and did not require surgery. It would appear that these patients were not in general as ill as those with > 50% pancreatic necrosis. In the latter group, imipenem did not show benefit in preventing infection, and the mortality was equally high in both groups.

At the present time, imipenem should not be given to all patients with pancreatic necrosis. First, specialists in infectious disease have expressed concern that organisms resistant to imipenem will develop if imipenem is widely used, and have also expressed concern regarding the high cost of this antibiotic. Second, patients with pancreatic necrosis who are not experiencing organ failure have an excellent prognosis, whether or not the necrosis is secondarily infected [53, 79, 86].

In a second randomized prospective nonblinded study, patients with necrotizing pancreatitis received either cefuroxime intravenously or no antibiotic treatment within 24 h of admission [87]. There was no decrease in secondary pancreatic infections among patients who received cefuroxime, but there were fewer urinary tract infections experienced by this group. Despite the apparent lack of improvement in secondary pancreatic infection, there were statistically fewer deaths among patients who received the antibiotic. While this result would seem to favor the use of early antibiotic treatment in acute necrotizing pancreatitis, this result is confounded by the fact that 73% of patients randomized to the nonantibiotic group eventually received antibiotics for various reasons at a mean of 6 days after admission. Further, antibiotic treatment was changed in 67% of patients who originally received cefuroxime. In addition, more patients in the nonantibiotic group than in the antibiotic group received operative intervention on the pancreas for reasons that are not clear. (In all, 10 patients with infected necrosis and 11 with sterile necrosis received operative intervention. The reason for surgery among the 11 with sterile necrosis was not made clear.) Hence, because of these confounding variables, the results of the study are difficult to interpret.

In a third study, intestinal decontamination with oral norfloxacin, colistin, and amphotericin in a randomized prospective but nonblinded study among patients with necrotizing pancreatitis did not confer a statistically significant reduction in mortality [69]. Patients with severe pancreatitis by both CT scan (Balthazar-Ranson grades D or E [see Table 9.4]) and early prognostic signs (Imrie score ≥ 3 [see Table 9.6]) had a very high mortality whether they received antibiotics or not (31% vs. 55%). As in the previous study, patients who did not receive antibiotics underwent operative intervention on the pancreas more frequently than those who received antibiotics, but the reason for this difference is not clear.

In summary, additional studies will be required to determine the role of prophylactic antibiotics in prevention of pancreatic infection. Ideally, these studies should be double-blinded in order to prevent the possibility of bias. In addition, a decision should be made to standardize the treatment of sterile necrosis. While it remains controversial as to whether patients with severe sterile necrosis should undergo early surgical debridement or prolonged aggressive medical treatment with delayed surgical debridement if required after 4–6 weeks [49], a decision should be reached regarding these two options such that all patients with sterile necrosis receive identical treatment.

11.1.2
Medical Management of Mild Pancreatitis

11.1.2.1
Supportive Care

According to the conclusions reached at the Atlanta symposium, pancreatitis is considered mild when predictors of severity such as Ranson's signs and APACHE-II scores are low and there are no systemic complications [9, 19]. Under these circumstances, if clinical improvement is sustained, CT scan in general is not required. Even if CT scan is obtained and reveals the presence of necrotizing pancreatitis, the absence of organ dysfunction would substantiate the fact that the episode of pancreatitis is indeed mild as long as clinical improvement was sustained.

In mild pancreatitis, the main goal of treatment is supportive care [7, 92]. It is particularly important to ensure adequate fluid replacement. Even in mild pancreatitis, the combination of vomiting, diaphoresis and third-space losses may result in significant loss of intravascular volume. If hypovolemia occurs, there may eventually be compromise of the microcirculation of the pancreas that could result in necrotizing pancreatitis. The clinician is well advised to utilize a metabolic flow sheet to assess fluid status and provide appropriate fluid replacement. Fluid balance with careful intake and output measurement should be reassessed at least every 8 h during the first few days of illness in order to ensure adequate fluid replacement.

11.1.2.2
Other Measures

In general, abdominal pain can be relieved by parenteral meperidine in doses of 50–100 mg intramuscularly every 3–4 h as needed. If pain is severe, a narcotic agent can be given parenterally with the use of patient-controlled anesthesia (PCA pump). By this method, adequate dosages of narcotics are administered as needed by an infusion pump with availability of *breakthrough* doses. The amount of narcotic agent and frequency of administration can be preset to avoid indiscriminate usage. The dosage should be adjusted on a daily basis based on the needs of the patient. While morphine may increase the tone of the sphincter of Oddi, there is no evidence that the use of this narcotic agent for relief of pain intensifies the disease process.

A nasogastric tube was once thought to be helpful for the purposes of *resting the pancreas*. The theory was that even the basal secretion of gastric acid would stimulate some pancreatic secretion and by doing so might intensify the inflammatory reaction. More recently, there have been several studies that have concluded that a nasogastric tube is not beneficial in mild pancreatitis [88, 92]. In similar fashion, the use of an H_2-receptor blocking agent or a protein pump inhibitor is not beneficial. Accordingly, unless there is gastric or intestinal ileus or intractable nausea and vomiting, nasogastric tube should not be employed [92].

Antibiotic therapy does not play a useful role to mild pancreatitis. The use of antibiotics should be utilized to treat infections such as pulmonary, biliary, or urinary, but not as a prophylactic agent in mild pancreatitis.

11.1.2.3
Refeeding

The timing of refeeding is a source of concern to clinicians. As yet, there have been no randomized prospective trials which have documented the optimal time to offer oral intake. In general, refeeding can be cautiously begun when abdominal tenderness has subsided and there has been marked subsidence of abdominal pain such that a narcotic agent is no longer needed. Additional helpful signs prior to refeeding are the presence of bowel sounds and expression of hunger on the part of the patient. It is probably not necessary to wait for return of serum amylase to normal. Indeed, in many patients, serum amylase or lipase are abnormal even at the time of discharge [58].

In mild pancreatitis, oral refeeding usually commences by the 3rd–7th day of hospitalization. While an H_2-receptor blocking agent or proton pump inhibitor may reduce the secretion of gastric acid in response to food and by doing may reduce the stimulation of pancreatic fluid, there is no evidence that these agents are beneficial in preventing an exacerbation of symptoms. There is also no evidence that pharmacologic strategy to reduce secretion of pancreatic enzymes is beneficial. In general, small feedings are suggested. Since foods that consist mostly of carbohydrate seem to stimulate the pancreas less than foods containing fat and protein [91], it is generally suggested that diet consist mostly of carbohydrates. However, there are no data in man to support the benefit of a particular diet during refeeding.

11.1.3
Medical Management of Severe Pancreatitis

As outlined by the conclusions of the Atlanta symposium, severe pancreatitis is characterized by unfavorable predictors of severity (including high APACHE-II scores and high Ranson's signs) and by the development of systemic complications [19, 92]. Systemic complications include shock with a systolic blood pressure <90 mm Hg, pulmonary insufficiency with an arterial pO_2 of ≤ 60 mm Hg, renal failure with creatinine >2 mg/dl and gastrointestinal bleeding with >500 ml/24 h [8, 9, 19]. Among patients with unfavorable predictors of severity and/or evidence of systemic complications, the likelihood is that the patient has necrotizing pancreatitis. Dynamic contrast-enhanced CT scan has proven to be accurate in distinguishing interstitial pancreatitis from necrotizing pancreatitis [4, 5, 17, 22, 38, 63]. Local complications such as necrotizing pancreatitis, pancreatic pseudocyst, and pancreatic abscess will be covered in Sect. 11.2.

Additional early signs that are helpful in recognizing that the pancreatitis is severe include:

- Hemoconcentration with a hematocrit $>50\%$. This abnormality signifies that there has been massive third-space losses with profound hypovolemia requiring urgent fluid resuscitation
- Oliguria with urine output <50 ml/h. This finding reinforces the need for vigorous fluid resuscitation
- Tachycardia with pulse >120 beats/min. Tachycardia may be caused by hypovolemia, catabolic effects of tissue injury in the retroperitoneum, or systemic effects including pulmonary complications
- Encephalopathy and coma, which may be caused by general systemic toxicity of circulating enzymes and toxins, injurious effects of pancreatic enzymes on tissue in the central nervous system, or metabolic abnormalities such as systemic acidosis. Patients with encephalopathy at admission have a high mortality [23]

In the presence of unfavorable early signs, specific evidence of organ dysfunction, or danger signals such as those listed above, the patient should be transferred to a specialized unit such as an intensive care unit for coordinated care under the direction of a multidisciplinary team with representatives from the departments of medicine (including gastroenterology and pulmonology), surgery, and radiology (Table 11.2).

Table 11.2. Medical management of severe pancreatitis

- Fluid resuscitation
- Respiratory care
- Cardiovascular care
- Relief of pain
- Limitation of systemic complications
- Treatment of infection
- Treatment of metabolic complications
- Nutritional support

11.1.3.1
Fluid Resuscitation

It is essential to provide adequate replacement of intravascular volume. Fluid resuscitation counteracts hypotension and renal insufficiency, and helps protect the microcirculation of the pancreas. Altogether too frequently, the quantity of intravenous replacement that is required for these purposes is underestimated. During the first several days, fluid resuscitation may require in excess of 5–6 l each day and at times in excess of 10 l to maintain an adequate intravascular volume. A careful flow sheet that includes intake and output and vital signs provides some guidance as to the adequacy of fluid resuscitation. However, when fluid needs are considerable and the patient is seriously ill, there is a requirement for measurements provided by a central venous pressure catheter or Swan-Ganz catheter in order to gauge the adequacy of fluid resuscitation and to ensure that large volumes of intravenous fluid do not result in congestive heart failure. The use of a Swan-Ganz catheter is particularly advised when fluid requirements are substantial, when cardiovascular status is unstable, or when respiratory function is deteriorating. Because the retroperitoneal inflammatory process leads not only to a loss of large quantities of fluid but also seepage of albumin from the circulation, it is advisable to include colloid as part of the fluid resuscitation especially if serum albumin falls to less than 2 g/l.

It appears that a hematocrit of approximately 30% provides optimal viscosity of red blood cells that enhances the flow of blood in the microcirculation of the pancreas [50, 55]. If the hematocrit decreases to levels below 25%–30%, packed red blood cells should be infused to maintain a hematocrit of approximately 30%.

11.1.3.2
Respiratory Care

Hypoxemia in severe pancreatitis may be caused by atelectasis, pneumonia, congestive heart failure, pleural effusions, progressive fatigue, and after the first several days, the development of adult respiratory distress syndrome (ARDS). Respiratory injury in acute pancreatitis may result from the damaging effects of phospholipase A_2 from the pancreas as well as from enzymes which are secreted by activated white blood cells that damage pulmonary capillaries and membranes of alveolar cells [85]. Measurement of blood gases should be obtained at frequent intervals in severe pancreatitis in order to detect the presence of hypoxemia and acidosis. Measurements of oxygen saturation with a pulse oximeter should be obtained continuously to alert the clinician to the possibility of hypoxemia. When hypoxemia is documented, oxygen can be provided by nasal prongs or by mask. If hypoxemia cannot be corrected by these methods, endotracheal intubation and assisted ventilation should be provided. The physician should be alert to the development of fatigue and provide assisted ventilation at an early stage in order to prevent pancreatic tissue hypoxia.

It is important to distinguish hypoxemia caused by congestive heart failure (which is manifested by an increasing pulmonary artery wedge pressure) from a pulmonary event such as ARDS (which is manifested by a normal pulmonary artery wedge pressure). ARDS requires assisted ventilation with positive end-expiratory pressure. While this is a serious complication and occasionally leads to refractory pulmonary failure and death, this condition usually improves after several days and is potentially totally reversible.

11.1.3.3
Cardiovascular Care

Cardiac complications include congestive heart failure, cardiac arrhythmia, myocardial infarction, and cardiogenic shock and are treated by appropriate pharmacologic strategy in an intensive care unit. Deterioration of renal function attributed to hypovolemia requires treatment with vigorous fluid resuscitation. Acute tubular necrosis requires either peritoneal dialysis or hemodialysis.

11.1.3.4
Relief of Pain

Pain may be excruciating in acute pancreatitis. If meperidine in a dosage of 75–100 mg administered intramuscularly or intravenously every 3–4 h is not effective, the patient should be allowed the use of a narcotic agent administered by the technique of patient-controlled anesthesia (PCA) in order to ensure adequate pain relief. It is essential that the physician review the need for narcotic medications daily and, if necessary, several times each day to provide adequate analgesia and to prevent excessive use of narcotic agents.

11.1.3.5
Limitation of Systemic Complications

As indicated earlier in this chapter, reduction of pancreatic secretion and inhibition of inflammatory mediators in circulation have not been effective in limiting systemic complications. A nasogastric tube is helpful when there is intestinal or gastric ileus or when there is a threat of aspiration. Thus far, the use of peritoneal lavage to remove activated pancreatic enzymes and toxins within ascitic fluid before these substances can be reabsorbed into the circulation and produce toxicity has also been ineffective [92].

In one multicenter, randomized clinical trial, the use of peritoneal lavage for 3 days showed no benefit when compared to a control group that did not receive lavage [72]. However, this result may have been influenced by some methodologic considerations. First, peritoneal lavage was delayed for 36 h from the onset of symptoms. Second, a diagnostic lavage was required for the purposes of assessing prognosis before patients entered the study. This diagnostic lavage may have actually provided treatment to the control group. Third, since not all patients underwent a diagnostic lavage, it is possible that some patients did not have ascites. If the value of lavage is to flush ascitic fluid that contains enzymes from the peritoneal cavity, it is important in analyzing results to have known whether ascites was present.

While the role of peritoneal lavage at this time remains unproven, it would be of interest to initiate a new study utilizing patients who are seriously ill (on the basis of unfavorable early prognostic signs and/or organ dysfunction), are shown to have a significant amount of ascites (by abdominal ultrasound), and are proven to have a considerable amount of enzymes within the ascites (by percutaneous aspiration).

Another potential method of removing activated pancreatic enzymes is by irrigation of the lesser sac or anterior pararenal space if CT scan reveals a large fluid collection in either area. Potentially, the percutaneous insertion of one or more catheters in these areas with lavage technique might be beneficial for patients with refractory shock and/or progressive respiratory insufficiency. Thus far, there have been no formal studies that have evaluated the safety and benefit of this technique. Because there is a potential for introducing infection, percutaneous drainage, if utilized at all, should be restricted to patients who are experiencing profound organ dysfunction despite maximal therapy.

As indicated earlier in this chapter, ERCP is recommended within the first 2–3 days among patients with gallstone pancreatitis who are exhibiting evidence of biliary sepsis and among patients with severe gallstone pancreatitis who are experiencing severe organ dysfunction. If stones are visualized in the common bile duct, they should be removed.

11.1.3.6
Treatment of Infection

Pancreatic infection rarely occurs in interstitial pancreatitis unless the patient is seriously ill [49] but may occur in 20%–50% of patients with necrotizing pancreatitis [12, 14, 79, 86]. Infection in necrotizing pancreatitis is either a spreading infection of devitalized tissue in the retroperitoneum (termed *infected necrosis*) or a localized abscess [16, 35]. Among patients with infected necrosis, approximately 50% develop infection within the first 2 weeks of illness [12, 43]. A pancreatic abscess may not occur until after the first month of illness [16, 35]. In 3 studies thus far [69, 79, 87], the use of prophylactic antibiotics helped in decreasing the incidence of pancreatic infection in only one [79]. Pancreatic infection can be documented by guided percutaneous aspiration with bacteriologic sampling for Gram stain and culture [12, 43] and occasionally by the presence of retroperitoneal air visualized on CT scan. When infection is documented, antibiotics should be prescribed. Infected necrosis should be treated by prompt surgical debridement [8, 73]. An abscess can usually be treated successfully by pigtail catheter drainage or by surgical drainage [8, 16, 35].

11.1.3.7
Metabolic Complications

During the first several days of severe pancreatitis, there may be transient hyperglycemia that normalizes as the inflammatory process subsides. For this reason, insulin should be administered with great caution and at widely spaced intervals of at least 6 h.

Hypocalcemia may occur on the basis of a reduction in nonionized or ionized calcium [1,6]. A reduction of nonionized calcium is usually associated with loss of serum albumin from the circulation as a result of tissue inflammation and third-space losses. Since a reduction of nonionized calcium from the circulation is not associated with symptoms, it requires no specific therapy. As serum albumin increases, either as a result of infusion of albumin or clinical improvement, serum nonionized calcium is restored to normal.

Reduction in serum ionized calcium may lead to neuromuscular irritability. Theories to explain a decrease in ionized calcium include: deposition of nonionized calcium within areas of fat necrosis; associated hypomagnesemia; or metabolic abnormalities involving the inhibition of parathormone secretion, refractoriness of bone to stimulation by parathormone, or complexing of ionized calcium with fatty acids in serum [1,6].

In the absence of hypomagnesemia, a reduction in ionized calcium should be treated with intravenous calcium gluconate if there are signs or symptoms of neuromuscular irritability. Before initiating treatment with intravenous calcium, it should be ascertained that the patient is not hypokalemic and is not receiving treatment with digitalis. Under these circumstances, a rapid infusion of intravenous calcium could result in a serious cardiac arrhythmia because calcium that is infused binds to myocardial receptors thereby displacing potassium and intensifying the harmful effects of hypokalemia on the heart [6].

When coexisting hypomagnesemia causes a reduction of ionized calcium, the replacement of magnesium intravenously should restore serum calcium to normal. Magnesium depletion may be caused by vomiting, loss of magnesium in urine, or deposition of magnesium in areas of fat necrosis [6].

11.1.3.8
Nutritional Support

In mild pancreatitis, oral intake can usually be restored within 3–7 days of hospitalization, and total parenteral nutrition is not required. In severe pancreatitis, patients may be without oral nourishment for 3–6 weeks and should receive nutritional support in the form of total parenteral nutrition (TPN) that is initiated within the first few days of hospitalization. TPN can reverse the catabolic features in severe pancreatitis and may also help in improving mortality [80, 90]. It would appear that lipids can be administered safely in TPN solutions if serum triglycerides do not increase significantly. Serum triglyceride should be measured daily while using a source of lipids in TPN. If serum triglycerides are increased to ≥ 500 mg%, lipids should be eliminated from the solution.

In severe pancreatitis, there are no uniform guidelines as to when to initiate oral feeding. In general, once TPN has been initiated, it is usually maintained for 2–3 weeks. Hence, under ordinary circumstances, the clinician should strongly consider oral alimentation after approximately 21 days of hospitalization. If at that time abdominal pain and tenderness have subsided, organ dysfunction has improved, and the patient is experiencing bowel function and is hungry, it is reasonable to initiate oral intake in small feedings. There may be a theoretical advantage in initiating oral intakes with carbohydrates rather than fat or protein, which appear to stimulate pancreatic secretion to a greater extent.

The clinician may be reluctant to initiate oral intake if the CT scan still shows considerable inflammation. An abnormal CT scan should not by itself preclude the initiation of oral intake. Available evidence thus far indicates that resolution of inflammatory changes on CT scan may take several months [58]. Indeed, following severe acute pancreatitis, the majority of patients at discharge continue to show convincing abnormalities on CT scan [58]. Abnormalities on CT scan [58] and ERCP [89] and abnormalities of pancreatic function [89] may persist indefinitely following an episode of acute pancreatitis. Hence, the decision to refeed is primarily based on clinical judgment.

11.2
Treatment of Local Complications

The 3 most serious local complications of acute pancreatitis are pancreatic necrosis, pancreatic pseudocyst, and pancreatic abscess. A fourth is smoldering unresolved acute pancreatitis.

11.2.1
Necrotizing Pancreatitis

Necrotizing pancreatitis takes place in approximately 20% of cases of acute pancreatitis [86]. Pancreatic necrosis should be suspected when early predictors of severity such as Ranson's scores are ≥ 6, APACHE-II scores are ≥ 14, or when specific laboratory tests such as C-reactive protein are elevated [8, 25, 30, 46, 65, 94, 97, 100], and/or when there is evidence of severe systemic complications such as shock, renal failure, or respiratory failure [8, 19, 79, 86]. As indicated in the previous chapters, the best way to confirm a diagnosis of pancreatic necrosis is with dynamic contrast-enhanced CT scan [4, 5, 17, 22, 38, 63] (see Figs. 9.4, 9.5, 9.7, 9.8).

The intensity of treatment of necrotizing pancreatitis depends on the clinical course of the patient. In the absence of organ failure and other manifestations of systemic toxicity, patients should be maintained on intravenous fluid replacement until such time as clinical judgment indicates that it is reasonable to offer oral nourishment (see Sects. 11.1.2.3, 11.1.3.9). In general, guidelines for medical management in acute pancreatitis should not be influenced by the unexpected finding of necrosis on CT scan in a patient who is essentially asymptomatic. If refeeding should lead to an exacerbation of abdominal pain, intravenous fluid should be continued for an arbitrary 5–7 additional days (see Sect. 11.2.2.7).

Patients with pancreatic necrosis who have evidence of organ failure and persisting systemic toxicity usually require total parenteral nutrition for at least 2 weeks. Systemic toxicity includes unresolved pain, persistent fever and leukocytosis or persistent tachycardia (pulse > 100 beats/min). Usually after 14–21 days, evidence of organ failure and systemic toxicity subside. At this time, even if CT scan continues to show impressive inflammatory changes, it is reasonable to commence oral feeding if the patient no longer requires narcotic agents for pain, bowel sounds have returned, and the patient is hungry (see Sect. 11.1.2.3).

However, if organ dysfunction and systemic toxicity persist during the initial 7–14 days of illness, the patient either has secondary infection of the pancreas (i.e., infected necrosis) or severe sterile necrosis.

11.2.1.1
Infected Necrosis of the Pancreas

Secondary infection of the pancreas has for many years been a dreaded complication of acute pancreatitis [43]. Before CT scanning became available, it was not uncommon to treat patients with severe pancreatitis medically for at least 4–6 weeks before resorting to surgery as a last effort to save the life of a seriously ill and possibly moribund patient. In most instances, the necrotic tissue that was debrided was infected, the patient invariably required multiple reexplorations for debridement of residual infected tissue. Mortality was generally > 50%. The delay in surgical intervention was thought to be an important factor in the high mortality.

Now that pancreatic necrosis can be readily visualized by dynamic contrast-enhanced CT scan, surgeons are better prepared to perform pancreatic debridement in two situations. The first is if there is documentation of secondary infection of the pancreas. This information can be provided by CT-guided percutaneous aspiration with bacteriological sampling for Gram stain and culture [12, 43]. The documentation of pancreatic infection usually leads to surgical debridement within 24 h. The second is persistence of systemic toxicity among patients with severe sterile necrosis [8, 49, 73]. (That is, patients who have undergone CT-guided percutaneous aspiration, and Gram stain and culture have been found to be negative for microorganisms.) The rationale of surgery in severe sterile necrosis will be covered in Sect. 11.2.1.2.

The majority of patients with infected necrosis have unresolved systemic complications including respiratory failure (Table 11.3) [86]. Usually, white blood count is $\geq 20\,000/mm^3$, with temperature 101–103 °F (38.3–39.4 °C) [43]. In the absence of air bubbles, there is no particular feature on dynamic contrast-enhanced CT scan that permits the distinction between infected necrosis and severe sterile necrosis (see Fig. 9.8).

When pancreatic infection is suspected on the basis of unresolved organ failure and/or persisting systemic toxicity, guided percutaneous aspiration with bacteriological sampling should be performed by a radiologist trained in interventional technique. Needle aspirates should be obtained from areas of necrosis using a 20–22 gauge

Table 11.3. When to suspect pancreatic infection

- Necrotizing pancreatitis
- Persistence of systemic complications
  Organ failure
  Increased white blood cell count and/or temperature
- Air in the anterior pararenal space

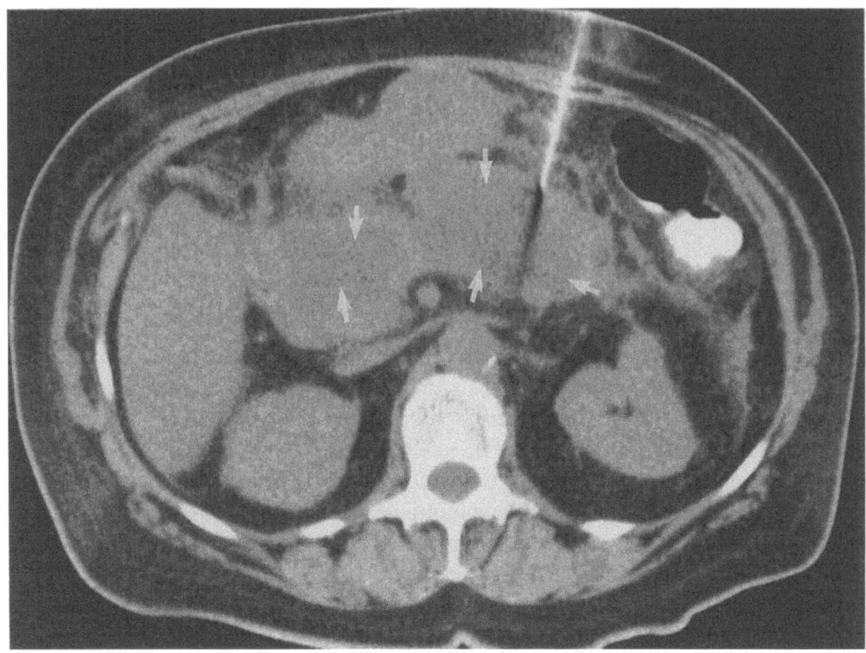

Fig. 11.1 a. Infected necrosis. Unenhanced CT scan in this 65-year-old woman who 2 months earlier had undergone an uneventful laparoscopic cholecystectomy following an episode of gallstone pancreatitis. Because of the sudden onset of chills, fever, and abdominal pain, she was admitted on the prior day to another hospital where dynamic contrast-enhanced CT scan revealed considerable pancreatic necrosis. Large areas of low-attenuation material can be appreciated even on this unenhanced CT scan (*arrows*). The needle is seen to advance into one of the areas

needle via a route designated by CT scan that avoids colon (see Figs. 9.5, 9.7). Because of the importance of not transgressing the colon and thereby risking the inoculation of colonic flora into the retroperitoneum, all patients should receive oral contrast routinely to opacify the colon. Fluid obtained by guided percutaneous aspiration should be hand-carried immediately to the bacteriology laboratory for Gram stain and culture (for aerobic and anaerobic bacteria and fungi) (Fig. 11.1 a, b).

In our experience during the past 15 years with guided percutaneous aspiration among 104 patients strongly suspected of harboring pancreatic infection, 51 (49%) have been documented to have pancreatic infection on the basis of a positive culture [12]. In all but 4 instances, Gram stain also revealed organisms. Hence, Gram stain has proven to be very reliable as an early indicator of the presence of pancreatic infection. There was no instance of a positive Gram stain followed by a negative culture.

On the basis of this experience, we have learned that pancreatic infection occurred in approximately 50% within the first 14 days and 71% within the first 21 days [12, 43]. Hence, pancreatic infection takes place relatively early in severe acute pancreatitis. The majority of infections were caused by *Klebsiella*, *E. coli*, or *Staphylococcus aureus*. There were only 2 infections caused by a candida species. In 86% of infections, only

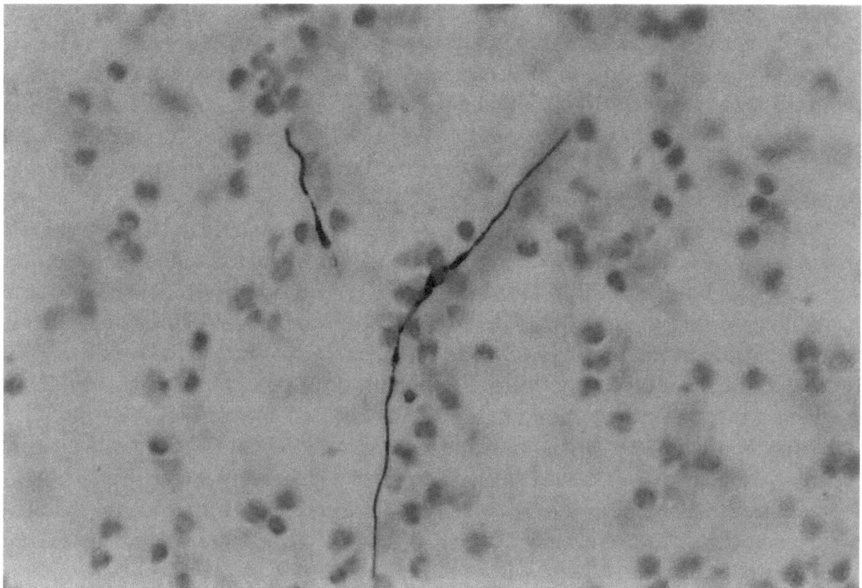

Fig. 11.1 b. Infected necrosis. Gram stain of pancreatic exudate shows pseudohyphae of candidal organisms with characteristic beading morphology in an aspirate containing abundant inflammatory cells. Culture revealed the presence of candida albicans. The patient underwent pancreatic debridement. The debrided tissue revealed the presence of the same candida species. She made an uneventful recovery

1 organism was recovered. The reason may be the fact that aspirations were done relatively early in the course of the illness before the appearance of opportunistic organisms. Finally, while the overall rate of infection during the past 15 years was 49%, it appears that the rate of infection has decreased from 60% in the first seven years to 34% in the past eight years. The explanation may be the use of potent antibiotics that may prevent the development of secondary pancreatic infection (Table 11.4).

In our experience, there have been no complications [12, 43]. Thus, CT-guided percutaneous aspiration is a safe, accurate method of diagnosing pancreatic infection. The accuracy of this technique probably relates to the fact that necrotic tissue in the retroperitoneum is diffusely infected such that it is unlikely that an aspiration from

Table 11.4. Pancreatic infection: major features

- *Klebsiella*, *E. coli*, and *Staphylococcus aureus* are the most common pathogens
- Pancreatic infection is usually unimicrobial
- Pancreatic infection usually occurs early in acute pancreatitis
- Prevalence appears to be decreasing
- Can be diagnosed safely and accurately by guided percutaneous aspiration (GPA)
- Gram stain of GPA is invariably positive

one area would be sterile whereas that from another would be infected. Indeed, when retroperitoneal fluid and necrotic pancreatic tissue have been subjected to bacteriological analysis at the time of debridement, both the fluid component and the necrotic tissue have been shown to contain bacteria. In comparison, in situations in which the preoperative percutaneous aspiration was sterile (thereby identifying the process as sterile rather than infected necrosis), neither the fluid nor the necrotic material obtained at surgery have contained bacteria [11].

Without the use of guided percutaneous aspiration, there is no reliable preoperative technique of distinguishing severe sterile pancreatitis from infected necrosis. First, patients with both sterile and infected necrosis may exhibit identical hemodynamic instability. Second, there are no individual blood tests or battery of blood tests that accurately distinguish infected from sterile necrosis. Third, white blood count and temperatures are identical among patients with both conditions [43]. Fourth, while many patients with ≥ 6 positive Ranson's signs have infected necrosis, some do not [5]. In addition, approximately 10% of patients with necrotizing pancreatitis who have only 0–2 positive Ranson's signs have been documented to harbor pancreatic infection [5].

Once percutaneous aspiration has identified the presence of organisms, surgical debridement should be performed (Fig. 11.2 a–f) [14, 20, 40, 71]. In many instances, more than one surgical debridement will be required to eliminate the major portion of infected pancreatic and peripancreatic tissue. The surgeon exercises great care in gentle finger dissection of necrotic tissue in order to avoid bleeding. As part of the surgical exploration, the surgeon inspects the areas in the right and left gutters lateral to the colon in order to eliminate pockets of infection that may be sequestered in these areas. There are three main surgical approaches that can be utilized:

- Aggressive debridement with external drainage in the form of Jackson Pratt drains and stuffed Penrose drains. In this technique, the abdomen is closed completely
- Aggressive debridement with placement of several soft drains into the retroperitoneum for the purposes of continuous lavage with physiologic fluid in order to continue to rinse out infected debris. With this technique, the abdomen is also closed
- Aggressive debridement with the abdomen left open with suitable packing. The presumed advantage of this technique is the ability to perform a reexploration with greater ease, even in the intensive care unit without need for transfer to an operating room

Experienced surgeons have achieved good results with all three techniques. It is difficult to compare the results of these three techniques because published surgical series include patients with different indications for surgery and severity of illness. Furthermore, these three techniques have not been subjected to a randomized prospective trial in a multihospital collaborative protocol. Overall mortality is 10%–48% [8, 12, 14, 15, 35, 79, 84, 86].

The availability of percutaneous techniques of therapy has raised the question as to whether radiologic techniques should be utilized in the treatment of infected necrosis. In general, even large catheters cannot remove infected necrotic tissue, which may be distributed widely throughout the retroperitoneum and has a solid or semisolid consistency that cannot generally pass through the indwelling catheters [8]. On rare

Fig. 11.2a–c. Pancreatic ductal disruption; infected necrosis. a Dynamic contrast-enhanced CT scan performed on a 62-year-old woman with smoldering pancreatitis reveals an area of nonenhancement in the body of the pancreas consistent with necrosis and/or loculated fluid (*horizontal black arrow*) and loculated fluid collections in the lesser sac and in the anterior pararenal space (*vertical arrows*). Because of persistent pain preventing oral alimentation, a ductal disruption was suspected. b ERCP reveals two areas of extravasation of contrast in the body of the pancreas (*arrows*). There is slight narrowing of the main pancreatic duct in the area of the extravasations. Other than this, the main pancreatic duct and side branches appear normal. A stent was placed through the ampulla of Vater into the main pancreatic duct and positioned beyond the area of disruptions, thereby preventing further extravasation of pancreatic fluid. c Dynamic contrast-enhanced CT scan performed after the insertion of the stent reveals extensive fluid in the lesser sac and anterior pararenal space (*vertical arrows*). The stent is visible within the pancreatic duct (*horizontal arrow*). The stent was removed 2 weeks later

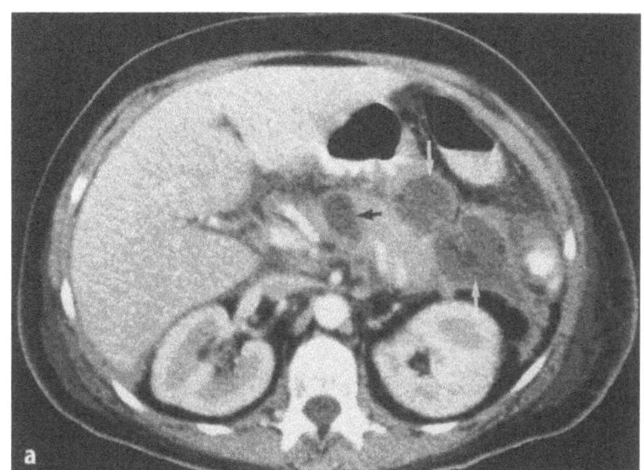

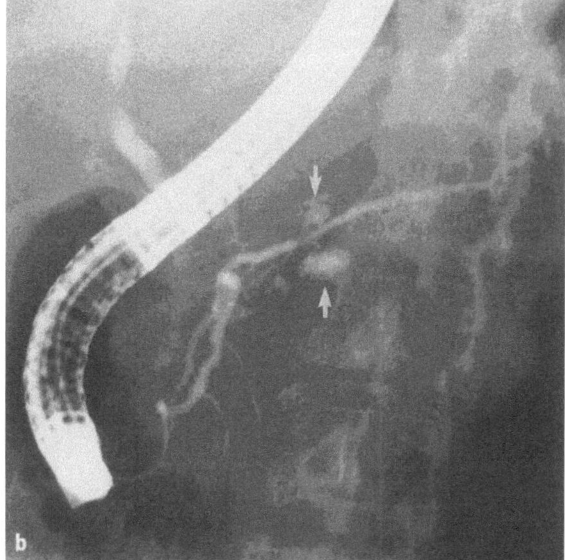

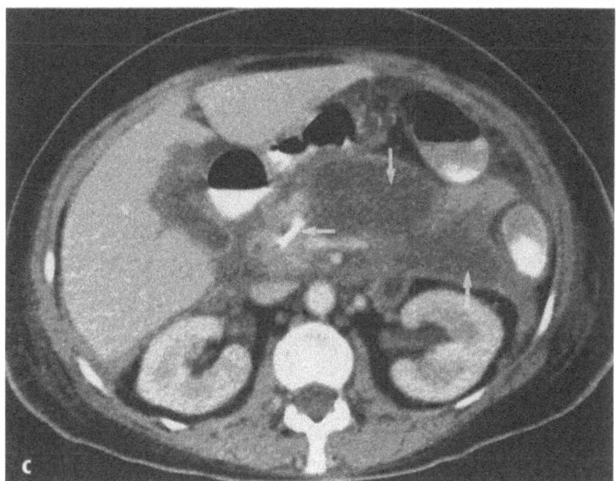

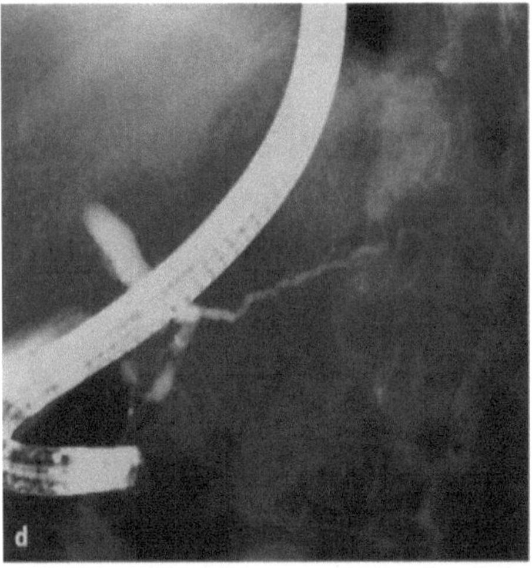

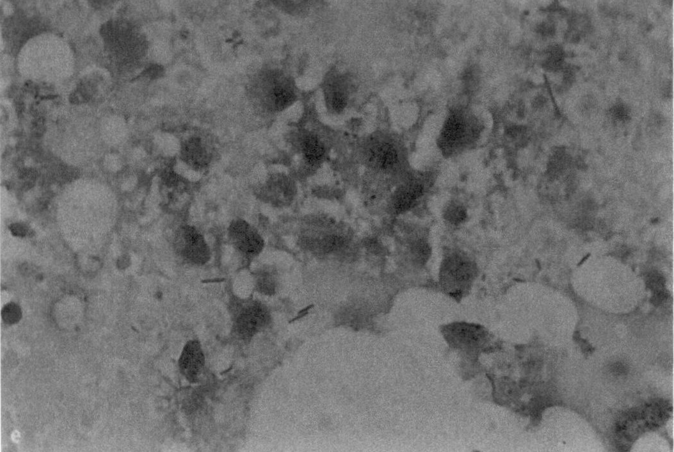

Fig. 11.2 d, e. Pancreatic ductal disruption; infected necrosis. **d** Follow-up ERCP reveals no further extravasation of fluid. However, fever, leukocytosis, and abdominal pain persisted. Guided percutaneous aspiration revealed the presence of Gram-negative bacilli. **e** Gram stain of guided percutaneous aspirate. There are abundant Gram-negative bacilli which on culture proved to be E. coli. The patient underwent surgical debridement of peripancreatic and pancreatic infected necrosis. Gram stain and culture of fluid and necrotic debris in the operating room revealed the same organism

occasion, it may be advisable to utilize catheter drainage for 12–36 h in a patient who is critically ill and in shock. Under these circumstances, the catheters may eliminate a sufficient amount of infected fluid such that debridement can then be carried out more safely. However, in one series, the use of percutaneous technique was shown to delay surgical intervention without achieving noticeable benefit and was therefore deemed in general to be unhelpful [84].

A final problem after successful debridement of infected necrosis is the development of a pancreatic fistula to the gastrointestinal tract or to skin [49]. A fistula involv-

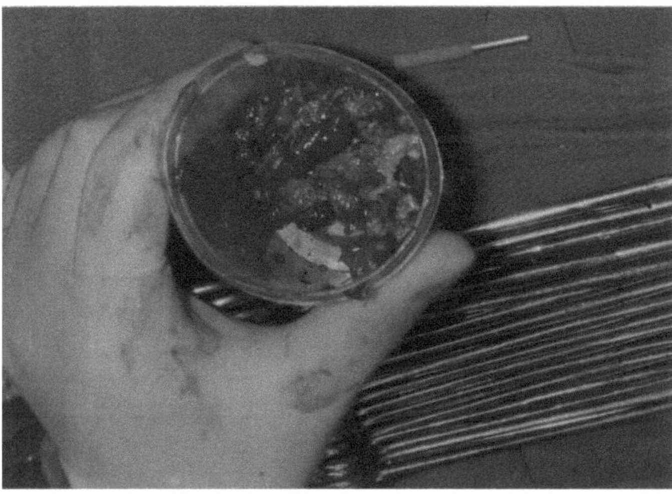

Fig. 11.2f. Pancreatic ductal disruption; infected necrosis. Infected necrosis debrided at surgery. The patient made an uneventful recovery. The placement of a stent across a ductal disruption has proven to be an effective way of healing a ductal disruption. In most instances, this treatment leads to clinical improvement of unresolved pancreatitis. However, in the presence of pancreatic or peripancreatic necrosis, insertion of a stent into the pancreatic duct may lead to infection

ing the colon requires proximal decompression in the form of a colostomy; one involving the duodenum or stomach may require prolonged total parenteral nutrition. A pancreatic fistula to the skin usually becomes clinically apparent when amylase-rich fluid is seen to exit via indwelling drainage catheters placed near the pancreatic area. The basis of this type of fistula is presumably disruption of pancreatic ducts, either as part of the necrotizing process or possibly as a complication of the debridement itself. The volume of pancreatic juice is usually small, and within several weeks a pancreatic fistula to the skin usually closes spontaneously. Sandostatin administered subcutaneously in a dosage of 50–200 µg every 8 h may be helpful in closing a pancreatic fistula.

Patients with infected necrosis of the pancreas usually require a prolonged expensive hospitalization. Patients are frequently demoralized and debilitated by this lengthy illness. However, there is information that the quality of life following recovery from this devastating illness can be excellent [36].

11.2.1.2
Sterile Necrosis of the Pancreas

In the absence of systemic complications, sterile necrosis of the pancreas is clinically mild, and the mortality should be close to zero [53, 86]. In the presence of systemic complications, mortality is high [53, 86]. In one series characterized by high Ranson's and APACHE-II scores in the first 48 h, mortality was 38% [53]. Options for medical treatment depend on clinical status (Fig. 11.3).

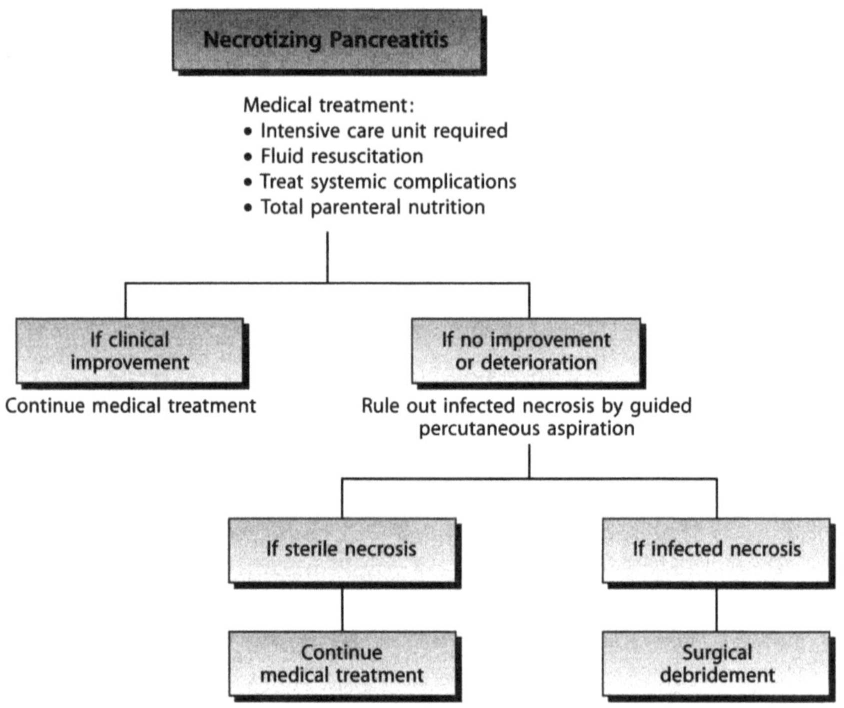

Fig. 11.3. Management of severe necrotizing pancreatitis

11.2.1.2.1
Necrotizing Pancreatitis With Clinical Improvement

If there is improvement in organ failure and systemic toxicity, medical treatment should be continued. Total parenteral nutrition may be required. When organ failure subsides, oral alimentation can be initiated (see Sect. 11.1.2.3).

11.2.1.2.2
Necrotizing Pancreatitis Without Clinical Improvement

If there is no clinical improvement during the first 7–10 days, and if organ failure persists or intensifies, the patient has either severe sterile necrosis or infected necrosis. At some point during the first 7–10 days, CT-guided percutaneous aspiration for Gram stain and culture should be obtained to exclude the presence of infected necrosis (see Figs. 9.5, 9.7). In most instances, unless there is precipitous deterioration of the patient, aspiration need not be performed during the initial 5–7 days. An important reason is that even if pancreatic tissue is infected, it usually has not demarcated sufficiently from viable tissue in the form of a necrotic coagulum that can be debrided adequately early in the course of infected necrosis. During the few days that may be

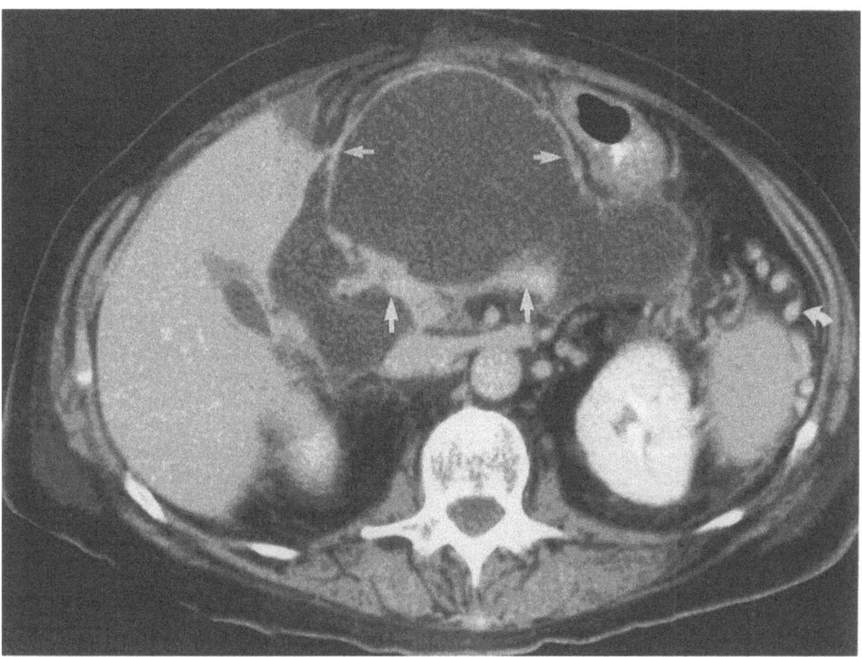

Fig. 11.4. Sterile necrosis associated with a pancreatic pseudocyst. Dynamic contrast-enhanced CT scan performed on a 71-year-old woman with gallstone pancreatitis reveals a paucity of normally enhancing pancreas (*vertical arrows*). The pancreatic body and tail are replaced by a low-attenuation multiloculated mass that extends anteriorly into the lesser sac compressing the stomach. This mass appears to have a well-formed enhancing capsule (*horizontal arrows*). This mass extends into a perihepatic location. Splenic vein thrombosis was present with numerous perisplenic venous collaterals (*curved arrow*). This appearance conforms to a Balthazar-Ranson severity index of 10 (4 points for grade E pancreatitis and 6 points for > 50% pancreatic necrosis). While the appearance of the encapsulated fluid is consistent with a pseudocyst, the paucity of normal pancreatic parenchyma indicates that this patient also has severe necrotizing pancreatitis. The encapsulated structure is composed of both fluid in the lesser sac and the necrotic pancreas. Because of persistent pain and inability to eat after 6 weeks, she underwent surgical treatment. This consisted of debridement of a considerable amount of necrotic pancreas, evacuation of fluid, and surgical anastomosis of the capsule to the posterior wall of the stomach. She made an uneventful recovery. This is an example of necrotizing pancreatitis in association with a pancreatic pseudocyst. Evacuation of the fluid by the radiologic insertion of a catheter, the endoscopic creation of a cystgastrostomy, or a surgical cystgastrostomy without elimination of necrosis predisposes to infection of the residual necrotic pancreas

required for a necrotic coagulum to form, the use of systemic antibiotics should protect the patient against a serious bloodstream infection associated with infected necrosis. It is therefore recommended that patients with pancreatic necrosis and organ failure be placed on potent broad-spectrum antibiotic coverage. The use of antibiotics in this fashion has not been shown to impair the accuracy of percutaneous aspiration for bacteriologic sampling [43].

If guided percutaneous aspiration does not reveal the presence of bacteria, options for treatment would include continuation of medical therapy or debridement of severe

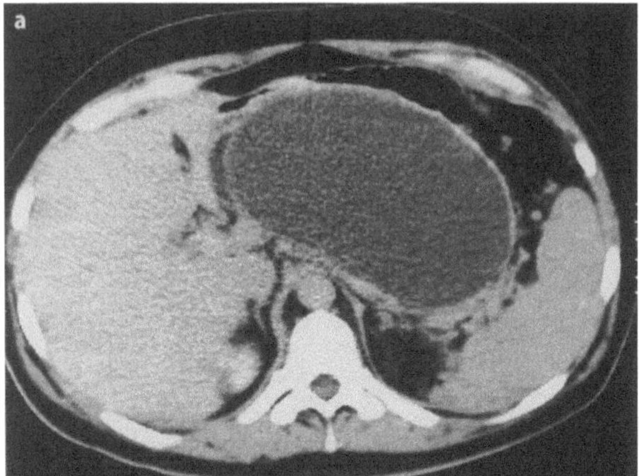

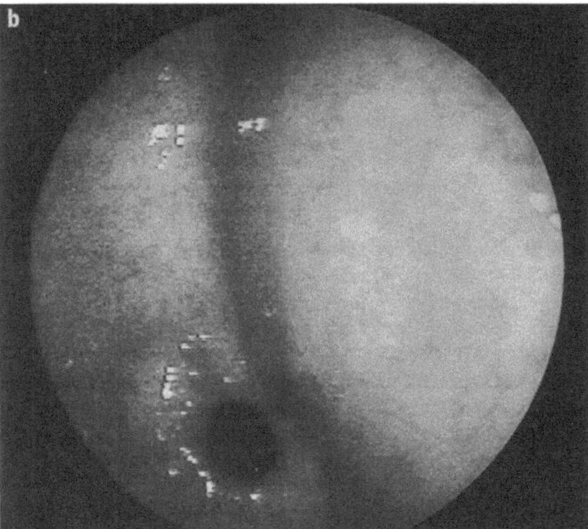

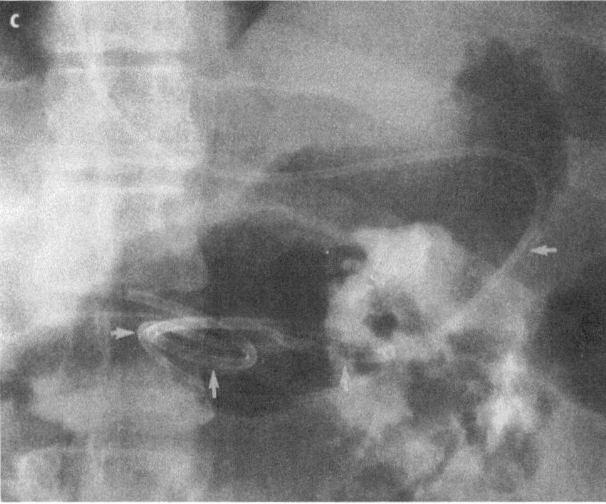

Fig. 11.5 a–c. Sterile necrosis associated with a pancreatic pseudocyst. **a** Dynamic contrast-enhanced CT scan performed 8 weeks after clinical recovery of a 34-year-old man with idiopathic pancreatitis reveals absence of enhancement of the body and tail of the pancreas. Replacing the body and tail is a large encapsulated low-attenuation mass extending into the lesser sac compressing the stomach anteriorly. This is an example of a large pancreatic pseudocyst that has at its base extensive necrosis of the body and tail of the pancreas. Because of persistent abdominal pain pertaining to oral intake, an attempt was made to treat this condition with an endoscopic cystgastrostomy. **b** Endoscopic view of the antrum of the stomach reveals a pylorus and a well-defined bulge indenting the stomach from the posterior aspect caused by the pancreatic pseudocyst. **c** Following the creation of an endoscopic cystgastrostomy, a considerable amount of cloudy sterile pancreatic fluid was evacuated. A double-pigtail catheter (*vertical arrows*) was inserted as well as a nasocystic catheter (*horizontal arrows*) for irrigation of the pancreatic area in an effort to dislodge and remove pancreatic material. The pancreatic material could not be removed. When the patient became febrile, he underwent surgical debridement of a considerable amount of pancreatic necrosis. His postoperative course was uneventful

sterile necrosis. Thus far, there have not been randomized prospective trials comparing medical with surgical treatment or comparing early with late surgical debridement among patients with severe sterile necrosis. It is probable that patients with severe sterile necrosis complicated by systemic complications have a high mortality whether or not early surgical debridement is carried out. While it remains unknown which is the better course of action, the consensus at present is that severe sterile necrosis should be managed medically for the first 3–4 weeks in the hope that the severe systemic toxicity will eventually resolve and the patient can be managed without need for surgery [49]. After 4–6 weeks, if surgery is required, it presumably can be done more safely because severe systemic toxicity has subsided.

There are several possible indications for surgery after 4–6 weeks. The first is lingering respiratory insufficiency requiring prolonged intubation and assisted ventilation. Failure to wean off of a respirator under these circumstances may be attributed to persisting intraabdominal inflammation. Following debridement and irrigation of the retroperitoneum, patients, in general, have shown improvement in respiratory status and have been able to be extubated. A second indication for late surgery is compression of stomach or other hollow viscus causing intractable nausea and thereby preventing establishment of oral intake. A third indication is recurrent pain with each attempt at oral intake of food (Figs. 11.4, 11.5 a–c). The explanation for pain appears to be the fact that loculated fluid in and around the necrotic pancreas is under great pressure. With oral intake, there is presumably additional pancreatic secretion that increases this pressure further. Following debridement, this pressure is alleviated, and the patient is then able to eat without pain.

In necrotizing pancreatitis, hospitalization can be lengthy. It is not unusual for a patient with severe necrotizing pancreatitis to be hospitalized for 2–3 months and even longer. At the time of surgery, it is helpful to insert a feeding jejunostomy in order to eliminate the need for total parenteral nutrition. Jejunostomy feeding can be continued in a rehabilitation center or at home until such time as the patient is able to resume oral intake.

11.2.2
Treatment of Pancreatic Pseudocyst

11.2.2.1
Medical Treatment

Until recently, a pseudocyst > 5 cm in size that has been present for at least 6 weeks has usually been decompressed surgically. The rationale has been a concern that a serious and even life-threatening complication might occur, such as bleeding, infection, or perforation. Recently, this approach has been challenged. First, earlier studies that had suggested a high complication rate of untreated pseudocysts did not have a complete follow-up of all cases. Second, 2 recent retrospective studies have provided information that an asymptomatic pseudocyst of any size does not require surgical intervention. In the few patients who developed serious symptoms, such as bleeding or infection, surgical intervention was then undertaken [98, 102]. In both studies, only

50%–60% of all patients with pseudocysts required operative intervention, either early because of severe pain or on rare occasion at a later interval. There was no mortality in either series among patients whose pseudocysts were treated medically. In fact, there was no mortality among patients who required surgery [98, 102].

Accordingly, many physicians are now more comfortable in the nonsurgical management of an asymptomatic pseudocyst. It is reasonable to obtain an abdominal ultrasound every 3 months in order to follow the size of the pseudocyst. Patients should be advised to report immediately any new symptoms such as chills and fever or abdominal pain.

There is no proven medical strategy for reducing the size of a pancreatic pseudocyst. While it is possible that measures that reduce the flow of pancreatic juice may in time diminish its size, there are no randomized prospective trials that have evaluated manipulation of diet, use of total parenteral nutrition, or a variety of medications that are capable of reducing the flow of pancreatic juice (such as Sandostatin, proton pump inhibitors, or H_2-blocking agents). A pseudocyst that is symptomatic can be treated by surgical, radiologic, or endoscopic means. Thus far, there have been no randomized prospective trials comparing the cost and effectiveness of these methods of therapy.

11.2.2.2
Surgical Treatment

The traditional method of pseudocyst drainage is surgical. The two standard surgical approaches are cystogastrostomy and cystoduodenostomy if there is firm attachment of the pseudocyst wall with broad adherence to duodenum or stomach, respectively. If the pseudocyst does not have this anatomic proximity, a Roux-en-Y cystojejunostomy is usually performed. Alternatively, if the pseudocyst is located in the tail of the pancreas, a resection of the tail including the cyst can be performed. If the pseudocyst is burrowing into the hilum of the spleen, a splenectomy may also be required (Fig. 11.6).

If a pseudocyst is grossly infected, some surgeons would prefer not to perform an internal anastomosis and instead would drain the pseudocyst externally. When this is performed, a fistula may take place, but it usually close within several months. The administration of Sandostatin subcutaneously may help in closing a fistula. An alternative method for a frankly infected pseudocyst would be percutaneous catheter drainage. A third option would be to proceed with an anastomosis such as a cystogastrostomy, as long as the contents of the pseudocyst can be rinsed at the time of surgery.

Mortality following surgical drainage of pancreatic pseudocyst depends largely on the presence of organ dysfunction or comorbid disease. In recent series, mortality has varied between 0% and 6% [83, 98, 102]. If a patient is at unacceptable surgical risk, nonsurgical options for decompression should be pursued. Recurrence rates following internal anastomosis are in the 15% range [83]. There are two possible explanations for the apparent development of a pseudocyst following successful internal drainage. The first is the possibility that the patient initially had 2 pseudocysts and that one was not visualized at surgery and was not decompressed. The second is that a sole pseudocyst was decompressed but then recurred. Recurrence of a pseudocyst is most apt to take place if there is blockage of the main pancreatic duct downstream from the sur-

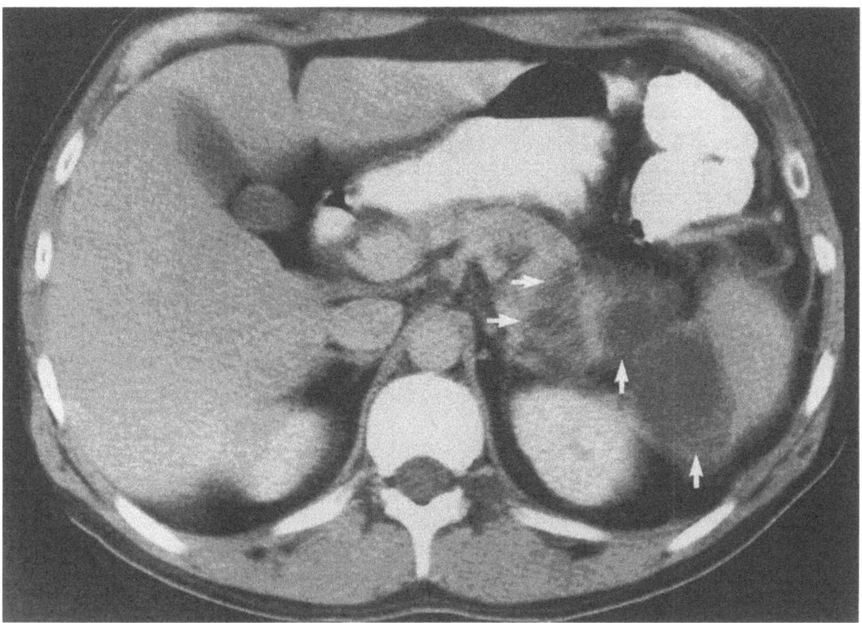

Fig. 11.6. Sterile necrosis with pseudocyst extending into the spleen. Dynamic contrast-enhanced CT scan shows areas of nonenhancement in the tail of the pancreas (*horizontal arrows*) with relatively normal enhancement of the body of the pancreas. There are pseudocysts that extend into the splenic hilum (*upper vertical arrow*) and into the spleen in a subcapsular location (*lower vertical arrow*). This patient had recovered from an acute episode of acute pancreatitis but was experiencing severe left upper quadrant pain. He underwent a distal pancreatectomy and splenectomy and made a complete recovery

gical internal anastomosis. In this circumstance, the increased pressure in the pancreatic duct persists, and there is further leakage of pancreatic juice in the vicinity of the initial pseudocyst.

It is now recommended that patients undergo preoperative ERCP to determine whether there is blockage of the main pancreatic duct. If there is, the surgeon might well consider a resection of the pseudocyst rather than an internal anastomosis. If an internal drainage remains the better option, the surgeon may take special care to create a large opening in the anastomosis of the pseudocyst wall and the loop of hollow viscus that is utilized.

11.2.2.3
Radiologic Treatment

Both sterile and infected pseudocysts can be effectively drained with percutaneous catheter drainage [4, 13, 28, 37, 44, 96]. Success of this technique requires a team of radiologists that is dedicated to patient care. The radiologists should make daily rounds at the bedside to insure optimal care of the catheter. In addition, radiology should be on-call at all times to help in the assessment and treatment of complications such as infection. Infection may take place if particulate material blocks the catheter creating stasis of fluid in the pseudocyst. A valuable clue to this possibility in the context of chills and fever is a markedly reduced flow through the catheter itself. Should this take place, it may be necessary to exchange the catheter over a wire. Alternatively, one might consider cautious instillation of a small amount of fluid via the catheter.

If there is persistent flow, Sandostatin in a dosage of 50–200 µg subcutaneously every 8 h may help in diminishing the flow [13].

The catheter should be left in place until the drainage each day diminishes to a very scant amount. When this occurs, a follow-up CT scan should be obtained to be absolutely sure that the pseudocyst has been fully decompressed. A reduction of flow might take place if there is blockage of the tube or if there is migration of the tube outside the pseudocyst wall.

Reports have generally noted success with percutaneous catheter drainage of pseudocysts [13, 28, 39, 44, 96]. Percutaneous catheter drainage is likely to fail if there is obstruction of the main pancreatic duct [2]. For this reason, an ERCP should be obtained prior to the decision to attempt catheter drainage. If the main pancreatic duct fills completely without filling of a pseudocyst, the presumption is that the pseudocyst is in continuity with a secondary or tertiary duct and that percutaneous catheter drainage will succeed. Similarly, if contrast material is seen to enter the pseudocyst, it is likely that catheter drainage will have a high likelihood of success because pancreatic fluid will have the opportunity to travel antegrade towards the duodenum via the main pancreatic duct. However, if there is obstruction to flow of the main pancreatic duct such that the pseudocyst does not fill, percutaneous catheter drainage should not be attempted, because pancreatic ductal obstruction will continue to prevent pancreatic fluid from flowing into the duodenum, and there is likely to be a permanent pancreatic fistula draining via the catheter [2, 99]. While there appears to be logic to this formulation and algorithms have been developed which have utilized results of ERCP to determine the type of pseudocyst decompression that should be employed [2, 99], there have been no randomized prospective trials which have assessed the impact of pancreatic ductal obstruction on success of various modalities of pseudocyst drainage.

11.2.2.4
Endoscopic Treatment

There are two endoscopic methods that have been utilized to drain a pancreatic pseudocyst [27, 41, 51, 64]. First, if the pseudocyst is broadly impacted against the wall of the stomach (or duodenum), endoscopic cystogastrostomy (or cystoduodenostomy) can be performed with insertion of a double pigtail catheter between the cyst and hollow viscus in order to facilitate evacuation of fluid out of the pseudocyst [41, 51, 64]. Some endoscopists also insert a nasocystic drain in order to be able to provide irrigation of the cyst should there be evidence of infection (Fig. 11.5 a–c). Second, if the pseudocyst is in continuity with the main pancreatic duct, a stent can be inserted directly into the duct and then into the pseudocyst itself in order to facilitate evacuation of fluid from the pseudocyst into the duodenum and promote healing [27]. After 3–4 weeks, a CT scan should be obtained. If there is closure of the pseudocyst, the double pigtail catheter (or pancreatic ductal stent) can then be removed.

Because an endoscopically placed stent may in time induce ductal changes similar to those of chronic pancreatitis, this technique should be utilized for no longer than a few weeks or should perhaps be reserved for a pseudocyst in the head of the pancreas.

The most important complication of endoscopic drainage of a pseudocyst is bleeding. Increasingly, endoscopic ultrasound is being utilized to help in the localization of a pseudocyst and to be sure that there are no large vessels in the area considered for drainage. A second complication is infection should the double pigtail catheter be occluded with inspissated material.

If ERCP prior to the procedure shows a blockage of the main pancreatic duct, there might be a concern that an endoscopic cystogastrostomy might fail, especially if the anastomosis is small. Thus far, as mentioned above, there have not been prospective studies that have evaluated the impact of ductal obstruction on the success of endoscopic drainage.

Since failure of radiologic and endoscopic drainage of pancreatic pseudocysts increases morbidity and prolongs hospitalization [83], these therapies should be performed at centers that have experienced radiologists and endoscopists that have particular interest in the treatment of pancreatic pseudocysts.

11.2.2.5
Pancreatic Pseudocysts Associated With Pancreatic Necrosis

Pancreatic pseudocysts extend for the most part outside the confines of the pancreas and wall off within the lesser sac, or some other location in proximity with the pancreas. On occasion, a pancreatic pseudocyst occurs in association with considerable pancreatic necrosis. The coexistence of pancreatic necrosis can be easily visualized by a careful inspection of dynamic contrast-enhanced CT scan. When there is pancreatic necrosis in association with a pancreatic pseudocyst, it is likely that there is considerable necrotic debris from the necrotic pancreas itself at the base of the pseudocyst (Figs. 11.4, 11.5 a–c). In time, the necrotic debris probably liquefies. However, it is very difficult to determine by CT scan whether a relatively homogenous appearing low-attenuation area within the pancreas contains liquid, solid necrosis, or both. Endoscopic ultrasound, or magnetic resonance imaging (MRI) as an alternative, might facilitate this distinction.

The importance of associated pancreatic necrosis is, as follows. If either endoscopic or percutaneous catheter drainage is performed, neither technique can readily evacuate particulate necrotic material. As a result, there is a high likelihood of infection, which may then require surgical debridement [47]. Surgeons have learned to recognize this condition, and at the time of surgical drainage, insert a probing finger deep into a pseudocyst in order to retrieve necrotic debris before completing the anastomosis. Accordingly, at the present time, it appears safer to offer surgical decompression of a pseudocyst associated with a substantial amount of pancreatic necrosis than to attempt decompression by either endoscopic or radiologic means.

11.2.2.6
Pancreatic Abscess

A pancreatic abscess is a collection of frank pus in the vicinity of the pancreas. It usually occurs 4–6 weeks after the onset of acute pancreatitis. The pathophysiology may be either secondary infection of a sequestrum of sterile necrosis or secondary infection of a pseudocyst. It may also occur if drains are inserted in the retroperitoneum following pancreatic surgery.

Clinical presentation is dominated by chills, fever, leukocytosis, and at times, abdominal discomfort. CT scan may show a poorly marginated low-density mass that at times contains diffuse air bubbles. The options for treatment include percutaneous catheter drainage and surgical drainage. The mortality of a pancreatic abscess appears to be less than that of infected necrosis of the pancreas. At the time of discovery of the abscess, the patient usually no longer has evidence of organ failure or systemic toxicity.

11.2.2.7
Smoldering Pancreatitis

The concept of smoldering pancreatitis implies that an episode does not fully subside and that the patient continues to experience abdominal pain and tenderness that precludes oral feeding. Alternatively, abdominal pain and tenderness may subside for several days but then recurs with additional attempts at oral feeding. Ordinarily, the sequence suggests a complication of pancreatitis. The most common complications that would explain smoldering pancreatitis include an unresolved episode with persisting peripancreatic inflammatory changes that can be visualized on CT scan, a pseudocyst, the development of pancreatic necrosis, or disruption or stenosis of the main pancreatic duct.

Treatment of ongoing pancreatitis may require total parenteral nutrition for 1–2 weeks. Treatment of a new pancreatic pseudocyst can be percutaneous, endoscopic, or surgical.

Treatment of pancreatic necrosis associated with unresolved pain usually requires surgical debridement.

A disruption of the pancreatic duct with extravasation of fluid into peripancreatic tissue can be documented by ERCP (see Fig. 11.2 a–f) [29, 57]. Insertion of a transpapillary pancreatic duct stent to the area or just beyond the area of extravasation frequently allows the disruption to heal (Fig. 11.7 a–d). When the stent is removed 3–4 weeks later, repeat ERCP frequently confirms healing such that the stent can be removed. While there is a possibility of inducing changes of chronic pancreatitis, this complication is not likely to occur with the use of a stent for only a few weeks. In addition, this form of therapy has less morbidity than surgical resection. An alternative form of treatment for disruption, however, would be resection of the area beyond the disruption.

Rather than ductal obstruction, an alternative finding on ERCP would be a stricture with diffuse dilatation of the main and secondary pancreatic ducts upstream (a finding that is characteristic of obstructive pancreatitis). Surgical resection of the pancreas beyond the stricture is the treatment of choice. The role of pancreatic stenting and/or balloon dilatation of a stricture in this circumstance is untested.

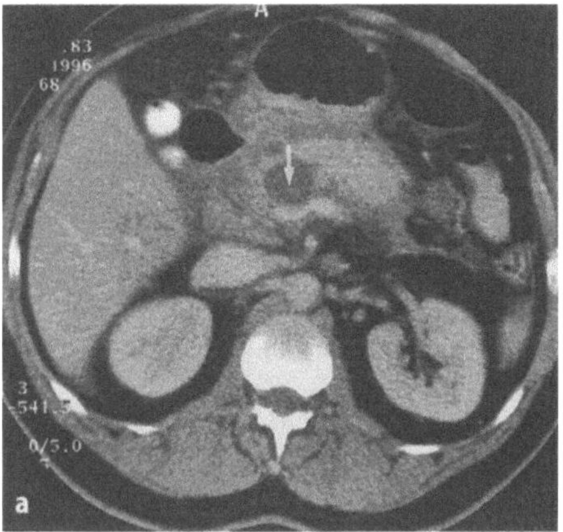 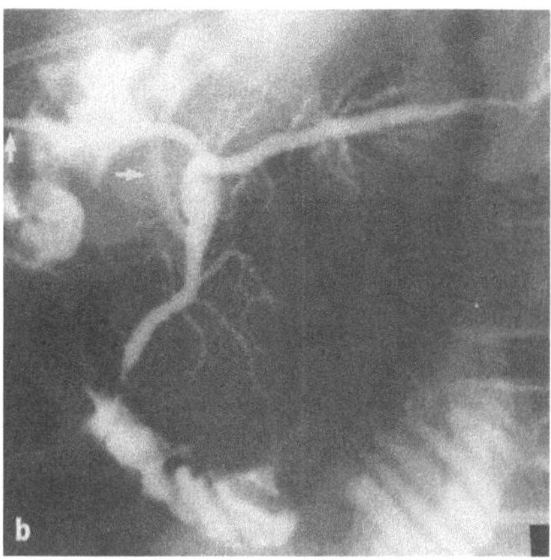

Fig. 11.7 a, b. Pancreas divisum with ductal disruption. **a** Dynamic contrast-enhanced CT scan in a 38-year-old patient with recurrent episodes of pancreatitis reveals an area of nonenhancement of the body of the pancreas consistent with fluid and/or necrosis (*arrow*). Otherwise, enhancement of the pancreatic parenchyma is uniform. There are inflammatory changes surrounding the pancreas. At other levels, a large fluid collection in the gastrohepatic ligament was noted. Because of intractable pain, pigtail catheters were inserted into the fluid collection of the gastrohepatic ligament and into the intrapancreatic fluid collection. Both drained amylase-rich clear fluid. Following insertion of the catheter, pain was completely relieved. **b** Injection of contrast via the intrapancreatic drainage catheter (*arrows*) fills the dorsal pancreatic duct, confirming the presence of a ductal disruption which led to the development of the intrapancreatic fluid collection and the large collection in the gastrohepatic ligament. The dorsal pancreatic duct is enlarged in caliber. The pancreatic side branches are dilated throughout the neck, body, and tail of the pancreas. Contrast is seen to flow into the duodenum via the dorsal papilla. A prior ERCP revealed filling of a small ventral duct consistent with pancreas divisum, but the accessory papilla could not be identified. The recurrent episodes of pancreatitis were thought attributable to stenosis of the dorsal duct as it entered the duodenum leading to a ductal disruption and the development of the intrapancreatic fluid collection demonstrated in Fig. 11.7 a

11.3
Treatment of Systemic Complications

11.3.1
Shock

Treatment of hypovolemic shock requires an estimation of the amount of fluid needed within 24 h to compensate for excessive third-space losses, losses through nasogastric suction, and perspiration. Measurements provided by a central venous pressure catheter or a Swan-Ganz catheter are best for gauging adequacy of fluid resuscitation and the capacity of the heart to tolerate large volumes of fluid [10]. During the first several days, daily replacement of 2–4 l/24 h are usually necessary in edematous pancreatitis. In the severe forms of the disease, daily replacement of fluid often exceeds 5–6 l and at times more than 10 l. If only a small amount of fluid has to be replaced, this can be done by infusion of 5% glucose or isotonic electrolyte solutions. If fluid losses are greater and require more than 3–4 l/24 h, this indicates a severe loss of protein. In this case, 500–1000 ml of 5% human albumin solution can be utilized, which is

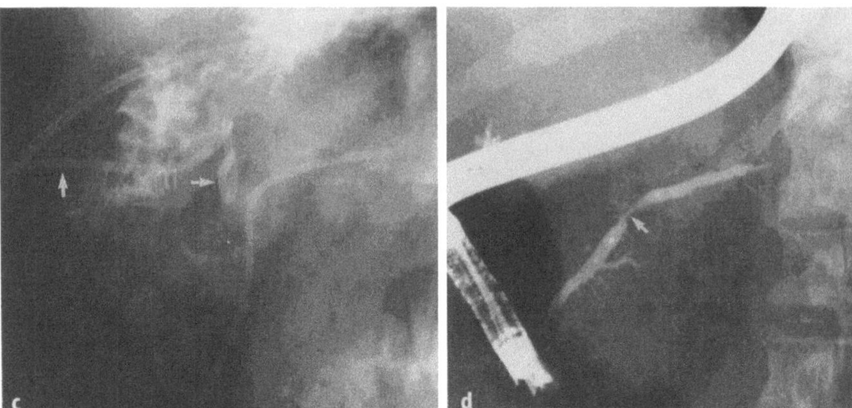

Fig. 11.7 c, d. Pancreas divisum with ductal disruption. **c** With the aid of intravenous secretin for identification of the dorsal papilla, the dorsal duct was accessed, dorsal duct sphincterotomy was performed, and a pancreatic stent was inserted beyond the disruption of the pancreatic duct at the genu. The pigtail catheter can once again be seen (*arrows*). A second catheter can also be seen that had drained a second collection of pancreatic fluid. Following insertion of the stent, the patient was able to eat without discomfort. There was no further extravasation of pancreatic juice, and after 1 week, the two catheters were removed. Pancreatic infection did not take place, presumably because of the absence of significant peripancreatic and pancreatic necrosis. **d** One month later, the stent was removed, and repeat ERCP shows a narrowing in the main pancreatic duct at the area of the previous disruption (*arrow*). The tip of the catheter utilized to instill contrast is seen just proximal to the stricture. There is no extravasation of contrast material. There is mild dilatation of the main pancreatic duct beyond the area of stenosis. The patient has remained asymptomatic for the past 9 months

one of the oldest treatments for acute pancreatitis [31–33]. If there is retroperitoneal hemorrhage, blood or packed red cells are also required. A hematocrit of approximately 30%–32% appears to be optimal in terms of viscosity of red cells within the microcirculation of the pancreas [56]. Whether volume replacement fluids (dextrane or HAES [hydroxyethyl starch] solution), or albumin solutions (human albumin versus fresh plasma) is effective in acute pancreatitis, is still an open question. A multicenter clinical trial for low-volume fresh-frozen plasma showed no beneficial effect on the course of the disease [66].

Rapid and adequate infusion therapy in severe acute pancreatitis is of utmost importance. If circulatory shock (systolic arterial blood pressure < 80 mm Hg for more than 10–15 min) occurs in spite of sufficient volume replacement, catecholamines should be utilized (dopamine in circulation-stimulating dosage or noradenalin). Shock in acute pancreatitis may resemble early septic-toxic shock: Cardiac index and pulmonary right-to-left shunt are increased whereas systemic blood pressure and especially peripheral vascular resistance are diminished. When clinical signs of sepsis occur (rectal temperature > 38.5 °C, metabolic acidosis, thrombocytes < 100 000/µl, leukocytes > 12 000/µl and/or positive blood culture), and when necrosis of the pancreas is found on contrast-enhanced CT, early application of Imipenem has been shown to lower significantly the rate of infection and septic complications [79], but not the rate of surgery and the mortality rate.

11.3.2
Renal Insufficiency

When renal insufficiency develops despite sufficient volume replacement under control of central venous pressure, a loop diuretic (e.g., furosemide 40–120 mg/day) should be used. If impairment of renal function persists, dopamine infusion (renal dosage: 1–2 µg/kg body weight/min) is indicated. In animal experiments, such a dosage has been found to stimulate pancreatic secretion [95]. However, in humans, such a dopamine dosage does not influence exocrine pancreatic secretion [59]. In progressive renal insufficiency, dialysis procedure is indicated (hemodialysis, hemofiltration, or peritoneal dialysis).

11.3.3
Respiratory Insufficiency

Arterial blood gas analysis should be performed in each case of severe acute pancreatitis and should be repeated in the initial phase of severe acute pancreatitis every 12–24 h. Alternatively, continuous or intermittent pulse oximetry should be utilized. This should be done even if there are no clinical signs and symptoms of respiratory failure [82].

When there is hypoxemia (arterial pO_2 <70 mm Hg), humidified oxygen should be provided by mask or nasal prongs. If hypoxemia persists or if arterial pO_2 falls below 60 mm Hg under room atmosphere, and if there is increasing fatigue due to ventilatory efforts on the part of the patient that within a short interval of time would compromise adequate ventilation, endotracheal intubation and assisted ventilation should be provided.

It has to be decided whether hypoxemia is caused by ARDS (pulmonary artery wedge pressure normal) or by congestive heart failure (pulmonary artery wedge pressure increased). In both cases, assisted ventilation with positive end-expiratory pressure is necessary [48].

Pleural effusions, which may also contribute to respiratory insufficiency, usually vanish spontaneously when the inflammatory process of the gland subsides. Only in rare cases of large pleural effusions, puncture of the intrapleural space and evacuation of the pleural effusion is necessary for decompressing the lung.

11.3.4
General Systemic Therapy (Removal of Activated Pancreatic Enzymes)

One dreams of being able to treat acute pancreatitis by preventing or stopping pancreatic enzyme activation. Promising results using aprotinin [93] could not be confirmed in subsequent trials [42, 70, 75]. New synthetic protease inhibitors showed beneficial effects in animal experiments [62]. However, in subsequent human trials, a significant effect on mortality rate was not found [26, 45, 101].

To remove activated pancreatic enzymes and toxins contained within ascitic fluid before these can be reabsorbed into the circulation, peritoneal lavage has been recommended. In rats, where peritoneal lavage has free access to the animal's pancreas, continuous peritoneal dialysis had a significant effect on length and rate of survival [60, 61]. Although in a large controlled clinical trial peritoneal lavage had no significant effect on mortality rate [72], the question whether peritoneal lavage can be helpful is not definitely answered.

11.4
Treatment of Metabolic Complications

11.4.1
Hyperglycemia

Hyperglycemia occurs frequently in the early stage of severe acute pancreatitis. However, blood glucose levels normalize as the inflammatory process subsides. When blood glucose levels exceed 250 mg/dl, regular (amorphous) insulin should be administered cautiously in small dosages and usually in intervals of at least 6–8 h.

11.4.2
Hypocalcemia

Hypocalcemia may occur due to a decrease in nonionized or ionized calcium. A decrease in nonionized calcium is caused by loss of albumin from the systemic circulation. It will return to normal when serum albumin levels increase during treatment.

A reduction in ionized calcium is rare and may be associated with signs of neuromuscular irritability. It is due to a deposition of ionized calcium within areas of fat necrosis and to the development of hypomagnesemia. A reduction in ionized calcium not associated with a reduction in magnesium levels can be treated with intravenous calcium gluconate. A 10-ml ampule of 10% calcium gluconate can be administered intravenously in 1000 ml of replacement fluid during a 4- to 6-h interval. Additional amounts of calcium may be infused over a similar time frame until clinical improvement. Since a 10-ml ampule contains 1 g of calcium gluconate but only 93 mg of calcium and since approximately 400 mg of dietary calcium is absorbed daily, calcium replacement provided by this amount of calcium glucanate is not excessive. In an emergency situation, 2 ampules (10 ml each) of 10% calcium gluconate can be safely administered in a 10- to 15-min period if the clinician is certain that the patient is not hypokalemic and is not receiving treatment with digitalis. In either situation, rapid intravenous application of calcium may induce fatal arrhythmia because infused calcium binds with myocardial receptors and may intensify potential harmful effects of hypokalemia on the heart [10].

11.4.3
Hypomagnesemia

Magnesium levels may decrease due to vomiting, loss of magnesium in urine, and deposition of magnesium in areas of fat necrosis. In this rare condition, magnesium infusion (2-ml ampule of 50% magnesium sulfate in 1000 ml of replacement fluid) should be given during 4 to 6 h. One ampule of magnesium sulfate contains only 8 mEq of magnesium, which is slightly less than the amount of dietary magnesium that is absorbed on a daily basis from the small intestine. In severe magnesium deficiency, 2 ampules can be safely administered. If magnesium deficiency is extreme and renal function is normal, it is safe to dilute 5 ampules (40 mEq) of 50% magnesium sulfate in 500 ml of replacement fluid and infuse it slowly during a 6-h interval. Under this treatment, both serum calcium and magnesium levels should increase.

11.5
Treatment of Extrapancreatic Complications

11.5.1
Obstruction of Common Bile Duct, Duodenum, Colon, and Ureter

The obstruction of the common bile duct, duodenum, colon, and ureter may be due to the inflammatory swelling of the gland and/or the development of a large pancreatic pseudocyst. Usually, obstruction decreases with the reduction of the inflammatory process. However, in rare cases surgical intervention is necessary.

11.5.1.1
Pancreatic Pseudocyst

Since the introduction of ultrasound for follow-up of patients with acute pancreatitis it has been known that the development of pancreatic pseudocysts is a frequent event. Pancreatic pseudocysts with <6 cm in diameter are usually asymptomatic. Larger pancreatic pseudocysts may lead to the above mentioned obstructions and, possibly due to the intracystic pressure, contribute to the pain in these patients (see Fig. 9.6). In these cases, ultrasound- or CT-guided puncture may relieve both pain and obstruction, but this may be only temporarily because of the probable refilling of the pancreatic pseudocyst.

An uncomplicated, asymptomatic pancreatic pseudocyst <6 cm in diameter does not require therapeutic procedures and should not delay the beginning of oral food intake. When bleeding occurs from eroded vessels within the cystic wall, immediate embolism of the involved vessel or surgical treatment is necessary. Asymptomatic larger pancreatic pseudocysts should also be left alone as long as they are symptom-free. Spontaneous resolution has been described in 28%–40% of the cases [3, 21].

11.5.2
Gastrointestinal Bleeding

In severe acute pancreatitis, acid-induced lesions of the upper gastrointestinal tract should be prevented by application of H_2-antagonists or a proton-pump inhibitor. In case of bleeding from ulcerations in the stomach or the duodenum, endoscopic intervention is necessary. In the rare cases of gastrointestinal bleeding in acute pancreatitis due to erosion of vessels, either in the neighborhood of necrosis or in the wall of a pancreatic pseudocyst, immediate embolism of the involved vessel or surgical treatment is necessary.

References

1. Agarwal N, Pitchumoni CS (1993) Acute pancreatitis: a multisystem disease. Gastroenterologist 1:115–128
2. Ahearne PM, Baillie JM, Cotton PB, Baker ME, Meyers WC, Pappas TN (1992) An endoscopic retrograde cholangiopancreatography (ERCP)-based algorithm for the management of pancreatic pseudocysts. Am J Surg 163:111–116
3. Aranha GV, Prinz RA, Esguerra AC, Greenlee HB (1983) The nature and course of cystic pancreatic lesions diagnosed by ultrasound. Arch Surg 118:486–488
4. Balthazar EJ, Freeny PC, vanSonnenberg E (1994) Imaging and intervention in acute pancreatitis. Radiology 193:297–306
5. Balthazar EJ, Robinson DL, Megibow AJ, Ranson JHC (1990) Acute pancreatitis: value of CT in establishing prognosis. Radiology 174:331–336
6. Banks PA (1982) Metabolic complications of pancreatitis. In: Bradley III EL (ed) Complications of Pancreatitis. Medical and Surgical Management. W.B. Saunders Comp., Philadelphia–London etc, pp 176–202
7. Banks PA (1994) Acute pancreatitis: conservative management. Dig Surg 11:220–225
8. Banks PA (1994) Acute pancreatitis: medical and surgical management. Am J Gastroenterol 89: S78–S85
9. Banks PA (1994) A new classification system for acute pancreatitis. Am J Gastroenterol 89: 151–152
10. Banks PA (1995) Acute pancreatitis. In: Haubrich WS, Schaffner F, Berk JE (eds) Bockus Gastroenterology, vol. 4, 5th edn. W.B. Saunders Comp., Philadelphia–London–Toronto etc, pp 2888–2917
11. Banks PA, Gerzof SG, Chong FK, Worthington MG, Doos WG, Sullivan JG, Johnson WC (1990) Bacteriologic status of necrotic tissue in necrotizing pancreatitis. Pancreas 5:330–333
12. Banks PA, Gerzof SG, Langevin RE, Silverman SG, Sica GT, Hughes MD (1995) CT-guided aspiration of suspected pancreatic infection. Bacteriology and clinical outcome. Int J Pancreatol 18: 265–270
13. Barkin JS, Reiner DK, Deutsch E (1991) Sandostatin for control of catheter drainage of pancreatic pseudocyst. Pancreas 6:245–248
14. Bassi C (1994) Infected pancreatic necrosis. Int J Pancreatol 16:1–10
15. Beger HG, Bittner R, Block S, Büchler M (1986) Bacterial contamination of pancreatic necrosis. A prospective clinical study. Gastroenterology 91:433–438
16. Bittner R, Block S, Büchler M, Beger HG (1987) Pancreatic abscess and infected pancreatic necrosis. Different local septic complications in acute pancreatitis. Dig Dis Sci 32:1082–1087
17. Block S, Maier W, Bittner R, Büchler M, Malfertheiner P, Beger HG (1986) Identification of pancreas necrosis in severe acute pancreatitis: imaging procedures versus clinical staging. Gut 27: 1035–1042
18. Bockman DA (1992) Microvasculature of the pancreas. Relation to pancreatitis. Int J Pancreatol 12:11–21
19. Bradley III EL (1993) A clinically based classification system for acute pancreatitis. Summary of the International Symposium on Acute Pancreatitis, Atlanta, Ga, September 11 through 13, 1992. Arch Surg 128:586–590
20. Bradley III EL (1994) Necrosectomy in acute pancreatitis. J HBP Surg 2:152–154
21. Bradley III EL, Clements JL Jr, Gonzalez AC (1979) The natural history of pancreatic pseudocysts: a unified concept of management. Am J Surg 137:135–141

22. Bradley III EL, Murphy F, Ferguson C (1989) Prediction of pancreatic necrosis by dynamic pancreatography. Ann Surg 210:495–504
23. Buggy BP, Nostrant TT (1983) Lethal pancreatitis. Am J Gastroenterol 78:810–814
24. Büchler M, Malfertheiner P, Frieß H, Isenmann R, Vanek E, Grimm H, Schlegel P, Friess T, Beger HG (1992) Human pancreatic tissue concentration of bactericidal antibiotics. Gastroenterology 103:1902–1908
25. Büchler M, Malfertheiner P, Schoetensack C, Uhl W, Beger HG (1986) Sensitivity of antiproteases, complement factors and C-reactive protein in detecting pancreatic necrosis. Results of a prospective clinical study. Int J Pancreatol 1:227–235
26. Büchler M, Malfertheiner P, Uhl W, Schölmerich J, Stöckmann F, Adler G, Gaus W, Rolle K, Beger HG, German Pancreatitis Study Group (1993) Gabexate mesilate in human acute pancreatitis. Gastroenterology 104:1165–1170
27. Catalano MF, Geenen JE, Schmalz MJ, Johnson GK, Dean RS, Hogan WJ (1995) Treatment of pancreatic pseudocysts with ductal communication by transpapillary pancreatic duct endoprosthesis. Gastrointest Endosc 42:214–218
28. Criado E, De Stefano AA, Weiner TM, Jaques PF (1992) Long term results of percutaneous catheter drainage of pancreatic pseudocysts. Surg Gynecol Obstet 175:293–298
29. Devière J, Bueso H, Baize M, Azar C, Love J, Moreno E, Cremer M (1995) Complete disruption of the main pancreatic duct: endoscopic management. Gastrointest Endosc 42:445–451
30. Domínguez-Muñoz JE, Carballo F, García MJ, de Diego JM, Gea F, Yangüela J, de la Morena J (1993) Monitoring of serum proteinase-antiproteinase balance and systemic inflammatory response in prognostic evaluation of acute pancreatitis. Results of a prospective multicenter study. Dig Dis Sci 38:507–513
31. Elliott DW (1955) The mechanism of benefit derived from concentrated human serum albumin in experimental acute pancreatitis. Surg Forum 5:384–390
32. Elliott DW (1957) Treatment of acute pancreatitis with albumin and whole blood. Arch Surg 75:573–580
33. Elliott DW, Zollinger RM, Moore R, Ellison EH (1955) The use of human serum albumin in the management of acute pancreatitis. Experimental and clinical observations. Gastroenterology 28:563–587
34. Fan S-T, Lai ECS, Mok FPT, Lo C-M, Zheng S-S, Wong J (1993) Early treatment of acute biliary pancreatitis by endoscopic papillotomy. N Engl J Med 328:228–232
35. Fedorak IJ, Ko TC, Djuricin G, McMahon M, Thompson K, Prinz RA (1992) Secondary pancreatic infections: are they distinct clinical entities? Surgery 112:824–831
36. Fenton-Lee D, Imrie CW (1993) Pancreatic necrosis: assessment of outcome related to quality of life and cost of management. Br J Surg 80:1579–1582
37. Fink AS, Hiatt JR, Pitt HA, Bennion RS, DeSouza LR, McCoy RD, Meyer JH, Thompson JE Jr, Webster JL, Wilson SE (1988) Indolent presentation of pancreatic abscess. Experience with 100 cases. Arch Surg 123:1067–1972
38. Freeny PC (1993) Incremental dynamic bolus computed tomography of acute pancreatitis. Int J Pancreatol 13:147–158
39. Freeny PC, Lewis GP, Traverso LW, Ryan JA (1988) Infected pancreatic fluid collections: percutaneous catheter drainage. Radiology 167:435–441
40. Frey CF (1994) How I do it – Necrosectomy in acute pancreatitis. J HBP Surg 2:155–158
41. Funnell IC, Bornman PC, Krige JEJ, Beningfield SJ, Terblanche J (1994) Endoscopic drainage of traumatic pancreatic pseudocyst. Br J Surg 81:879–881
42. Gauthier A, Gillet M, Di Costanzo J, Camelot G, Maurin P, Sarles H (1978) Étude controlée multicentrique de l'aprotinine et du glucagon dans le traitement des pancréatites aiguës. Gastroenterol Clin Biol 2:777–784
43. Gerzof SG, Banks PA, Robbins AH, Johnson WC, Spechler SJ, Wetzner SM, Snider JM, Langevin RE, Jay ME (1987) Early diagnosis of pancreatic infection by computed tomography-guided aspiration. Gastroenterology 93:1315–1320
44. Gerzof SG, Johnson WC, Robbins AH, Spechler SJ, Nabseth DC (1984) Percutaneous drainage of infected pancreatic pseudocysts. Arch Surg 119:888–893
45. Goebell H (1988) Multicenter double-blind study of gabexate-mesilate (Foy), given intravenously in low dose in acute pancreatitis. Digestion 40:83 (abstr)

46. Gross V, Schölmerich J, Leser H-G, Salm R, Lausen M, Rückauer K, Schöffel U, Lay L, Heinisch A, Farthmann EH, Gerok W (1990) Granulocyte elastase in assessment of severity of acute pancreatitis. Comparison with acute-phase proteins, C-reactive protein, α_1-antitrypsin, and protease inhibitor α_2-macroglobulin. Dig Dis Sci 35:97–105
47. Hariri M, Slivka A, Carr-Locke DL, Banks PA (1994) Pseudocyst drainage predisposes to infection when pancreatic necrosis is unrecognized. Am J Gastroenterol 89:1781–1784
48. Hayes MF Jr, Rosenbaum RW, Zibelman M, Matsumoto T (1974) Adult respiratory distress syndrome in association with acute pancreatitis. Evaluation of positive end expiratory pressure ventilation and pharmacologic doses of steroid. Am J Surg 127:314–319
49. Ho HS, Frey CF (1995) Gastrointestinal and pancreatic complications associated with severe pancreatitis. Arch Surg 130:817–823
50. Hotz HG, Schmidt J, Ryschich EW, Foitzik T, Buhr HJ, Warshaw AL, Herfarth C, Klar E (1995) Isovolemic hemodilution with dextran prevents contrast medium induced impairment of pancreatic microcirculation in necrotizing pancreatitis of the rat. Am J Surg 169:161–166
51. Howell DA, Holbrook RF, Bosco JJ, Muggia RA, Biber BP (1993) Endoscopic needle localization of pancreatic pseudocysts before transmural drainage. Gastrointest Endosc 39:693–698
52. Jenkins SA, Berein A (1995) Review article: the relative effectiveness of somatostatin and octreotide therapy in pancreatic disease. Aliment Pharmacol Ther 9:349–361
53. Karimgani I, Porter KA, Langevin RE, Banks PA (1992) Prognostic factors in sterile pancreatic necrosis. Gastroenterology 103:1636–1640
54. Kingsnorth AN, Galloway SW, Formela LJ (1995) Randomized, double-blind phase II trial of Lexipafant, a platelet-activating factor antagonist, in human acute pancreatitis. Br J Surg 82:1414–1420
55. Klar E, Foitzik T, Buhr H, Messmer K, Herfarth C (1993) Isovolemic hemodilution with dextran 60 as treatment of pancreatic ischemia in acute pancreatitis. Clinical practicability of an experimental concept. Ann Surg 217:369–374
56. Klar E, Messmer K, Warshaw AL, Herfarth C (1990) Pancreatic ischaemia in experimental acute pancreatitis: mechanism, significance and therapy. Br J Surg 77:1205–1210
57. Kozarek RA, Ball TJ, Patterson DJ, Freeny PC, Ryan JA, Traverso LW (1991) Endoscopic transpapillary therapy for disrupted pancreatic duct and peripancreatic fluid collections. Gastroenterology 100:1362–1370
58. Lankisch PG, Haseloff M, Becher R (1994) No parallel between the biochemical course of acute pancreatitis and morphologic findings. Pancreas 9:240–243
59. Lankisch PG, Koop H (1978) Dopamin-Wirkung auf die basale Pankreassekretion. Dtsch Med Wochenschr 103:391–392
60. Lankisch PG, Koop H, Winckler K, Schmidt H (1979) Continuous peritoneal dialysis as treatment of acute experimental pancreatitis in the rat. II. Analysis of its beneficial effect. Dig Dis Sci 24:117–122
61. Lankisch PG, Koop H, Winckler K, Schmidt H (1979) Continuous peritoneal dialysis as treatment of acute experimental pancreatitis in the rat. I. Effect on length and rate of survival. Dig Dis Sci 24:111–116
62. Lankisch PG, Pohl U, Göke B, Otto J, Wereszczynska-Siemiatkowska U, Gröne H-J, Rahlf G (1989) Effect of FOY-305 (camostate) on severe acute pancreatitis in two experimental animal models. Gastroenterology 96:194–199
63. Larvin M, Chalmers AG, McMahon MJ (1990) Dynamic contrast enhanced computed tomography: a precise technique for identifying and localising pancreatic necrosis. Br Med J 300:1425–1428
64. Lawson JM, Baillie J (1995) Endoscopic therapy for pancreatic pseudocysts. Gastrointest Endosc Clin North Am 5:181–193
65. Leese T, Shaw D, Holliday M (1988) Prognostic markers in acute pancreatitis: can pancreatic necrosis be predicted? Ann R C Surg Engl 70:227–232
66. Leese T, Thomas WM, Holliday M, Attard A, Watkins M, Neoptolemos JP, Hall C (1991) A multicentre controlled clinical trial of high-volume fresh frozen plasma therapy in prognostically severe acute pancreatitis. Ann R C Surg Engl 73:207–214
67. Lefer AM, Martin J (1970) Origin of myocardial depressant factor in shock. Am J Physiol 218:1423–1427

68. Luengo L, Vicente V, Gris F, Coronas JM, Escuder J, Gomez JR, Castellote JM (1994) Influence of somatostatin in the evolution of acute pancreatitis. A prospective randomized study. Int J Pancreatol 15:139–144
69. Luiten EJT, Hop WCJ, Lange JF, Bruining HA (1995) Controlled clinical trial of selective decontamination for the treatment of severe acute pancreatitis. Ann Surg 222:57–65
70. M.R.C. Multicentre Trial of Glucagon and Aprotinin (1977) Death from acute pancreatitis. Lancet 2:632–635
71. Matsuno S, Takeda K, Sunamura M, Kobari M (1994) How I do it – Necrosectomy in acute pancreatitis. Open drainage with diverting ileostomy for acute necrotizing pancreatitis. J HBP Surg 2:159–162
72. Mayer AD, McMahon MJ, Corfield AP, Cooper MJ, Williamson RCN, Dickson AP, Shearer MG, Imrie CW (1985) Controlled clinical trial of peritoneal lavage for the treatment of severe acute pancreatitis. N Engl J Med 312:399–404
73. McFadden DW, Reber HA (1994) Indications for surgery in severe acute pancreatitis. Int J Pancreatol 15:83–90
74. McKay CJ, Imrie CW, Baxter JN (1993) Somatostatin and somatostatin analogues – are they indicated in the management of acute pancreatitis? Gut 34:1622–1626
75. Medical Research Council Multicentre Trial (1980) Morbidity of acute pancreatitis: the effect of aprotinin and glucagon. Gut 21:334–339
76. Messori A, Rampazzo R, Scroccaro G, Olivato R, Bassi C, Falconi M, Pederzoli P, Martini N (1995) Effectiveness of gabexate mesilate in acute pancreatitis. A metaanalysis. Dig Dis Sci 40:734–738
77. Neoptolemos JP, Carr-Locke DL, London NJ, Bailey IA, James D, Fossard DP (1988) Controlled trial of urgent endoscopic retrograde cholangiopancreatography and endoscopic sphincterotomy versus conservative treatment for acute pancreatitis due to gallstones. Lancet 2:979–983
78. Paran H, Neufeld D, Mayo A, Shwartz I, Singer P, Kaplan O, Skornik Y, Klausner J, Freund U (1995) Preliminary report of a prospective randomized study of octreotide in the treatment of severe acute pancreatitis. J Am Coll Surg 181:121–124
79. Pederzoli P, Bassi C, Vesentini S, Campedelli A (1993) A randomized multicenter clinical trial of antibiotic prophylaxis of septic complications in acute necrotizing pancreatitis with imipenem. Surg Gynecol Obstet 176:480–483
80. Pisters PWT, Ranson JHC (1992) Nutritional support for acute pancreatitis. Surg Gynecol Obstet 175:275–284
81. Ranson JHC, Berman RS (1990) Long peritoneal lavage decreases pancreatic sepsis in acute pancreatitis. Ann Surg 211:708–718
82. Ranson JHC, Turner JW, Roses DF, Rifkind KM, Spencer FC (1974) Respiratory complications in acute pancreatitis. Ann Surg 179:557–566
83. Rao R, Fedorak I, Prinz RA (1993) Effect of failed computed tomography-guided and endoscopic drainage on pancreatic pseudocyst management. Surgery 114:843–849
84. Rattner DW, Legermate DA, Lee MJ, Mueller PR, Warshaw AL (1992) Early surgical débridement of symptomatic pancreatic necrosis is beneficial irrespective of infection. Am J Surg 163:105–110
85. Rinderknecht H (1994) Genetic determinants of mortality in acute necrotizing pancreatitis. Int J Pancreatol 16:11–15
86. Roscher R, Beger HG (1987) Bacterial infection of pancreatic necrosis. In: Beger HG, Büchler M (eds) Acute Pancreatitis. Springer, Berlin–Heidelberg, pp 314–317
87. Sainio V, Kemppainen E, Puolakkainen P, Taavitsainen M, Kivisaari L, Valtonen V, Haapiainen R, Schröder T, Kivilaakso E (1995) Early antibiotic treatment in acute necrotising pancreatitis. Lancet 346:663–667
88. Sarr MG, Sanfey H, Cameron JL (1986) Prospective, randomized trial of nasogastric suction in patients with acute pancreatitis. Surgery 100:500–504
89. Seidensticker F, Otto J, Lankisch PG (1995) Recovery of the pancreas after acute pancreatitis is not necessarily complete. Int J Pancreatol 17:225–229
90. Sitzmann JV, Steinborn PA, Zinner MJ, Cameron JL (1989) Total parenteral nutrition and alternate energy substrates in treatment of severe acute pancreatitis. Surg Gynecol Obstet 168:311–317
91. Solomon TE (1995) Physiology of the exocrine pancreas. In: Haubrich WS, Schaffner F, Berk JE (eds) Bockus Gastroenterology, 5th edn. W.B. Saunders Comp., Philadelphia–London etc, pp 2821–2834

92. Steinberg W, Tenner S (1994) Acute pancreatitis. N Engl J Med 330:1198–1210
93. Trapnell JE, Rigby CC, Talbot CH, Duncan EHL (1974) A controlled trial of Trasylol in the treatment of acute pancreatitis. Br J Surg 61:177–182
94. Uhl W, Büchler M, Malfertheiner P, Martini M, Beger HG (1991) PMN-elastase in comparison with CRP, antiproteases, and LDH as indicators of necrosis in human acute pancreatitis. Pancreas 6:253–259
95. Valenzuela JE, Defilippi C, Diaz G, Navia E, Merino Y (1977) Effect of dopamine (DPM) on human gastric and pancreatic secretion. Gastroenterology 72:1144 (abstr)
96. vanSonnenberg E, Wittich GR, Casola G, Brannigan TC, Karnel F, Stabile BE, Varney RR, Christensen RR (1989) Percutaneous drainage of infected and noninfected pancreatic pseudocysts: experience in 101 cases. Radiology 170:757–761
97. Vesentini S, Bassi C, Talamini G, Cavallini G, Campedelli A, Pederzoli P (1993) Prospective comparison of C-reactive protein level, Ranson score and contrast-enhanced computed tomography in the prediction of septic complications of acute pancreatitis. Br J Surg 80:755–757
98. Vitas GJ, Sarr MG (1992) Selected management of pancreatic pseudocysts: operative versus expectant management. Surgery 111:123–130
99. Weltz C, Pappas TN (1995) Pancreatography and the surgical management of pseudocysts. Gastrointest Endosc Clin North Am 5:269–279
100. Wilson C, Heads A, Shenkin A, Imrie CW (1989) C-reactive protein, antiproteases and complement factors as objective markers of severity in acute pancreatitis. Br J Surg 76:177–181
101. Yang C-Y, Chang-Chien C-S, Liaw Y-F (1987) Controlled trial of protease inhibitor gabexelate mesilate (FOY) in the treatment of acute pancreatitis. Pancreas 2:698–700
102. Yeo CJ, Bastidas JA, Lynch-Nyhan A, Fishman EK, Zinner MJ, Cameron JL (1990) The natural history of pancreatic pseudocysts documented by computed tomography. Surg Gynecol Obstet 170:411–417

12 Acute Pancreatitis: Prognosis

12.1
Introduction

The prognosis of a given attack of acute pancreatitis depends on multiple factors, e.g., etiology, number of previous attacks, and severity. Severity of the disease is established by clinical, biochemical, and imaging procedure scores. Mortality rate strongly depends on the presence or absence of necrosis, pancreatic infection, and the development of systemic complications. Long-term prognosis depends on the development of late sequelae, i.e., of the development of pancreatic duct changes, exo- and endocrine pancreatic insufficiency, and pancreatic pseudocysts. The quality of life will also be affected. Finally, the relapse rate in patients with acute pancreatitis is of interest, since recent studies have shown that the progression of acute to chronic pancreatitis is closely related to the incidence and severity of acute attacks [6].

12.2
Etiology

Whether a particular etiology of acute pancreatitis leads to a more severe course of the disease is a frequent topic of discussion. However, two studies have shown that etiology is not decisive for the prognosis of acute pancreatitis (Table 12.1) [71, 93, 125].

Table 12.1. Etiology in relation to mortality

Etiology	Patients		Mortality	
	(n)	(%)	(n)	(%)
Biliary tract disease	227	38	13	6
Alcohol	177	29	13	7
Other	65	11	3	5
Unknown	133	22	8	6
Total	602	100	37	6

Differences not significant

12.3
Initial or Repeated Episodes

The initial episode of acute pancreatitis is most likely to have severe complications and fatal outcome. In an earlier series, 12% of patients died after the second attack [108]. Subsequent attacks had no serious morbidity or any mortality. In an epidemiological study of acute pancreatitis in a defined German population, 25 (18%) of 141 patients with a first attack of acute pancreatitis had at least one subsequent attack, and 8 (6%) of all patients had two or more. Mortality rate was 10% (14/141) for the first attack of acute pancreatitis, 8% (2/25) for the first relapse and zero for all subsequent relapses. Relapses occurred more frequently in alcoholics [9].

12.4
Severity

12.4.1
General

Severity of acute pancreatitis depends on the presence of systemic complications and pancreatic necrosis. Numerous studies have dealt with clinical, biochemical, and imaging procedure scores to evaluate whether acute pancreatitis is severe or not. Unfortunately, most of these parameters cannot be estimated on admission or, if so, they may be falsely normal on admission, since acute pancreatitis is a dynamic process, and severity of complications may not have been fully established on admission.

12.4.2
Clinical Parameters

Initial studies suggested that the prognosis for acute pancreatitis among elderly patients was unfavorable [24, 103, 111]. A more recent study involving more than 600 patients who experienced a mortality rate of 6.1%, has shown that age is not a decisive prognostic factor [71].

A careful history concerning alcohol consumption yields important information. Patients who have consumed >1000 g pure alcohol during the week prior to admission have a higher mortality and complication rate [60]. However, this is only true for the first epidose of alcoholic pancreatitis, and not for recurrent attacks.

Clinical assessment of acute pancreatitis can correctly predict severity in mild cases as early as 8 h after admission; within 48 h, clinical assessment is better than Ranson and Imrie criteria [97]. In severe acute pancreatitis, however, clinical assessment is less effective after 8 h, improves after 24 h and 48 h, and is then equivalent to the biochemical parameters (see Table 9.2) [97]. Schölmerich et al. [114] developed a clinical score for acute pancreatitis using daily bedside examination (Table 12.2). The score enabled the group to predict the subsequent course of disease in 80% of the patients from the first hospital day onwards, and in more than 90% on day 4. Thus, bedside

Table 12.2. Clinical score in acute pancreatitis (daily bedside examination) [114]

Skin color	Normal/pale or red/icterus	0/1/2
Temperature	Normal/37.5–38.0 °C/ > 38 °C	0/1/2
Consciousness	Normal/somnolence/coma	0/1/2
Abdominal pain (need for analgesics)	None/mild/severe	0/1/2
Abdominal guarding	None/mild/severe	0/2/2
Bowel sounds	Normal/reduced/none	0/1/2
		12

evaluation of patients may be the standard against which other more sophisticated imaging or laboratory techniques should be measured. Further studies are required.

Obesity, best estimated by using the body mass index (BMI) (calculated as weight in kilograms, divided by height in meters squared), has been shown to be an important prognostic factor in acute pancreatitis [46, 64, 78, 105]. The presence of body wall ecchymosis in acute pancreatitis has been found to be associated with a mortality rate of 35% [35] (see Table 9.1).

12.4.3
Biochemical Severity Predictors

12.4.3.1
Scoring Systems

12.4.3.1.1
Ranson's Prognostic Criteria

The prognostic signs of Ranson et al. [108] (see Table 9.5) are applied worldwide. This group identified 11 objective tests of prognostic significance. One of them is age (> 55 years), 4 of 5 that are measured at the time of admission are laboratory findings indicating intensity of the inflammatory process. The 6th, measured within the first 48 h of admission, reflect the impact of third-space losses and systemic complications. A decrease in hematocrit of > 10 percentage points (indicating that hemoconcentration caused by third-space loss has been overcome by appropriate fluid resuscitation within the first 48 h), a serum calcium level < 8 mg/dl (reflecting loss of unionized calcium from the circulation associated with loss of serum albumin), and an estimated fluid sequestration > 6 l reflect severe third-space losses. An increase of blood urea nitrogen, a decrease of arterial pO_2, and evidence of metabolic acidosis reflect systemic complications, especially renal failure, respiratory failure, and cardiovascular instability. Ranson [107] modified his list of signs for patients with gallstones in whom he found no correlation between arterial oxygen tension and prognosis. In addition, these signs for patients with biliary induced acute pancreatitis take into account that such patients are usually older and may be diabetic (see Table 9.5).

The original signs (see Table 9.5), but not the modified signs for patients with biliary acute pancreatitis, have been used worldwide in clinical trials to assess the severity of acute pancreatitis. When there are 2 or fewer positive Ranson signs, almost all patients survive; with 3–5 positive signs, mortality is 10%–20%, with 6 or more positive signs, in excess of 50%. Patients with 3 or more Ranson's signs have a high frequency rate of systemic complications and are more likely to develop pancreatic necrosis, which is usually infected when 6 or more positive signs are present [10, 11, 16, 27, 30, 34, 80, 81, 117, 119, 130]. The clinical application of Ranson's signs are subject to the following clinical limitations [13]:

- A full 48 h of observation is required to measure fluid sequestration (i.e., the difference between intravenous fluid intake and the output of fluid in urine and nasogastric aspirate).
- In addition, some of the remaining signs may not be detectable until near the end of the 48-h period. A delay of 48 h to establish severity has its disadvantages, i.e., therapy may not be maximized within the first few hours to prevent complications.

12.4.3.1.2
Imrie's Prognostic Criteria

Imrie et al. [54] suggested a slight modification of Ranson's criteria for centers where acute pancreatitis of biliary etiology predominates [19, 102]. Severe acute pancreatitis was indicated with 3 or more of the 9 prognostic factors (see Table 9.6) [19, 102].

12.4.3.1.3
Bank's Prognostic Criteria

Bank et al. [12] divided the risk factors into broad categories including cardiac, pulmonary, renal, metabolic, hematologic, neurologic, and hemorrhagic complications (Table 12.3) [12]. If no clinical criteria were positive, mortality rate was 2%. Whereas if 1 or more criteria were positive, mortality was 56%. Mortality was similar for patients with 6 or more positive Ranson's signs. The required 48-h interval is again a drawback. The second drawback is that some of the risk factors are the very complications one would like to prevent in acute pancreatitis, e.g., shock and adult respiratory distress syndrom (ARDS).

Table 12.3. Bank's prognostic criteria [12]

Cardiac	Shock, tachycardia > 130, arrhythmia, ECG changes
Pulmonary	Dyspnea, rales, pO_2 < 60 mm Hg, adult respiratory distress syndrome (ARDS)
Renal	Urine output < 50 ml/h, rising blood urea nitrogen and/or creatinine
Metabolic	Low or falling calcium, pH, albumin decrease
Hematological	Falling hematocrit, diffuse intravascular coagulation (low platelets, split products)
Neurological	Irritability, confusion, localizing signs
Hemorrhagic disease	− on signs or peritoneal tap
Tense distension	− severe ileus, fluid $+ +$
Interpretation:	$\geq 1 =$ severe (potentially lethal) disease

12.4.3.1.4
Agarwal's and Pitchumoni's Simplified Prognostic Criteria

Agarwal and Pitchumoni [3] (Table 12.4) separated the prognostic criteria into 4 categories: cardiac, pulmonary, renal, and metabolic derangement. The presence of one or more criteria correctly identifies patients with complications; however, these criteria also require 48 h. In the absence of any simplified prognostic criteria, complication rate was 7.5%, whereas one or more prognostic criteria indicated a complication rate of 48%. A similar complication rate was found in patients with 3 to 5 Ranson's signs.

Table 12.4. Simplified prognostic criteria according to Agarwal and Pitchumoni [3]

	During initial 48 h		
Cardiac	Blood pressure	< 90 mm Hg;	
	tachycardia	> 130/min	
Pulmonary	Dyspnea; pO_2	< 60 mm Hg	
Renal	Urine output	< 50 ml/h	
Metabolic	Calcium	< 8 mg/dl;	
	Albumin	< 3.2 g/dl	

12.4.3.1.5
Hong Kong Criteria

Fan et al. [42] reported that blood urea of > 4.7 mmol/l (28.2 mg/dl) and/or glucose higher than 11 mmol/l (198 mg/dl) at the time of admission to hospital detect severe acute pancreatitis with a sensitivity and specificity comparable with Imrie's multifactor scoring system. They recommended this alternative approach because of its simplicity and the ability to predict the severity at the time of admission [42]. Furthermore, the Hong Kong group showed that their criteria had an overall accuracy comparable with those of the APACHE-II (Acute Physiology and Chronic Health Evaluation) scores (cutoff level > 11) [40].

However, in a comparative study, Imrie's group [52] showed that the Hong Kong criteria were less accurate than both their own criteria for identifying severe attacks of acute pancreatitis and clinical assessment after 48 h.

12.4.3.1.6
APACHE-II Scores

The APACHE-II illness grading system assesses points of severity on the basis of age, chronic health status, and a quantitative measure of the degree of abnormality of 12 physiologic variables (Table 12.5) [65]. This system has been used to assess severity in a variety of clinical situations, including, in recent years, acute pancreatitis. APACHE-II scores on admission, at 48 h, and at the time of surgery have been helpful in identifying high risk patients [34, 64, 82, 117, 130]. Patients with APACHE-II scores of 9 or less within the first 48 h survived, whereas those with APACHE-II scores of 13 and more had a high likelihood of a fatal outcome. Daily measurement of APACHE-II scores is recommended to determine whether scores remain at 9 or below.

Table 12.5. The APACHE-II severity of disease classification system (see also Table 9.7). According to [65]

1. **Physiologic points**
   - Temperature
   - Mean arterial pressure
   - Heart rate
   - Respiratory rate
   - Oxygenation (arterial pO_2)
   - Arterial pH
   - Serum sodium
   - Serum potassium
   - Serum creatinine
   - Hematocrit
   - White cell count
   - Glasgow coma score
2. **Age points**
3. **Chronic health points**
   - Liver
   - Cardiovascular
   - Respiratory
   - Renal
   - Immunocompromised

12.4.3.1.7
Comparison of Multiple-Parameter Prognostic Systems

Several studies have compared various multiple-parameter scoring systems and concluded that there is no ideal prognostic system with 100% sensitivity and specificity. A most recent prospective multicenter study including 719 episodes of acute pancreatitis comparing Ranson's, Imrie's and APACHE-II scores and predicting organ system failure and fluid collections defined by the Atlanta criteria showed that APACHE-II scores were the most accurate and rapid of these systems [23].

12.4.3.2
Peritoneal Lavage for Prognosis

In a number of studies, prognosis has been based on peritoneal lavage performed on admission. Recovery of any volume of peritoneal fluid with a dark color or recovery of > 20 ml of free intraperitoneal fluid of any color is associated with severe acute pancreatitis [31, 33, 94, 96, 97, 104]. Because this method is invasive, it has not found wide application.

12.4.3.3
Single Markers

Arterial pO_2 which is included in most of the scoring systems should be measured on admission in suspected severe acute pancreatitis and during follow-up to diagnose acute respiratory failure. A decrease of arterial pO_2 from 70 or above to < 60 mm Hg has been shown to be associated with a distinctly raised mortality (5.9% versus 13.2%) [57].

Low *serum amylase* levels upon admission were found diagnostic of advanced pancreatic necrosis [1, 2], later confirmed upon surgery or postmortem in selected cases [132]. However, when correlated with contrast-enhanced computed tomography (CT) results, high, not low, amylase and lipase levels were shown to indicate severe acute pancreatitis [77].

Measurement of *C-reactive protein* (CRP) distinguishes necrotizing pancreatitis from interstitial pancreatitis in a number of studies [28, 77, 95, 106, 129], but it usually takes 2 days to reach maximal CRP levels, and raised CRP levels in patients with pancreatic necrosis are not present until the 4th day [59].

Measurements of *catalytic phospholipase A* activity [17, 27], *trypsinogen activation peptide* [50], *granulocyte elastase* [37, 49, 124, 126], *pancreatitis-associated protein* [58], and *interleukin-6* [85, 127], have been used to differentiate between interstitial and necrotic pancreatitis with considerable success. However, these methods are seldomly available outside specialized gastroenterological units.

Earlier studies have shown that methemalbumin is able to differentiate between hemorrhagic and interstitial pancreatitis, but false-positive results are possible [47, 76]. In acute pancreatitis, the detection of methemalbumin indicates hemorrhagic pancreatitis and the same risk of mortality and the development of complications as more than 4 Ranson's signs [79].

12.4.4
Imaging Procedures

A poor correlation exists between ultrasonographic findings and the clinical course as well as the diagnosis of necrotizing pancreatitis [20, 84].

The contrast-enhanced CT using simultaneous administration of oral and intravenous injection of contrast media gives the most accurate picture of damage of the pancreas in the course of acute pancreatitis and the local complication of the disease. The results correlate well with the prognosis of the disease [10, 11, 30, 110]. A CT grading has been developed by the Balthazar group for intra- and extrapancreatic changes due to pancreatitis and measuring the amount of necrosis (see Table 9.4) [10, 11].

There is a distinct correlation between lack of contrast enhancement and pancreatic necrosis [62]. However, sensitivity and specificity depend on the extent of necrosis, i.e., sensitivity and specificity are lower in minor necrotic areas [91]. False-positive results may be obtained when acute pancreatitis is superimposed on chronic pancreatitis involving areas of fibrosis, and false-negative results may be obtained when tests are performed early in the course of the disease [91]. Sepsis occurs more frequently among patients who have > 30% necrosis than among those with ≤ 30% [68]. The frequency of infection of pancreatic necrosis is directly correlated with the extent of such necrosis [15].

It is believed that the necessity for contrast-enhanced CT in case of acute pancreatitis should be reserved for severe cases [30, 88]. Furthermore, comparative studies have not shown the superiority of CT criteria over modified Imrie's criteria scores [87].

At present, it is controversial whether intravenous contrast medium can worsen acute necrotizing pancreatitis in animal experiments [44, 63, 67, 113]. A first analysis of the effect of contrast-enhanced CT on the outcome of acute pancreatitis was done retrospectively and failed to show any influence of the contrast medium [98].

When the course of clinical symptoms, serum enzymes, and CT were compared, it was found that the imaging procedure does not reflect the return to normal of symptoms and pancreatic enzymes. Even 3 months after discharge, 23% of patients have an abnormal Balthazar CT score, ranging between 1 and 3 points (Fig. 12.1) [75].

This confirms an earlier study showing that pathological findings in acute pancreatitis remain even though clinical symptoms have disappeared [72].

Based on the present studies, the use of CT in acute pancreatitis can be recommended [45]. A CT is recommended in patients with clinical severe acute pancreatitis (based on prognostic criteria, such as Ranson's signs or APACHE-II scores) who do not manifest rapid clinical improvement within 72 h of conservative medical treatment. It is further indicated in patients who have demonstrated clinical improvement, but then manifest an acute change in their clinical status, indicating a complication, e.g., fever, pain, inability to tolerate oral food intake, hypotension, etc.

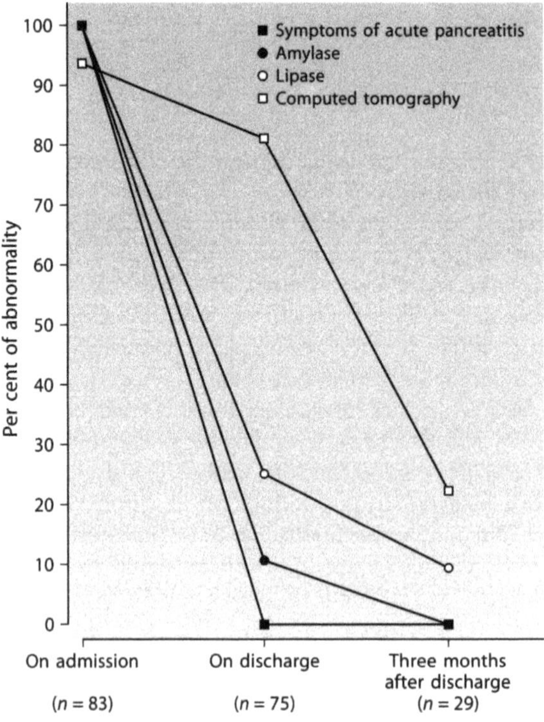

Fig. 12.1. Course of symptoms, serum amylase, lipase, and CT in patients with acute pancreatitis. One patient who was readmitted 3 months after discharge with acute pancreatitis, elevated enzymes, and normal CT was excluded. (From [75] with permission)

It should be noted, that an initially normal CT of the pancreas may become abnormal, that is, an initially normal CT does not necessarily indicate a good prognosis [75, 86].

Follow-up CTs should be done when the patient's clinical status suggests complications. Follow-up scans are recommended on day 7 to 10, when the initial scan has shown a Balthazar score between 3 and 10. Since important complications can develop without becoming clinically evident early on, e.g., notable evolution of a fluid collection into pseudocysts or development of an arterial pseudoaneurysm, a scan should be performed at the time of hospital discharge to confirm reasonable resolution of initial changes [5].

CT examinations may be beyond the scope of small hospitals. Therefore, the finding that pleural effusions and pulmonary infiltrates demonstrated on chest X-ray correlate well with the CT score, development of necrosis and pancreatic pseudocysts, and mortality rate, may be of help for these institutions [73, 74].

Dynamic contrast-enhanced magnetic resonance imaging (MRI) may be superior to CT. However, even if this could be confirmed in later studies, this type of imaging is of no clinical importance for small and medium-sized hospitals [83].

12.5
Systemic Complications

The development of systemic complications is associated with high mortality [61]. Whereas systemic complications may occur during the course of interstitial pancreatitis, they can usually be treated successfully with low mortality (see Sect. 10.2). An analysis of lethal complications of acute pancreatitis in 719 patients has shown that therapy should focus on the progression from respiratory failure to multiple organ system failures since mortality rises sharply, especially in the presence of pancreatic necrosis [51].

12.6
Mortality

Studies published during the last 5 decades (each with more than 100 patients) concerning the mortality rate among patients with acute pancreatitis show a decrease in mortality rate (Table 12.6) [70], probably due to the improvement of diagnosis of the disease and its complications and the development of intensive care therapy. Furthermore, endoscopy or surgery in biliary pancreatitis has decreased the mortality of this etiology [131].

In a recent survey from two German centers including 602 patients, mortality rate was 6.1% [70]. In another recent multicenter investigation of death from acute pancreatitis from the North-West Themse region for 631 patients, it was shown that mortality rate was 9%. 31% of the patients died within the first week, usually because of multisystem organ failure, 68% died after the first week of complications related to infection, comorbid conditions, or noninfected complications [92].

Table 12.6. Studies published during the last 5 decades with detailed data concerning the mortality rate of patients with acute pancreatitis [70]

Author(s)	Place of the investigation	Period	Patients (*n*)	Mortality rate (%)
Albo et al. [4]	San Francisco	1942–1961	133	25.0
Trapnell and Duncan [122]	Bristol	1950–1969	590	20.2
Krupp [66]	Basel	1952–1961	197	36.0
Black et al. [18]	Atlanta	1955–1964	250	23.0
Edlund et al. [39]	Göteborg	1956–1960	460	8.0
White et al. [128]	Seattle	1956–1965	358	12.0
Imrie [53]	Glasgow	1960–1970	140	21.4
Madsen and Schmidt [90]	Copenhagen	1960–1970	122	8.0
Jacobs et al. [61]	Boston	1963–1969	519	12.9
Satiani and Stone [112]	Atlanta	1966–1975	389	6.7
Lukash [89]	Bethesda	not mentioned	100	5.0
Ong et al. [101]	Hong Kong	1967–1976	311	9.6
Svensson et al. [118]	Göteborg	1968–1969	105	12.0
		1974–1975	204	3.0
Corfield et al. [32]	Bristol	1968–1979	638	19.6
Thomson [120]	Aberdeen	1968–1980	632	9.5
Olsen [100]	Oakland	1969–1970	100	6.0
Bourke et al. [21]	Nottingham	1969–1974	202	17.8
Buggy and Nostrant [25]	Michigan	1969–1979	410	7.8
Imrie and Blumgart [55]	Glasgow	1971–1974	191	11.0
Ranson and Spencer [109]	New York	1971–1977	450	7.1
Thomson et al. [121]	Aberdeen	1983–1985	359	7.8
Fan et al. [41]	Hong Kong	1983–1986	268	7.1
Fan et al. [40]	Hong Kong	1988–1991	176	6.0
Beaux et al. [14]	Edinburgh	1989–1993	279	6.1
Lankisch et al. [70]	Göttingen und Lüneburg	1980–1994	602	6.1
Total		1942–1994	8185	11.9

12.7
Late Morphological and Functional Consequences of the Pancreas

Although complete recovery of the pancreas after acute pancreatitis is still generally assumed, there are several mostly smaller studies using either direct [22, 38, 123] or indirect [48, 99] pancreatic function tests, that have reported a considerable percentage of patients with exocrine pancreatic insufficiency or permanent duct changes persisting for some time after acute pancreatitis attacks. Eventually, exocrine pancreatic insufficiency usually improves or returns to normal, whereas pancreatic duct changes are permanent [7, 8]. In 10% of patients, duct changes may be suggestive of obstructive or chronic pancreatitis. When patients were divided into those with alcohol- and biliary induced pancreatitis and evaluated on the basis of initial absence or presence of pancreatic necrosis, within 40 months, 95% of alcohol-induced and 81% of biliary induced pancreatitis still had morphological abnormalities upon imaging procedures. Up to 40 months later, in 91% of alcoholics, but in only 47% of the biliary patients, such abnormalities were still found. There were significantly more abnormal exocrine pancreatic function test results after alcoholic than biliary pancreatitis. A progression to chronic pancreatitis was not reported for these patients [26] but seems to be possible [6]. It is of practical importance to know that duct changes demonstrated by endoscopic retrograde cholangiopancreatography (ERCP) after acute pancreatitis may persist without any later signs and symptoms of acute or chronic pancreatitis [116].

After an acute attack of pancreatitis, pancreatic pseudocysts develop in 13%–18% of cases [69, 115]. Pancreatic pseudocysts occur more frequently in alcohol-induced pancreatitis [71]. However, patients with pancreatic pseudocysts caused by alcohol abuse had a more favorable prognosis than those with pseudocysts caused by preceding biliary acute pancreatitis in one study [56].

12.8
Quality of Life

There are only two studies concerning quality of life after acute pancreatitis. However, both show good long-term results, even after very severe acute pancreatitis [36, 43], thus justifying every therapeutic effort for these patients [29]. In the Finnish study [36], 65% of patients regained their full working capacity, and only 11% had to retire because of the complicated course of pancreatitis.

References

1. Abruzzo JL, Homa M, Houck JC, Coffey RJ (1958) Significance of the serum amylase determination. Ann Surg 147:921–930
2. Adams JT, Libertino JA, Schwartz SI (1968) Significance of an elevated serum amylase. Surgery 63:877–884
3. Agarwal N, Pitchumoni CS (1986) Simplified prognostic criteria in acute pancreatitis. Pancreas 1:69–73
4. Albo R, Silen W, Goldman L (1963) A critical clinical analysis of acute pancreatitis. Arch Surg 86:174–180
5. Alles AJ, Warshaw AL, Southern JF, Compton CC, Lewandrowski KB (1994) Expression of CA 72-4 (TAG-72) in the fluid contents of pancreatic cysts. A new marker to distinguish malignant pancreatic cystic tumors from benign neoplasms and pseudocysts. Ann Surg 219:131–134
6. Ammann RW, Muellhaupt B (1994) Progression of alcoholic acute to chronic pancreatitis. Gut 35:552–556
7. Angelini G, Cavallini G, Pederzoli P, Bovo P, Bassi C, Di Francesco V, Frulloni L, Sgarbi D, Talamini G, Castagnini A (1993) Long-term outcome of acute pancreatitis: a prospective study with 118 patients. Digestion 54:143–147
8. Angelini G, Pederzoli P, Caliari S, Fratton S, Brocco G, Marzoli G, Bovo P, Cavallini G, Scuro LA (1984) Long-term outcome of acute necrohemorrhagic pancreatitis. A 4-year follow-up. Digestion 30:131–137
9. Assmus C, Petersen M, Gottesleben F, Dröge M, Lankisch PG (1996) Epidemiology of acute pancreatitis in a defined German population. Digestion 57:217 (abstr)
10. Balthazar EJ, Ranson JHC, Naidich DP, Megibow AJ, Caccavale R, Cooper MM (1985) Acute pancreatitis: prognostic value of CT. Radiology 156:767–772
11. Balthazar EJ, Robinson DL, Megibow AJ, Ranson JHC (1990) Acute pancreatitis: value of CT in establishing prognosis. Radiology 174:331–336
12. Bank S, Wise L, Gersten M (1983) Risk factors in acute pancreatitis. Am J Gastroenterol 78:637–640

13. Banks PA (1995) Acute pancreatitis. In: Haubrich WS, Schaffner F, Berk JE (eds) Bockus Gastroenterology, vol. 4, 5th edn. W.B. Saunders Comp., Philadelphia-London-Toronto etc, pp 2888–2917
14. Beaux AC de, Palmer KR, Carter DC (1995) Factors influencing morbidity and mortality in acute pancreatitis; an analysis of 279 cases. Gut 37:121–126
15. Beger HG (1991) Surgery in acute pancreatitis. Hepatogastroenterology 38:92–96
16. Beger HG, Büchler M, Bittner R, Block S, Nevalainen T, Roscher R (1988) Necrosectomy and postoperative local lavage in necrotizing pancreatitis. Br J Surg 75:207–212
17. Bird NC, Goodman AJ, Johnson AG (1989) Serum phospholipase A2 activity in acute pancreatitis: an early guide to severity. Br J Surg 76:731–732
18. Black WS, Sutterfield TC, Martin JD Jr (1967) Acute pancreatitis. Am Surg 33:94–99
19. Blamey SL, Imrie CW, O'Neill J, Gilmour WH, Carter DC (1984) Prognostic factors in acute pancreatitis. Gut 25:1340–1346
20. Block S, Maier W, Clausen C, Büchler M, Malfertheiner P, Beger HG (1985) Diagnostik der nekrotisierenden Pankreatitis. Vergleich von Kontrastmittel-CT und Ultraschall in einer klinischen Studie. Dtsch Med Wochenschr 110:826–832
21. Bourke JB (1975) Variation in annual incidence of primary acute pancreatitis in Nottingham, 1969–74. Lancet 2:967–969
22. Bozkurt T, Maroske D, Adler G (1993) Exocrine pancreatic function after recovery from necrotizing pancreatitis. Hepatogastroenterology 40 (Suppl. I):60–64
23. Bradley III EL (1993) A clinically based classification system for acute pancreatitis. Summary of the International Symposium on Acute Pancreatitis, Atlanta, Ga, September 11 through 13, 1992. Arch Surg 128:586–590
24. Browder W, Patterson MD, Thompson JL, Walters DN (1993) Acute pancreatitis of unknown etiology in the elderly. Ann Surg 217:469–475
25. Buggy BP, Nostrant TT (1983) Lethal pancreatitis. Am J Gastroenterol 78:810–814
26. Büchler M, Hauke A, Malfertheiner P (1987) Follow-up after acute pancreatitis: morphology and function. In: Beger HG, Büchler M (eds) Acute Pancreatitis. Springer, Berlin–Heidelberg, pp 367–374
27. Büchler M, Malfertheiner P, Schädlich H, Nevalainen TJ, Friess H, Beger HG (1989) Role of phospholipase A_2 in human acute pancreatitis. Gastroenterology 97:1521–1526
28. Büchler M, Malfertheiner P, Schoetensack C, Uhl W, Scherbaum W, Beger HG (1986) Wertigkeit biochemischer und bildgebender Verfahren für Diagnose und Prognose der akuten Pankreatitis – Ergebnisse einer prospektiven klinischen Untersuchung. Z Gastroenterol 24:100–109
29. Carter DC (1993) Acute pancreatitis: the value of life. Br J Surg 80:1499–1500
30. Clavien P-A, Hauser H, Meyer P, Rohner A (1988) Value of contrast-enhanced computerized tomography in the early diagnosis and prognosis of acute pancreatitis. Am J Surg 155:457–466
31. Cooper MJ, Williamson RCN, Pollock AV (1982) The role of peritoneal lavage in the prediction and treatment of severe acute pancreatitis. Ann R C Surg Engl 64:422–425
32. Corfield AP, Cooper MJ, Williamson RCN (1985) Acute pancreatitis: a lethal disease of increasing incidence. Gut 26:724–729
33. Corfield AP, Cooper MJ, Williamson RCN, Mayer AD, McMahon MJ, Dickson AP, Shearer MG, Imrie CW (1985) Prediction of severity in acute pancreatitis: prospective comparison of three prognostic indices. Lancet 2:403–407
34. Demmy TL, Burch JM, Feliciano DV, Mattox KL, Jordan GL Jr (1988) Comparison of multiple-parameter prognostic systems in acute pancreatitis. Am J Surg 156:492–496
35. Dickson AP, Imrie CW (1984) The incidence and prognosis of body wall ecchymosis in acute pancreatitis. Surg Gynecol Obstet 159:343–347
36. Doepel M, Eriksson J, Halme L, Kumpulainen T, Höckerstedt K (1993) Good long-term results in patients surviving severe acute pancreatitis. Br J Surg 80:1583–1586
37. Domínguez-Muñoz JE, Carballo F, García MJ, de Diego JM, Gea F, Yangüela J, de la Morena J (1993) Monitoring of serum proteinase-antiproteinase balance and systemic inflammatory response in prognostic evaluation of acute pancreatitis. Results of a prospective multicenter study. Dig Dis Sci 38:507–513
38. Dormeyer HH, Neher M, Schönborn H, Röhrich H, Prellwitz W, Dennebaum R, Braun B, Baas U, Kümmerle F (1979) Langzeitergebnisse nach operativer Therapie der akuten hämorrhagisch-

nekrotisierenden Pankreatitis. Unter besonderer Berücksichtigung der endokrinen und exokrinen Pankreasfunktion. Dtsch Med Wochenschr 104:1670–1673
39. Edlund Y, Norbäck B, Risholm L (1968) Acute pancreatitis, etiology and prevention of recurrence. Follow-up study of 188 patients. Rev Surg 25:153–157
40. Fan S-T, Lai ECS, Mok FPT, Lo C-M, Zheng S-S, Wong J (1993) Prediction of the severity of acute pancreatitis. Am J Surg 166:262–269
41. Fan ST, Choi TK, Lai CS, Wong J (1988) Influence of age on the mortality from acute pancreatitis. Br J Surg 75:463–466
42. Fan ST, Choi TK, Lai ECS, Wong J (1989) Prediction of severity of acute pancreatitis: an alternative approach. Gut 30:1591–1595
43. Fenton-Lee D, Imrie CW (1993) Pancreatic necrosis: assessment of outcome related to quality of life and cost of management. Br J Surg 80:1579–1582
44. Foitzik T, Bassi DG, Schmidt J, Lewandrowski KB, Fernandez-del Castillo C, Rattner DW, Warshaw AL (1994) Intravenous contrast medium accentuates the severity of acute necrotizing pancreatitis in the rat. Gastroenterology 106:207–214
45. Freeny PC (1993) Incremental dynamic bolus computed tomography of acute pancreatitis. Int J Pancreatol 13:147–158
46. Funnell IC, Bornman PC, Weakley SP, Terblanche J, Marks IN (1993) Obesity: an important prognostic factor in acute pancreatitis. Br J Surg 80:484–486
47. Geokas MC, Rinderknecht H, Walberg CB, Weissman R (1974) Methemalbumin in the diagnosis of acute hemorrhagic pancreatitis. Ann Intern Med 81:483–486
48. Glasbrenner B, Büchler M, Uhl W, Malfertheiner P (1992) Exocrine pancreatic function in the early recovery phase of acute oedematous pancreatitis. Eur J Gastroenterol Hepatol 4:563–567
49. Gross V, Schölmerich J, Leser H-G, Salm R, Lausen M, Rückauer K, Schöffel U, Lay L, Heinisch A, Farthmann EH, Gerok W (1990) Granulocyte elastase in assessment of severity of acute pancreatitis. Comparison with acute-phase proteins, C-reactive protein, α_1-antitrypsin, and protease inhibitor α_2-macroglobulin. Dig Dis Sci 35:97–105
50. Gudgeon AM, Heath DI, Hurley P, Jehanli A, Patel G, Wilson C, Shenkin A, Austen BM, Imrie CW, Hermon-Taylor J (1990) Trypsinogen activation peptides assay in the early prediction of severity of acute pancreatitis. Lancet 335:4–8
51. Heath D, Alexander D, Wilson C, Larvin M, Imrie CW (1995) Which complications of acute pancreatitis are most lethal? A prospective multicentre clinical study of 719 episodes. Gut 36:A478 (abstr)
52. Heath DI, Imrie CW (1994) The Hong Kong criteria and severity prediction in acute pancreatitis. Int J Pancreatol 15:179–185
53. Imrie CW (1974) Observations on acute pancreatitis. Br J Surg 61:539–544
54. Imrie CW, Benjamin IS, Ferguson JC, McKay AJ, Mackenzie I, O'Neill J, Blumgart LH (1978) A single-centre double-blind trial of Trasylol therapy in primary acute pancreatitis. Br J Surg 65:337–341
55. Imrie CW, Blumgart LH (1975) Acute pancreatitis: a prospective study on some factors in mortality. Bull Soc Int Chir 34:601–603
56. Imrie CW, Buist LJ, Shearer MG (1988) Importance of cause in the outcome of pancreatic pseudocysts. Am J Surg 156:159–162
57. Imrie CW, Ferguson JC, Murphy D, Blumgart LH (1977) Arterial hypoxia in acute pancreatitis. Br J Surg 64:185–188
58. Iovanna JL, Keim V, Nordback I, Montalto G, Camarena J, Letoublon C, Lévy P, Berthézène P, Dagorn J-C (1994) Serum levels of pancreatitis-associated protein as indicators of the course of acute pancreatitis. Gastroenterology 106:728–734
59. Isenmann R, Büchler M, Uhl W, Malfertheiner P, Martini M, Beger HG (1993) Pancreatic necrosis: an early finding in severe acute pancreatitis. Pancreas 8:358–361
60. Jaakkola M, Sillanaukee P, Löf K, Koivula T, Nordback I (1994) Amount of alcohol is an important determinant of the severity of acute alcoholic pancreatitis. Surgery 115:31–38
61. Jacobs ML, Daggett WM, Civetta JM, Vasu MA, Lawson DW, Warshaw AL, Nardi GL, Bartlett MK (1977) Acute pancreatitis: analysis of factors influencing survival. Ann Surg 185:43–51
62. Johnson CD, Stephens DH, Sarr MG (1991) CT of acute pancreatitis: correlation between lack of contrast enhancement and pancreatic necrosis. Am J Roentgenol 156:93–95

63. Kaiser AM, Grady T, Gerdes D, Saluja M, Steer ML (1995) Intravenous contrast medium does not increase the severity of acute necrotizing pancreatitis in the opossum. Dig Dis Sci 40:1547–1553
64. Karimgani I, Porter KA, Langevin RE, Banks PA (1992) Prognostic factors in sterile pancreatic necrosis. Gastroenterology 103:1636–1640
65. Knaus WA, Draper EA, Wagner DP, Zimmerman JE (1985) APACHE II: a severity of disease classification system. Critical Care Med 13:818–829
66. Krupp S (1963) Die Pancreatitis. Ätiologie, Alters- und Geschlechtsverteilung, Therapie und Mortalität an Hand von 361 Fällen. Helv Chir Acta 30:367–400
67. Kusske AM, Patel AG, Toyama MT, Reber PU, Ashley SW, Reber HA (1995) Intravenous contrast does not effect the severity of experimental acute hemorrhagic pancreatitis. Gastroenterology 108:A368 (abstr)
68. Laccetti M, Rabitti PG, Manes G, Picciotto FP, Esposito P, Uomo G (1993) Relationship between the extent of pancreatic necrosis and sepsis in acute pancreatitis. Results of a prospective study. Eur J Gastroenterol Hepatol 5:871–873
69. Lankisch PG, Assmus C, Petersen M, Gottesleben F, Dröge M (1995) Epidemiology of acute pancreatitis in a defined German population. Pancreas 11:437 (abstr)
70. Lankisch PG, Burchard-Reckert S, Petersen M, Lehnick D, Schirren CA, Köhler H, Stöckmann F, Peiper HJ, Creutzfeldt W (1996) Morbidity and mortality in 602 patients with acute pancreatitis seen between the years 1980–1994. Z Gastroenterol 34:371–377
71. Lankisch PG, Burchard-Reckert S, Petersen M, Lehnick D, Schirren CA, Stöckmann F, Köhler H (1996) Etiology and age have only a limited influence on the course of acute pancreatitis. Pancreas 13:344–349
72. Lankisch PG, Buschmann-Kaspari H, Otto J, Schröder K, Koop H (1990) Correlation of pancreatic enzyme levels with the patient's recovery from acute edematous pancreatitis. Klin Wochenschr 68:565–569
73. Lankisch PG, Dröge M, Becher R (1994) Pleural effusions: a new negative prognostic parameter for acute pancreatitis. Am J Gastroenterol 89:1849–1851
74. Lankisch PG, Dröge M, Becher R (1996) Pulmonary infiltrations. Sign of severe acute pancreatitis. Int J Pancreatol 19:113–115
75. Lankisch PG, Haseloff M, Becher R (1994) No parallel between the biochemical course of acute pancreatitis and morphologic findings. Pancreas 9:240–243
76. Lankisch PG, Koop H, Otto J, Oberdieck U (1978) Evaluation of methaemalbumin in acute pancreatitis. Scand J Gastroenterol 13:975–978
77. Lankisch PG, Petersen M, Gottesleben F (1994) High, not low, amylase and lipase levels indicate severe acute pancreatitis. Z Gastroenterol 32:213–215
78. Lankisch PG, Schirren CA (1990) Increased body weight as a prognostic parameter for complications in the course of acute pancreatitis. Pancreas 5:626–629
79. Lankisch PG, Schirren CA, Otto J (1989) Methemalbumin in acute pancreatitis: an evaluation of its prognostic value and comparison with multiple prognostic parameters. Am J Gastroenterol 84:1391–1395
80. Larvin M, Chalmers AG, McMahon MJ (1990) Dynamic contrast enhanced computed tomography: a precise technique for identifying and localising pancreatic necrosis. Br Med J 300:1425–1428
81. Larvin M, Chalmers AG, Robinson PJ, McMahon MJ (1989) Debridement and closed cavity irrigation for the treatment of pancreatic necrosis. Br J Surg 76:465–471
82. Larvin M, McMahon MJ (1989) APACHE-II score for assessment and monitoring acute pancreatitis. Lancet 2:201–205
83. Larvin M, Ward J, Robinson PJ, Chalmers AG, McMahon MJ (1995) Dynamic contrast enhanced magnetic resonance imaging is superior to dynamic computed tomography in acute pancreatitis. Gut 36:A478 (abstr)
84. Lees WR (1986) Ultrasound in acute pancreatitis. In: Malfertheiner P, Ditschuneit H (eds) Diagnostic Procedures in Pancreatic Disease. Springer, Berlin-Heidelberg, pp 21–31
85. Leser H-G, Gross V, Scheibenbogen C, Heinisch A, Salm R, Lausen M, Rückauer K, Andreesen R, Farthmann EH, Schölmerich J (1991) Elevation of serum interleukin-6 concentration precedes acute-phase response and reflects severity in acute pancreatitis. Gastroenterology 101:782–785

86. London NJM, Neoptolemos JP, Lavelle J, Bailey I, James D (1989) Serial computed tomography scanning in acute pancreatitis: a prospective study. Gut 30:397–403

87. London NJM, Neoptolemos JP, Lavelle J, Bailey I, James D (1989) Contrast-enhanced abdominal computed tomography scanning and prediction of severity of acute pancreatitis: a prospective study. Br J Surg 76:268–272

88. Lucarotti ME, Virjee J, Alderson D (1993) Patient selection and timing of dynamic computed tomography in acute pancreatitis. Br J Surg 80:1393–1395

89. Lukash WM (1967) Complications of acute pancreatitis. Unusual sequelae in 100 cases. Arch Surg 94:848–852

90. Madsen OG, Schmidt A (1979) Acute pancreatitis. A study of 122 patients with acute pancreatitis observed for 5–15 years. World J Surg 3:345–352

91. Malfertheiner P, Domínguez-Muñoz JE (1993) Prognostic factors in acute pancreatitis. Int J Pancreatol 14:1–8

92. Mann DV, Hershman MJ, Hittinger R, Glazer G (1994) Multicentre audit of death from acute pancreatitis. Br J Surg 81:890–893

93. Martini M, Büchler M, Uhl W, Malfertheiner P, Friess H, Beger HG (1990) Etiology is not a prognostic factor in acute pancreatitis. Digestion 46:159 (abstr)

94. Mayer AD, McMahon MJ (1985) The diagnostic and prognostic value of peritoneal lavage in patients with acute pancreatitis. Surg Gynecol Obstet 160:507–512

95. Mayer AD, McMahon MJ, Bowen M, Cooper EH (1984) C reactive protein: an aid to assessment and monitoring of acute pancreatitis. J Clin Pathol 37:207–211

96. McMahon MJ, Pickford IR, Playforth MJ (1980) Early prediction of severity of acute pancreatitis using peritoneal lavage. Acta Chir Scand 146:171–175

97. McMahon MJ, Playforth MJ, Pickford IR (1980) A comparative study of methods for the prediction of severity of attacks of acute pancreatitis. Br J Surg 67:22–25

98. McMenamin DA, Gates LK (1995) Retrospective analysis of the effect of contrast enhanced CT on the outcome of acute pancreatitis. Gastroenterology 108:A374 (abstr)

99. Mitchell CJ, Playforth MJ, Kelleher J, McMahon MJ (1983) Functional recovery of the exocrine pancreas after acute pancreatitis. Scand J Gastroenterol 18:5–8

100. Olsen H (1974) Pancreatitis. A prospective clinical evaluation of 100 cases and review of the literature. Am J Dig Dis 19:1077–1090

101. Ong GB, Lam KH, Lam SK, Lim TK, Wong J (1979) Acute pancreatitis in Hong Kong. Br J Surg 66:398–403

102. Osborne DH, Imrie CW, Carter DC (1981) Biliary surgery in the same admission for gallstone-associated acute pancreatitis. Br J Surg 68:758–761

103. Park J, Fromkes J, Cooperman M (1986) Acute pancreatitis in elderly patients. Pathogenesis and outcome. Am J Surg 152:638–642

104. Pickford IR, Blackett RL, McMahon MJ (1977) Early assessment of severity of acute pancreatitis using peritoneal lavage. Br Med J 2:1377–1379

105. Porter KA, Banks PA (1991) Obesity as a predictor of severity in acute pancreatitis. Int J Pancreatol 10:247–252

106. Puolakkainen P, Valtonen V, Paananen A, Schröder T (1987) C-reactive protein (CRP) and serum phospholipase A2 in the assessment of the severity of acute pancreatitis. Gut 28:764–771

107. Ranson JHC (1979) The timing of biliary surgery in acute pancreatitis. Ann Surg 189:654–663

108. Ranson JHC, Rifkind KM, Roses DF, Fink SD, Eng K, Spencer FC (1974) Prognostic signs and the role of operative management in acute pancreatitis. Surg Gynecol Obstet 139:69–81

109. Ranson JHC, Spencer FC (1978) The role of peritoneal lavage in severe acute pancreatitis. Ann Surg 187:565–575

110. Rotman N, Chevret S, Pezet D, Mathieu D, Trovero C, Cherqui D, Chastang C, Fagniez P-L, The French Association for Surgical Research (1994) Prognostic value of early computed tomographic scans in severe acute pancreatitis. J Am Coll Surg 179:538–544

111. Sankari M, Agarwal N, Pitchumoni CS (1994) Acute pancreatitis in the elderly. Gastroenterology 106:A320 (abstr)

112. Satiani B, Stone HH (1979) Predictability of present outcome and future recurrence in acute pancreatitis. Arch Surg 114:711–716

113. Schmidt J, Hotz HG, Foitzik T, Ryschich E, Buhr HJ, Warshaw AL, Herfarth C, Klar E (1995) Intravenous contrast medium aggravates the impairment of pancreatic microcirculation in necrotizing pancreatitis in the rat. Ann Surg 221:257–264
114. Schölmerich J, Heinisch A, Leser H-G (1993) Diagnostic approach to acute pancreatitis: diagnosis, assessment of etiology and prognosis. Hepatogastroenterology 40:531–537
115. Schulze S, Baden H, Brandenhoff P, Larsen T, Burcharth F (1986) Pancreatic pseudocysts during first attack of acute pancreatitis. Scand J Gastroenterol 21:1221–1223
116. Seidensticker F, Otto J, Lankisch PG (1995) Recovery of the pancreas after acute pancreatitis is not necessarily complete. Int J Pancreatol 17:225–229
117. Stanten R, Frey CF (1990) Comprehensive management of acute necrotizing pancreatitis and pancreatic abscess. Arch Surg 125:1269–1275
118. Svensson J-O, Norbäck B, Bokey EL, Edlund Y (1979) Changing pattern in aetiology of pancreatitis in an urban Swedish area. Br J Surg 66:159–161
119. Teerenhovi O, Nordback I, Eskola J (1989) High volume lesser sac lavage in acute necrotizing pancreatitis. Br J Surg 76:370–373
120. Thomson HJ (1985) Acute pancreatitis in North and North-East Scotland. J R Coll Surg Edinb 30:104–110
121. Thomson SR, Hendry WS, McFarlane GA, Davidson AI (1987) Epidemiology and outcome of acute pancreatitis. Br J Surg 74:398–401
122. Trapnell JE, Duncan EHL (1975) Patterns of incidence in acute pancreatitis. Br Med J 2:179–183
123. Tympner F, Domschke W, Rösch W, Koch H, Demling L (1976) Verlauf der hydrokinetischen und ekbolen Pankreasfunktion nach akuter Pankreatitis. Z Gastroenterol 14:684–687
124. Uhl W, Büchler M, Malfertheiner P, Martini M, Beger HG (1991) PMN-elastase in comparison with CRP, antiproteases, and LDH as indicators of necrosis in human acute pancreatitis. Pancreas 6:253–259
125. Uhl W, Isenmann R, Curti G, Vogel R, Beger HG, Büchler MW (1996) Influence of etiology on the course and outcome of acute pancreatitis. Pancreas 13:335–343
126. Viedma JA, Pérez-Mateo M, Agulló J, Domínguez JE, Carballo F (1994) Inflammatory response in the early prediction of severity in human acute pancreatitis. Gut 35:822–827
127. Viedma JA, Pérez-Mateo M, Domínguez JE, Carballo F (1992) Role of interleukin-6 in acute pancreatitis. Comparison with C-reactive protein and phospholipase A. Gut 33:1264–1267
128. White TT, Murat JE, Morgan A (1968) Pancreatitis I. Review of 733 cases of pancreatitis from three Seattle hospitals. Northwest Med 67:374–378
129. Wilson C, Heads A, Shenkin A, Imrie CW (1989) C-reactive protein, antiproteases and complement factors as objective markers of severity in acute pancreatitis. Br J Surg 76:177–181
130. Wilson C, Heath DI, Imrie CW (1990) Prediction of outcome in acute pancreatitis: a comparative study of APACHE II, clinical assessment and multiple factor scoring systems. Br J Surg 77:1260–1264
131. Wilson C, Imrie CW, Carter DC (1988) Fatal acute pancreatitis. Gut 29:782–788
132. Winslet M, Hall C, London NJM, Neoptolemos JP (1992) Relation of diagnostic serum amylase levels to aetiology and severity of acute pancreatitis. Gut 33:982–986

13 Chronic Pancreatitis: Etiology

In most of the industrialized countries of the world, alcohol is the major etiological factor in the development of chronic pancreatitis. Gallstones, although a frequent cause of acute pancreatitis, almost never lead to chronic pancreatitis. There are other defined causes that make up a small proportion of cases (Table 13.1).

When the whole world is considered, tropical pancreatitis ranks as a major cause of chronic pancreatitis.

13.1
Alcohol-induced Chronic Pancreatitis

The increase in frequency of chronic pancreatitis in the industrialized countries parallels a marked increase in alcohol consumption [83].

A linear relation between alcohol consumption and the logarithmic risk for chronic pancreatitis has been demonstrated [23] (Fig. 13.1). Neither the type of alcoholic beverage nor the frequency of consumption (daily or only weekends) appear to have an influence on the development of chronic pancreatitis [73].

In contrast to the liver, the pancreas has no threshold for alcohol toxicity, although pancreatic sensitivity to alcohol seems to be greater in women than in men [23].

Table 13.1. Types and causes of chronic pancreatitis

- Alcohol-induced chronic pancreatitis
- Idiopathic pancreatitis (juvenile form? senile form?)
- Tropical pancreatitis
- Hereditary diseases of the pancreas
  Hereditary pancreatitis
  Cystic fibrosis?
- Obstructive chronic pancreatitis
- Congenital abnormalities
  Pancreas divisum
  Annular pancreas
  Ectopic pancreas
- Hyperparathyroidism
- Stress
- Radiation therapy
- Drugs

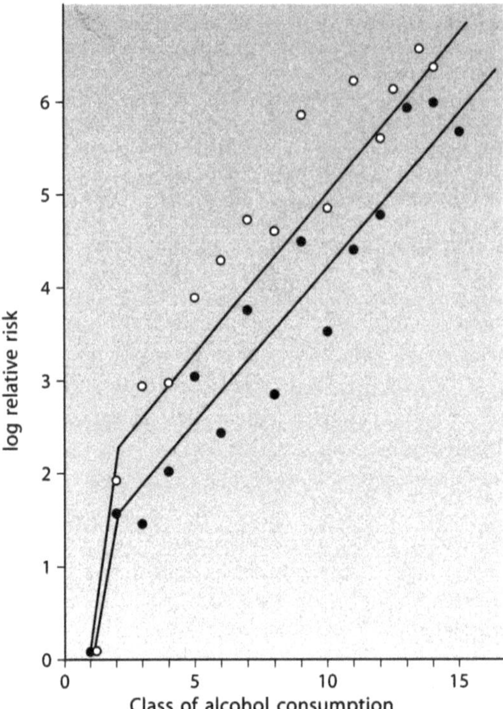

Fig. 13.1. Graphic representation of the log-relative risk as a function of alcohol consumption classes. International survey: lower line, estimated; closed circles, observed. Marseille survey: upper line, estimated; open circles, observed. (From [23] with permission)

Recently, a more rapid absorption of alcohol was demonstrated for women [30]. However, a significant association betweeen chronic pancreatitis and alcohol consumption was only found for men and not for women [84]. Consequently, the major cause of chronic pancreatitis may be different for men and women [21].

Although there is no doubt that alcohol is the major etiological factor behind chronic pancreatitis, it is still unclear why the majority of heavy drinkers do not develop chronic pancreatitis. It has been hypothesized that a diet high in fat and protein predisposes persons with high alcohol consumption to pancreatitis [23, 70, 73]. Both high (≥ 100 g/d) and low (≤ 85 g/d) consumption of fat are reported to be risk factors. However, this has not been confirmed in recent years for France, for the United States, and for Australia [55, 58, 67, 82].

Many alcoholics smoke, but a strong association between chronic pancreatitis and smoking cigarettes has been found only in men [10, 84]. Smokers have an increased risk of developing calcifications in chronic pancreatitis [19]. A recent multidimensional case-control study of dietary, alcohol, and tobacco habits in alcoholic men with chronic pancreatitis, however, showed the main predisposing or associated factor is a high caloric proportion of fat and protein intake. Type and quantity of alcohol, tobacco, and vitamins do not seem to play an important role [50].

Searches for human leukocyte antigens in patients with alcohol-induced chronic pancreatitis have shown both overrepresentation and underrepresentation of certain antigens [9, 27, 28, 33, 37, 42, 44], but no uniform picture has emerged.

α_1-antitrypsin deficiency [29, 56, 61] as well as antinuclear and pancreatic acinar cell antibodies [49, 60] have been proposed as additional etiological factors. However, large-scale studies have failed to prove this [45, 46, 68]. Furthermore, the incidence of antitissue antibodies is not higher in chronic pancreatitis as compared to cirrhosis [26].

13.2
Idiopathic Chronic Pancreatitis

Nonalcoholic chronic pancreatitis of unknown cause makes up 10%–30% of patients with chronic pancreatitis. Exocrine pancreatic insufficiency is said to develop less rapidly and calcifications are less frequently found in idiopathic than in alcohol-induced chronic pancreatitis [3].

Two subgroups have been reported: a juvenile and a senile form. The juvenile form is characterized by a mean age of about 25 years at the onset of symptoms, a painful clinical course, and an equal sex distribution [1]. Several other reports also seem to indicate that juvenile chronic pancreatitis is a special case [7, 25, 52, 79].

By contrast, manifestation of the senile form does not become clinically evident until the age of about 62 years, men predominate, the clinical course is mostly painless, and vascular disease is frequent [2].

13.3
Tropical Pancreatitis

A nonalcoholic form of chronic calcifying pancreatitis in tropical countries that has been observed mostly in children and young adults has been attributed at least in part to childhood malnutrition. The disease has been referred to in the literature as tropical pancreatitis, tropical calcific pancreatitis, nutritional pancreatitis, juvenile tropical pancreatitis syndrome, or fibrocalcific pancreatic diabetes [66].

The frequency of main symptoms such as pain, diabetes, and pancreatic calcifications is similar in alcoholic and tropical pancreatitis [20], although the etiologies differ.

At present, it cannot be explained why cases of tropical pancreatitis are concentrated in only certain geographic areas of a country, while kwashiorkor is seen throughout all regions. Micronutrient deficiencies and dietary toxins have been postulated as additional causes [64, 65]. In Kerala (India) and in southern parts of Nigeria, the tuber Manihot exculenta (cassava or tapioca) is consumed in large quantities as a staple in the diet. The hydrocyanic acid content of cassava is alleged to cause pancreatic injury. According to the oxidative stress concept for the development of chronic pancreatitis, cyanogens induce free radicals and deplete the scavenging enzymes. Evaluation of the micronutrient antioxidant status in the tropics has shown that the availability of β-carotene and ascorbic acid was low. It was suggested that culinary practices that erode the biological availabilities of both may predispose to pancreatic oxidative stress [13].

However, there is no direct clinical or experimental evidence to suggest that cassava causes chronic pancreatitis, and the etiology of tropical pancreatitis remains unknown [4, 59, 64, 66].

13.4
Hereditary Diseases of the Pancreas

13.4.1
Hereditary Pancreatitis

Only the characteristic onset at a young age and its autosomal-like propagation distinguishes it from other types of chronic pancreatitis (see Sect. 21.2.1).

13.4.2
Cystic Fibrosis

Recurrent pancreatitis may appear in some patients with cystic fibrosis [74]. It remains an open question whether these patients truly have chronic pancreatitis [76] (see Sect. 21.1.1).

13.5
Congenital Abnormalities Including Pancreas Divisum

Pancreas divisum, the most frequent ductal abnormality of the pancreas, occurs when the dorsal and the ventral pancreatic ducts fail to fuse. As a consequence, secretion from the larger part of the gland, the dorsal part, drains through the lesser papilla; secretion from the smaller section of the gland, the ventral part, drains through the major papilla. The clinical relevance of pancreas divisum for acute pancreatitis is controversial, and chronic pancreatitis related to pancreas divisum is distinctly uncommon [6, 69] (see Sect. 1.2.2).

Chronic pancreatitis associated with annular pancreas has been described in a few cases [22, 32, 36].

Furthermore, one report describes calcification of ectopic pancreas, similar to that in chronic pancreatitis [31] (see Sect. 1.2.3).

13.6
Obstructive Chronic Pancreatitis

Obstructive chronic pancreatitis may occur secondary to congenital or acquired stricture of the pancreatic duct, for example, after the healing of necrotic pseudocyst [48], or arising from duct-obstructing benign or malignant tumors [35, 38, 54, 72, 75], or after the formation of a scar between the head of the pancreas and the duodenum (i.e., groove pancreatitis) [5].

In recent years, an unusual dysplastic lesion of pancreatic ducts has been diagnosed with increasing frequency [53, 78]. A variety of names has been applied to this condition, including mucinous ductal ectasia, intraductal papillary-mucinous tumor, and intraductal mucin-hypersecreting neoplasm. This disorder originates from dysplastic pancreatic ductal epithelium, which secretes a copious amount of mucin. This is considered to be a precancerous lesion, and at the time of diagnosis at surgery, approximately 20%–30% have been found to be associated with invasive adenocarcinoma. The tumor is less aggressive than primary pancreatic ductal adenocarcinoma. The majority of patients have been elderly men who have experienced recurrent abdominal pain or episodes consistent with acute pancreatitis (including increases of serum amylase and lipase). Occasionally, patients have presented with evidence of exocrine pancreatic insufficiency.

Mucinous ductal ectasia is characterized on ultrasound and computed tomography (CT) scan by the presence of a markedly dilated main pancreatic duct which exhibits cystic features involving either a portion of the pancreas or the entire pancreas. At endoscopic retrograde cholangiopancreatography (ERCP), the ampulla is often markedly enlarged and distended by intraductal mucin. The orifice of the ampulla is frequently patulous, and thick mucinous material can be seen to extravasate from the ampulla either spontaneously or after gentle probing of the ampulla. Injection of contrast material may be very difficult because of the presence of thick mucin. ERCP shows either diffuse or segmental dilatation of the main pancreatic duct and the presence of amorphous intraductal filling defects caused by the presence of tenacious mucin. Cytologic examination of brush biopsy specimens may show the presence of malignant cells. Even if malignant cells are not present, it is not possible to know for sure whether malignant degeneration has already occurred. Because the condition is premalignant and may already be malignant at the time of investigation, the treatment of choice is surgical. If abnormalities on CT scan or ERCP provide evidence that the tumor is confined to the head or tail of the pancreas, either removal of the head of the gland (Whipple's operation) or distal pancreatectomy should be performed. When precise localization is uncertain by CT scan and ERCP, such as when there is diffuse dilatation of the main pancreatic duct, the treatment of choice is a total pancreatectomy in a patient whose general health permits extensive surgery [53].

13.7
Drug-induced Chronic Pancreatitis

A number of different drugs have been said to induce acute pancreatitis (see Sect. 5.5). Only a few case reports on patients treated with phenacetin [34], antihypertensive [81], and anticonvulsant drugs [62, 80] indicate that drugs may initiate chronic pancreatitis, too.

Some reports have also shown that occupational exposure to volatile gases is common among patients with idiopathic chronic pancreatitis. That this may be linked to chronic stimulation of cytochrome P450 (oxidative stress concept; see Sects. 6.4, 14.3) has been discussed [11, 12, 14, 24].

Further parallel studies on pathophysiology of chronic pancreatitis and environmental medicine are necessary.

13.8
Stress-induced Chronic Pancreatitis

Animal experiments have suggested that stress may play some role in the development of chronic pancreatitis [39–41, 77].

To determine whether the social class differences in chronic pancreatitis frequency may be explained by differences in physical activity at work, Breuer-Katschinski et al. [15] examined in a case-control study the effect of energy expenditure during work aside from smoking, alcohol intake, and social class. A high level of physical activity was found to be an independent risk factor for chronic pancreatitis apart from smoking and alcohol intake. The high risk among low social classes was accounted for by the energy expenditure during work, another form of stress. Further studies are required.

13.9
Radiation-induced Chronic Pancreatitis

Irradiation on the pancreas leads to progressive exocrine pancreatic insufficiency and histological changes of the pancreas compatible with a finding of chronic pancreatitis [63].

More than 70 years ago, atrophy of the acini and degeneration and necrosis of duct cells of the pancreas were described in patients who had experienced hepatic radiation injury [18]. Brick [16] described pancreatic fibrosis in young men who had received high-dose radiation for testicular tumors. Mitchell et al. [57] first discussed radiation pancreatitis as a clinical entity. More recently, additional patients with chronic pancreatitis very likely due to prior radiation therapy have been reported [17, 71]. A vascular process of the pancreas following radiotherapy for tumors in the neighborhood of the pancreas is regarded as the underlying pathogenetic mechanism [51].

13.10
Hyperparathyroidism

Chronic pancreatitis is an infrequent complication of hyperparathyroidism, occurring in about 1.5%–1.7% of hyperparathyroidism cases [8, 43]; the same frequency rate applies to the occurrence of hyperparathyroisdism (1.5%) in patients with chronic pancreatitis [47].

References

1. Ammann R (1976) Die idiopathische "juvenile" chronische Pankreatitis. Zum Problem der Beziehungen zwischen idiopathischer und alkohol-induzierter chronischer Pankreatitis. Dtsch Med Wochenschr 101:1789–1794
2. Ammann R, Sulser H (1976) Die "senile" chronische Pankreatitis – eine neue nosologische Einheit? Beobachtungen an 38 Fällen. Hinweise auf eine vaskuläre Ursache und Beziehungen zur primär schmerzlosen chronischen Pankreatitis. Schweiz Med Wochenschr 106:429–437

3. Ammann RW, Buehler H, Muench R, Freiburghaus AW, Siegenthaler W (1987) Differences in the natural history of idiopathic (nonalcoholic) and alcoholic chronic pancreatitis. A comparative long-term study of 287 patients. Pancreas 2:368–377

4. Balakrishnan V, Sauniere JF, Hariharan M, Sarles H (1988) Diet, pancreatic function, and chronic pancreatitis in South India and France. Pancreas 3:30–35

5. Becker V, Mischke U (1991) Groove pancreatitis. Int J Pancreatol 10:173–182

6. Bernard JP, Sahel J, Giovannini M, Sarles H (1990) Pancreas divisum is a probable cause of acute pancreatitis: a report of 137 cases. Pancreas 5:248–254

7. Beshlian K, Ryan JA Jr (1986) Pancreatitis in teenagers. Am J Surg 152:133–138

8. Bess MA, Edis AJ, van Heerden JA (1980) Hyperparathyroidism and pancreatitis. Chance or a causal association? JAMA 243:246–247

9. Betuel H, Selman M, Vachon A (1980) Pancréatites chroniques. Liaisons avec les antigènes H.L.A. Nouv Presse Med 9:42

10. Bourliere M, Barthet M, Berthezene P, Durbec JP, Sarles H (1991) Is tobacco a risk factor for chronic pancreatitis and alcoholic cirrhosis? Gut 32:1392–1395

11. Braganza JM (1983) Pancreatic disease: a casualty of hepatic "detoxification"? Lancet 2:1000–1003

12. Braganza JM, Jolley JE, Lee WR (1986) Occupational chemicals and pancreatitis: a link? Int J Pancreatol 1:9–19

13. Braganza JM, Schofield D, Snehalatha C, Mohan V (1993) Micronutrient antioxidant status in tropical compared with temperate-zone chronic pancreatitis. Scand J Gastroenterol 28:1098–1104

14. Braganza JM (ed) (1991) The pathogenesis of pancreatitis: based on a symposium held on 15 November 1990 at the University of Manchester under the auspices of the Pancreatic Society of Great Britain and Ireland. Manchester University Press, Manchester–New York

15. Breuer-Katschinski BD, Bracht J, Tietjen-Harms S, Goebell H (1996) Physical activity at work and the risk of chronic pancreatitis. Eur J Gastroenterol Hepatol 8:399–402

16. Brick IB (1955) Effects of million volt irradiation on the gastrointestinal tract. Arch Intern Med 96:26–31

17. Burbige EJ, Tarder GL, Belber JP (1977) Malabsorption following radiation therapy. Am J Gastroenterol 67:589–592

18. Case JT, Warthin AS (1924) The occurrence of hepatic lesions in patients treated by intensive deep roentgen irradiation. Am J Roentgenol 12:27–46

19. Cavallini G, Talamini G, Vaona B, Bovo P, Filippini M, Rigo L, Angelini G, Vantini I, Riela A, Frulloni L, Di Francesco V, Brunori MP, Bassi C, Pederzoli P (1994) Effect of alcohol and smoking on pancreatic lithogenesis in the course of chronic pancreatitis. Pancreas 9:42–46

20. Chari ST, Mohan V, Jayanthi V, Snehalatha C, Malathi S, Viswanathan M, Madanagopalan N (1992) Comparative study of the clinical profiles of alcoholic chronic pancreatitis and tropical chronic pancreatitis in Tamil Nadu, South India. Pancreas 7:51–58

21. DiMagno EP, Layer P, Clain JE (1993) Chronic pancreatitis. In: Go VLW, DiMagno EP, Gardner JD, Lebenthal E, Reber HA, Scheele GA (eds) The Pancreas: Biology, Pathobiology, and Disease, 2nd edn. Raven Press, New York, pp 665–706

22. Dowsett JF, Rode J, Russell RCG (1989) Annular pancreas: a clinical, endoscopic, and immunohistochemical study. Gut 30:130–135

23. Durbec JP, Sarles H (1978) Multicenter survey of the etiology of pancreatic diseases. Relationship between the relative risk of developing chronic pancreatitis and alcohol, protein and lipid consumption. Digestion 18:337–350

24. Døssing M, Jacobsen O, Rasmussen SN (1985) Chronic pancreatitis possibly caused by occupational exposure to organic solvents. Human Toxicol 4:237–240

25. Elitsur Y, Siddiqui SY, Sloven D, Rossi T, Afshani E, Lebenthal E (1989) Chronic pancreatitis with diffuse fibrosis in early childhood. Pancreas 4:504–510

26. Emanuelli G, Tappero G, Iuliano R, Dughera L, Gaia E (1989) Antitissue antibodies in chronic pancreatitis. Digestion 44:79–85

27. Fauchet R, Genetet B, Gosselin M, Gastard J (1979) HLA antigens in chronic alcoholic pancreatitis. Tissue Antigens 13:163–166

28. Forbes A, Schwarz G, Mirakian R, Drummond V, Chan C-K, Cotton PB, Bottazzo GF (1987) HLA antigens in chronic pancreatitis. Tissue Antigens 30:176–183

29. Freeman HJ, Weinstein WM, Shnitka TK, Crockford PM, Herbert FA (1976) Alpha1-antitrypsin deficiency and pancreatic fibrosis. Ann Intern Med 85:73–76

30. Frezza M, di Padova C, Pozzato G, Terpin M, Baraona E, Lieber CS (1990) High blood alcohol levels in women. The role of decreased gastric alcohol dehydrogenase activity and first-pass metabolism. N Engl J Med 322:95–99

31. Gamroth A, Fenn K (1989) Verkalkende Pankreasheterotopie im Bereich der kleinen Kurvatur des Magenkorpus. Fortschr Röntgenstr 150:738–739

32. Gilinsky NH, Lewis JW, Flueck JA, Fried AM (1987) Annular pancreas associated with diffuse chronic pancreatitis. Am J Gastroenterol 82:681–684

33. Gosselin M, Fauchet R, Genetet B, Gastard J (1978) Les antigènes HLA dans la pancréatite chronique alcoolique. Gastroenterol Clin Biol 2:883–886

34. Hangartner PJ, Bühler H, Münch R, Zaruba K, Stamm B, Ammann R (1987) Chronische Pankreatitis als wahrscheinliche Folge eines Analgetikaabusus. Schweiz Med Wochenschr 117:638–642

35. Heller SJ, Ferrari AP, Carr-Locke DL, Lichtenstein DR, Van Dam J, Banks PA (1996) Pancreatic duct stricture caused by islet cell tumors. Am J Gastroenterol 91:147–149

36. Itoh Y, Hada T, Terano A, Itai Y, Harada T (1989) Pancreatitis in the annulus of annular pancreas demonstrated by the combined use of computed tomography and endoscopic retrograde cholangiopancreatography. Am J Gastroenterol 84:961–964

37. Jalleh RP, Gilbertson JA, Williamson RCN, Slater SD, Foster CS (1993) Expression of major histocompatibility antigens in human chronic pancreatitis. Gut 34:1452–1457

38. Kahrilas PJ, Hogan WJ, Geenen JE, Stewart ET, Dodds WJ, Arndorfer RC (1987) Chronic recurrent pancreatitis secondary to a submucosal ampullary tumor in a patient with neurofibromatosis. Dig Dis Sci 32:102–107

39. Kaplan MH (1985) Stress, pancreatic perfusion, and acute pancreatitis: a unified concept of pathogenesis. Mt Sinai J Med 52:326–330

40. Kaplan MH (1986) Pathogenesis of pancreatitis: a unified concept. Int J Pancreatol 1:5–8

41. Kaplan MH, Wheeler WF, Kelly MJ (1983) Stress and diseases of the upper gut: II. Stress and pancreatic disease. Mt Sinai J Med 50:331–334

42. Keidar S, Teitelman U, Porath EB, Brook G, Naftali V (1987) Acute pancreatitis associated with rising cytomegalovirus titer. Israel J Med Sci 23:296–297

43. Koppelberg T, Bartsch D, Printz H, Hasse C, Rothmund M (1994) Die Pankreatitis beim primären Hyperparathyreoidismus (pHPT) ist eine Komplikation des fortgeschrittenen pHPT. Dtsch Med Wochenschr 119:719–724

44. Lankisch PG, Hierholzer E, Koop H, Kaboth U, Koch HF, Brunner E (1980) HLA-antigens in acute and chronic pancreatitis. Z Gastroenterol 18:524–526

45. Lankisch PG, Koop H, Seelig R, Seelig HP (1981) Antinuclear and pancreatic acinar cell antibodies in pancreatic diseases. Digestion 21:65–68

46. Lankisch PG, Koop H, Winckler K, Kaboth U (1978) a1-Antitrypsin in pancreatic diseases. Digestion 18:138–140

47. Lankisch PG, Löhr-Happe A, Otto J, Creutzfeldt W (1993) Natural course in chronic pancreatitis. Pain, exocrine and endocrine pancreatic insufficiency and prognosis of the disease. Digestion 54:148–155

48. Laugier R, Camatte R, Sarles H (1983) Chronic obstructive pancreatitis after healing of a necrotic pseudocyst. Am J Surg 146:551–557

49. Lendrum R, Walker G (1975) Serum antibodies in human pancreatic disease. Gut 16:365–371

50. Lévy P, Mathurin P, Roqueplo A, Rueff B, Bernades P (1995) A multidimensional case-control study of dietary, alcohol, and tobacco habits in alcoholic men with chronic pancreatitis. Pancreas 10:231–238

51. Lévy P, Menzelxhiu A, Paillot B, Bretagne JF, Fléjou JF, Bernades P (1993) Abdominal radiotherapy is a cause for chronic pancreatitis. Gastroenterology 105:905–909

52. Little JM, Tait N, Richardson A, Dubois R (1992) Chronic pancreatitis beginning in childhood and adolescence. Arch Surg 127:90–92

53. Loftus EV Jr, Olivares-Pakzak BA, Batts KP, Adkins MC, Stephens DH, Sarr MG, DiMagno EP, Members of the Pancreas Clinic, Pancreatic Surgeons of Mayo Clinic (1996) Intraductal papillary-mucinous tumors of the pancreas: clinicopathologic features, outcome, and nomenclature. Gastroenterology 110:1909–1918

54. Mathai V, Banerjee Jesudason SR, Muthusami JC, Kuruvilla R, Idikula J, Sada P (1994) Chronic pancreatitis caused by intraductal hydatic cysts of the pancreas. Br J Surg 81:1029
55. Mezey E, Kolman CJ, Diehl AM, Mitchell MC, Herlong HF (1988) Alcohol and dietary intake in the development of chronic pancreatitis and liver disease in alcoholism. Am J Clin Nutr 48:148–151
56. Mihas AA, Hirschowitz BI (1976) Alpha1-antitrypsin and chronic pancreatitis. Lancet 2:1032–1033
57. Mitchell CJ, Simpson FG, Davison AM, Losowsky MS (1979) Radiation pancreatitis: a clinical entity? Digestion 19:134–136
58. Montalto G, Cambon P, Bernard JP, Durbec JP, Sarles H (1992) Chronic pancreatitis in southern France. Evolution of dietary habits and natural history. Frequency of liver cirrhosis and other histological changes. Eur J Gastroenterol Hepatol 4:733–738
59. Narendranathan M, Cheriyan A (1994) Lack of association between cassava consumption and tropical pancreatitis syndrome. J Gastroenterol Hepatol 9:282–285
60. Neher M, Lemmel EM (1975) Antinukleäre Faktoren bei Patienten mit Pankreatitis "unklarer Ätiologie". Hinweis auf immunpathologische Genese? Dtsch Med Wochenschr 100:362–367
61. Novis BH, Young GO, Bank S, Marks IN (1975) Chronic pancreatitis and a1-antitrypsin. Lancet 2:748–749
62. Pezzilli R, Billi P, Melandri R, Broccoli PL, Fontana G (1992) Anticonvulsant-induced chronic pancreatitis. A case report. Ital J Gastroenterol 24:245–246
63. Pieroni PL, Rudick J, Adler M, Nacchiero M, Rybak BJ, Perlberg HJ Jr, Dreiling DA (1976) Effect of irradiation on the canine exocrine pancreas. Ann Surg 184:610–614
64. Pitchumoni CS (1984) Special problems of tropical pancreatitis. Clin Gastroenterol 13:941–959
65. Pitchumoni CS, Jain NK, Lowenfels AB, DiMagno EP (1988) Chronic cyanide poisoning: unifying concept for alcoholic and tropical pancreatitis. Pancreas 3:220–222
66. Pitchumoni CS, Scheele GA (1993) Interdependence of nutrition and exocrine pancreatic function. In: Go VLW, DiMagno EP, Gardner JD, Lebenthal E, Reber HA, Scheele GA (eds) The Pancreas: Biology, Pathobiology, and Disease, 2nd edn. Raven Press, New York, pp 449–473
67. Pitchumoni CS, Sonnenshein M, Candido FM, Panchacharam P, Cooperman JM (1980) Nutrition in the pathogenesis of alcoholic pancreatitis. Am J Clin Nutr 33:631–636
68. Rumessen JJ, Marner B, Thorsgaard Pedersen N, Permin H (1985) Autoantibodies in chronic pancreatitis. Scand J Gastroenterol 20:966–970
69. Sahel J, Cros R-C, Bourry J, Sarles H (1982) Clinico-pathological conditions associated with pancreas divisum. Digestion 23:1–8
70. Sarles H (1973) An international survey on nutrition and pancreatitis. Digestion 9:389–403
71. Sarles H (1992) Chronic pancreatitis and main pancreatic duct stricture following cobalt therapy. Eur J Gastroenterol Hepatol 4:509–510
72. Sarles H, Cambon P, Choux R, Payan MJ, Odaira S, Laugier R, Sahel J (1988) Chronic obstructive pancreatitis due to tiny (0.6 to 8 mm) benign tumors obstructing pancreatic ducts: report of three cases. Pancreas 3:232–237
73. Sarles H, Cros RC, Bidart JM, International Group for the Study of Pancreatic Diseases (1979) A multicenter inquiry into the etiology of pancreatic diseases. Digestion 19:110–125
74. Shwachman H, Lebenthal E, Khaw KT (1975) Recurrent acute pancreatitis in patients with cystic fibrosis with normal pancreatic enzymes. Pediatrics 55:86–95
75. Simpson WF, Adams DB, Metcalf JS, Anderson MC (1988) Nonfunctioning pancreatic neuroendocrine tumors presenting as pancreatitis: report of four cases. Pancreas 3:223–231
76. Stafford RJ, Grand RJ (1982) Hereditary disease of the exocrine pancreas. Clin Gastroenterol 11:141–170
77. Takano S, Kimura T, Yamaguchi H, Kinjo M, Nawata H (1992) Effects of stress on the development of chronic pancreatitis. Pancreas 7:548–555
78. Tenner S, Carr-Locke DL, Banks PA, Brooks DC, Van Dam J, Farraye FA, Turner JR, Lichtenstein DR (1996) Intraductal mucin-hypersecreting neoplasm "mucinous ductal ectasia": endoscopic recognition and management. Am J Gastroenterol 91:2548–2554
79. Trapnell JE (1990) Management of chronic relapsing pancreatitis in adolescents. World J Surg 14:48–52
80. Uden S, Acheson DWK, Reeves J, Worthington HV, Hunt LP, Brown S, Braganza JM (1988) Antioxidants, enzyme induction, and chronic pancreatitis: a reappraisal following studies in patients on anticonvulsants. Eur J Clin Nutr 42:561–569

81. Weaver GA (1987) Do antihypertensive agents cause chronic pancreatitis? J Clin Gastroenterol 9: 8–11
82. Wilson JS, Bernstein L, McDonald C, Tait A, McNeil D, Pirola RC (1985) Diet and drinking habits in relation to the development of alcoholic pancreatitis. Gut 26:882–887
83. Worning H (1990) Incidence and prevalence of chronic pancreatitis. In: Beger HG, Büchler M, Ditschuneit H, Malfertheiner P (eds) Chronic Pancreatitis. Springer, Berlin-Heidelberg, pp 8–14
84. Yen S, Hsieh CC, MacMahon B (1982) Consumption of alcohol and tobacco and other risk factors for pancreatitis. Am J Epidemiol 116:407–414

14 Chronic Pancreatitis: Pathophysiology

There is no one generally accepted concept for explaining the pathophysiology of chronic pancreatitis. Four major hypotheses have been proposed, that may to some extent explain the development of chronic pancreatitis, but further studies are required.

14.1
Concept of Primary Intraductal Obstruction

Histological features of alcoholic pancreatitis include sclerosis or fibrosis of the pancreas, disappearance of pancreatic parenchyma, an apparent increase in ductal structures, and in many cases intraductal stones.

The effect of alcohol on pancreatic secretion is different in alcoholics and nonalcoholics. In the latter group, drinking of alcohol increases secretion slightly, whereas intravenously given alcohol inhibits pancreatic secretion [23]. In comparison, alcoholics who consume more than 100 g alcohol/day, exhibit a decrease in bicarbonate concentration and volume of pancreatic secretion [22], followed by an increase of protein secretion [19, 21], a disturbed diffusion barrier, increased permeability between interstitial spaces [20], and enhanced diffusion of calcium into the ducts [13], where it precipitates in the alkaline juice. In combination, these changes lead to formation of protein plugs within pancreatic ductules that eventually calcify and obstruct the pancreatic ducts leading to periductal inflammation and fibrosis. Subsequently, areas of fibrosis coalesce and envelop larger areas of the pancreas [4].

According to the group led by Sarles [24, 25], chronic pancreatitis is caused by an inherited or acquired defect of the biosynthesis of lithostathine (formerly called pancreatic stone protein [PSP]) [26], that leads to decreased secretion of normal and increased secretion of abnormal lithostathine. Abnormal lithostathine is insoluble at the neutral pH of pancreatic juice and comprises the precipitates of fibrillar protein found in chronic pancreatitis. Recent studies have shown that the main constituent of pancreatic stones is $CaCo_3$ associated with an organic matrix containing lithostathine. The latter is present in pancreatic juice and inhibits precipitation of $CaCo_3$ in vitro [29]. Initially, discussion centered around why this protein was in the calculi if it inhibited their formation. Further studies by Dagorn [3] explained this by demonstrating that lithostathine is synthesized as a single protein but probably undergoes posttranslational modification and is secreted as 4 species of slightly different molecular weight (lithostathine S2–S5). Lithostathine then is hydrolyzed in pancreatic juice to 2 forms, H_1

and H_2. Lithostathine H_1 inhibits stone formation, but H_2 does not and is incorporated in pancreatic stones [3]. The same team has derived the complete sequence of prelithostathine messenger RNA [7], and Watanabe et al. [28] have characterized the structure of the gene.

Lithostathine H_2 and a second pancreatic protein GP_2 have been shown to have a strong tendency to self-associate in solution. Both lithostathine H_2 and GP_2 are found in pancreatic secretions. Lithostathine H_2-polypeptide has sequence homology with pancreatic thread protein. GP_2 has a considerable amount of sequence homology with Tamm-Horsfall protein [8], a major component of renal tubular casts. GP_2 is tightly attached to the inner membrane of secretory granules by a glycosyl-phosphotidylinositol linkage, but is cleaved from the membrane enzymatically and secreted into pancreatic juice [6]. More recently GP_2 was found to be an integral component of protein plugs in pancreatic juice in patients with alcohol-induced and idiopathic chronic pancreatitis. It was suggested that GP_2, the homologue to the renal cast protein uromodulin, may play a role in pancreatic plug formation similar to the role played by uromodulin in the pathogenesis of renal casts [5].

In clinical studies, decreased levels of lithostathine, at that time still called PSP, had been found in patients with chronic calcifying pancreatitis [16]. No differences between patients and controls were found in another study [27]. The conflicting data – perhaps in part due to a difference in methods – have been to date only partially explained [3]. Further biochemical and subsequent clinical studies are necessary.

In addition to abnormalities involving lithostathine and GP_2, there is an increase in viscosity due to increased protein secretion, an increase in calcium secretion and a decrease of citrate concentration in pancreatic juice in alcoholic dogs and chronic alcoholics. These abnormalities may contribute to the calcification process and thus to primary intraductal obstruction and to the development of alcoholic chronic pancreatitis [14, 15].

14.2
Concept of Primary Toxic-Metabolic Action of Alcohol

According to the team of Bordalo and Noronha [1, 2, 17, 18], fatty degeneration, loss of zymogen content of acinar cells, and periacinar fibrosis are seen in alcoholics at every stage of the disease. Changes in intracellular lipid metabolism, induced by alcohol and by its metabolites, could explain the fatty degeneration of acinar cells. They speculate, that as in the liver, these gross deposits of intracellular lipids and ethanol itself plus other factors could stimulate the resting fibroblasts causing the development of periacinar, perilobular and intralobular fibrosis. The majority of alcoholics, it is believed, never develop lesions beyond the stage of pancreatic fibrosis. However, in a few cases, the severity of periacinar fibrosis could result in cellular anoxia and necrosis, probably related to the impairment of parenchymal microcirculation. This process mainly located at the periphery would be responsible for the increasing fibrosis leading to the macronodular and later to the micronodular forms of chronic pancreatitis. These changes may occur without symptoms, e.g., pain, except when the ductal system becomes involved in the fibrotic distortion of the pancreatic architecture [1, 2, 17, 18].

In summary, the research team of Sarles and Dagorn [3, 24–26] believes that secretory changes occur first in the evolution of chronic pancreatitis (primary intraductal obstruction concept), whereas the group of Bordalo and Noronha [1, 2, 17, 18] considers secretory changes only secondary to morphological alterations (primary toxic-metabolic concept).

14.3
Concept of Oxidative Stress

This concept asserts a pathogenetic sequence as in acute pancreatitis (see Sect. 6.4).

Recurrent pancreatitis may be due to recurrent pancreatic oxidative stress, that eventually may lead to chronic pancreatitis.

14.4
Concept of Necrosis-Fibrosis Sequence

Klöppel and Maillet [10, 11] postulate a sequence of events that may connect acute with chronic pancreatitis. This sequence starts with interstitial fat necrosis and hemorrhage, including perilobular fibrosis. Perilobular fibrosis, in turn, may also distort the interlobular ducts, creating stenosis and dilatation. The ducts, once altered, hamper the normal flow of pancreatic secretions, thereby enabling the precipitation of proteins (protein plugs) and eventually their calcification (calculi). If duct obstruction becomes more extensive, the acinar cells upstream of such a stenosis disappear, leaving dense intralobular fibrosis (necrosis-fibrosis concept; Fig. 14.1 [11]).

This concept is also in response to two main questions about the development of chronic pancreatitis, e.g.: Why does biliary pancreatitis rarely, if ever, lead to chronic pancreatitis (Fig. 14.2), and why does alcoholic pancreatitis not always lead to chronic pancreatitis?

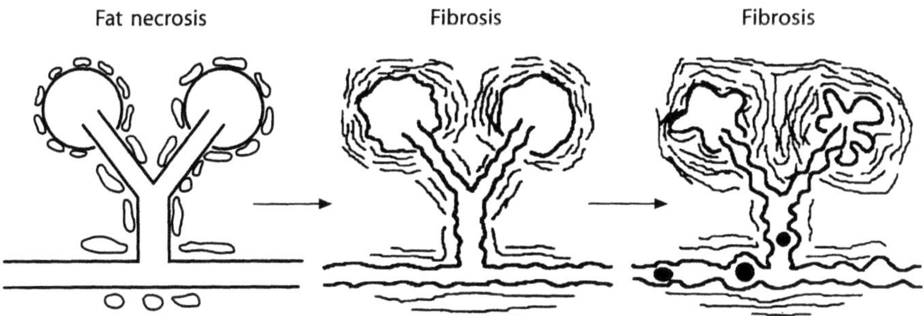

Fig. 14.1. Concept of necrosis-fibrosis. *Left:* Pancreatic lobule and duct surrounded by interstitial fat necrosis. *Center:* Pancreatic lobule encased by fibrosis that also involves the draining interlobular duct. *Right:* Pancreatic lobule partly replaced by intralobular fibrosis and encased by advanced perilobular fibrosis. The distorted draining duct is obstructed by calculi. (From [11] with permission)

Patients with acute biliary pancreatitis – according to this concept – have mostly mild acute pancreatitis, which is characterized by some spotty fat necrosis that barely involve the gland. Peripancreatic fat necrosis resolves without any alterations of the pancreas [12].

Patients with severe, nonbiliary acute pancreatitis are divided into 3 different groups [11]:

- In some patients with severe acute pancreatitis massive peripancreatic fat necrosis occurs but intrapancreatic areas are unaffected. In these patients an extrapancreatic pseudocyst will develop, but there is no progression to chronic pancreatitis.
- In a second group of patients with severe acute pancreatitis, peripancreatic necrosis is associated with some small foci of intrapancreatic necrosis. The sequelae of these lesions are extrapancreatic pseudocysts and small foci of scars within the pancreas. If the intrapancreatic fibrotic foci do not involve the main pancreatic duct and its direct branches, progression of the disease is unlikely to occur. It will, however, progress when the patient continues abusive alcohol consumption so that further

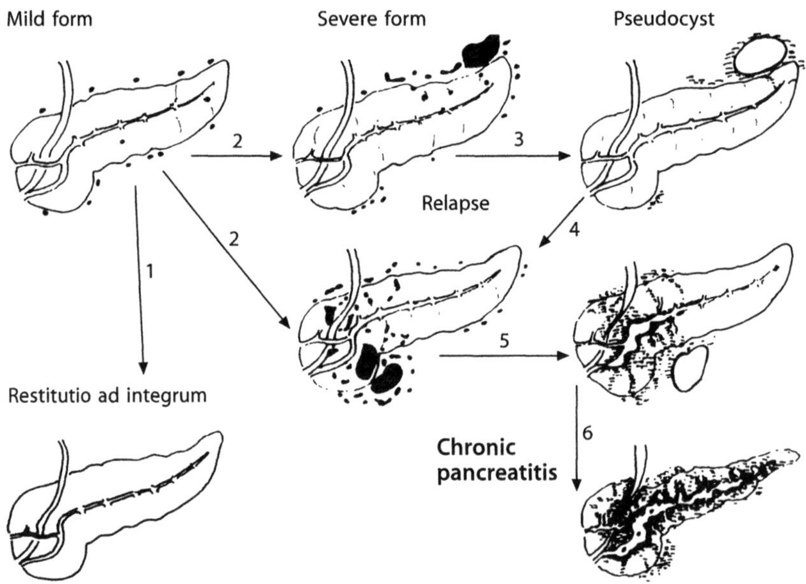

Fig. 14.2. Natural history of pancreatitis: Mild acute pancreatitis is characterized by spotty peripancreatic fat necrosis. 1 Resolution of the small peripancreatic fat necrosis results in restitutio ad integrum. 2 Mild acute pancreatitis may proceed to severe acute pancreatitis. 3 Severe acute pancreatitis with large confluent peripancreatic fat necrosis, but little intrapancreatic involvement, leads to an extrapancreatic pseudocyst. 4 Relapse of severe acute pancreatitis with intrapancreatic involvement. 5 Severe acute pancreatitis with extensive extra- and intrapancreatic foci of necrosis causes irreversible damage to the pancreas, inducing perilobular fibrosis and duct distortions. In addition, there may be extrapancreatic pseudocysts. 6 Early-stage chronic pancreatitis evolves into endstage chronic pancreatitis with severe duct changes, diffuse but still irregular fibrosis, and calculi. (From [10] with permission)

attacks of pancreatitis may occur. Continuous attacks tend to affect regions adjacent to the main pancreatic duct, resulting in alterations of the branches and eventually of the main pancreatic duct itself.

– In the third group of patients, large foci of intrapancreatic necrosis develop during the acute attack. In these patients chronic pancreatitis is most likely to develop even when alcohol consumption ceases. The clinical severity depends on whether the necrosis is mainly in the head of the pancreas or in the body and tail. When the head is the main target, the resulting duct obstruction causes dilatation of the main duct and its branches in the body and tail of the gland, and subsequently fibrosis. In these patients, apart from pain, exocrine and endocrine pancreatic insufficiency develop. When the damage is restricted to the body and/or tail, the patient, even when abstaining from alcohol, may suffer pain but will not develop pancreatic insufficiency, because normal tissue remains in the head of the pancreas [9–11].

References

1. Bordalo O, Baptista A, Dreiling D, Noronha M (1984) Early pathomorphological pancreatic changes in chronic alcoholism. In: Gyr KE, Singer MV, Sarles H (eds) Pancreatitis – Concepts and Classification. Elsevier Science Publ., Amsterdam, pp 57–60
2. Bordalo O, Goncalves D, Noronha M, Cristina ML, Salgadinho A, Dreiling DA (1977) Newer concept for the pathogenesis of chronic alcoholic pancreatitis. Am J Gastroenterol 68:278–285
3. Dagorn JC (1993) Lithostathine. In: Go VLW, DiMagno EP, Gardner JD, Lebenthal E, Reber HA, Scheele GA (eds) The Pancreas: Biology, Pathobiology, and Disease, 2nd edn. Raven Press, New York, pp 253–263
4. DiMagno EP, Layer P, Clain JE (1993) Chronic pancreatitis. In: Go VLW, DiMagno EP, Gardner JD, Lebenthal E, Reber HA, Scheele GA (eds) The Pancreas: Biology, Pathobiology, and Disease, 2nd edn. Raven Press, New York, pp 665–706
5. Freedman SD, Sakamoto K, Venu RP (1993) GP2, the homologue to the renal cast protein uromodulin, is a major component of intraductal plugs in chronic pancreatitis. J Clin Invest 92:83–90
6. Fukuoka S-I, Freedman SD, Scheele GA (1991) A single gene encodes membrane-bound and free forms of GP-2, the major glycoprotein in pancreatic secretory (zymogen) granule membranes. Proc Natl Acad Sci USA 88:2898–2902
7. Giorgi D, Bernard J-P, Rouquier S, Iovanna J, Sarles H, Dagorn J-C (1989) Secretory pancreatic stone protein messenger RNA. Nucleotide sequence and expression in chronic calcifying pancreatitis. J Clin Invest 84:100–106
8. Hoops TC, Rindler MJ (1991) Isolation of the cDNA encoding glycoprotein-2 (GP-2), the major zymogen granule membrane protein. Homology to uromudulin/Tamm-Horsfall protein. J Biol Chem 266:4257–4263
9. Klöppel G, Maillet B (1991) Pseudocysts in chronic pancreatitis: a morphological analysis of 57 resection specimens and 9 autopsy pancreata. Pancreas 6:266–274
10. Klöppel G, Maillet B (1991) Chronic pancreatitis: evolution of the disease. Hepatogastroenterology 38:408–412
11. Klöppel G, Maillet B (1992) The morphological basis for the evolution of acute pancreatitis into chronic pancreatitis. Virchows Arch [Pathol Anat] 420:1–4
12. Klöppel G, von Gerkan R, Dreyer T (1984) Pathomorphology of acute pancreatitis. Analysis of 367 autopsy cases and 3 surgical specimens. In: Gyr KE, Singer MV, Sarles H (eds) Pancreatitis – Concepts and Classification. Elsevier Science Publ., Amsterdam, pp 29–35
13. Layer P, Hotz J, Schmitz-Moormann HP, Goebell H (1982) Effects of experimental chronic hypercalcemia on feline exocrine pancreatic secretion. Gastroenterology 82:309–316
14. Lohse J, Pfeiffer A (1984) Duodenal total and ionised calcium secretion in normal subjects, chronic alcoholics, and patients with various stages of chronic alcoholic pancreatitis. Gut 25:874–880

15. Lohse J, Schmidt D, Sarles H (1983) Pancreatic citrate and protein secretion of alcoholic dogs in response to graded doses of caerulein. Pflügers Arch 397:141–143
16. Multigner L, Sarles H, Lombardo D, de Caro A (1985) Pancreatic stone protein. II. Implication in stone formation during the course of chronic calcifying pancreatitis. Gastroenterology 89: 387–391
17. Noronha M, Baptista A, Bordalo O (1984) Sequential aspects of pathology in chronic alcoholic disease of the pancreas. In: Gyr KE, Singer MV, Sarles H (eds) Pancreatitis – Concepts and Classification. Elsevier Science Publ., Amsterdam, pp 61–65
18. Noronha M, Salgadinho A, Ferreira de Almeida MJ, Dreiling DA, Bordalo O (1981) Alcohol and the pancreas. I. Clinical associations and histopathology of minimal pancreatic inflammation. Am J Gastroenterol 76:114–119
19. Planche NE, Palasciano G, Meullenet J, Laugier R, Sarles H (1982) Effects of intravenous alcohol on pancreatic and biliary secretion in man. Dig Dis Sci 27:449–453
20. Reber HA, Roberts C, Way LW (1979) The pancreatic duct mucosal barrier. Am J Surg 137: 128–134
21. Renner IG, Rinderknecht H, Valenzuela JE, Douglas AP (1980) Studies of pure pancreatic secretions in chronic alcoholic subjects without pancreatic insufficiency. Scand J Gastroenterol 15: 241–244
22. Sahel J, Sarles H (1979) Modifications of pure human pancreatic juice induced by chronic alcohol consumption. Dig Dis Sci 24:897–905
23. Sarles H (1975) Alcohol and the pancreas. Ann N Y Acad Sci 252:171–182
24. Sarles H (1984) Epidemiology and physiopathology of chronic pancreatitis and the role of the pancreatic stone protein. Clin Gastroenterol 13:895–912
25. Sarles H, Bernard JP, Johnson C (1989) Pathogenesis and epidemiology of chronic pancreatitis. Ann Rev Med 40:453–468
26. Sarles H, Dagorn JC, Giorgi D, Bernard JP (1990) Renaming pancreatic stone protein as "lithostathine". Gastroenterology 99:900–901
27. Schmiegel W, Burchert M, Kalthoff H, Roeder C, Bützow G, Grimm H, Kremer B, Soehendra N, Schreiber H-W, Thiele H-G, Greten H (1990) Immunochemical characterization and quantitative distribution of pancreatic stone protein in sera and pancreatic secretions in pancreatic disorders. Gastroenterology 99:1421–1430
28. Watanabe T, Yonekura H, Terazono K, Yamamoto H, Okamoto H (1990) Complete nucleotide sequence of human reg gene and its expression in normal and tumoral tissues. J Biol Chem 265: 7432–7439
29. Yamadera K, Moriyama T, Makino I (1990) Identification of immunoreactive pancreatic stone protein in pancreatic stone, pancreatic tissue, and pancreatic juice. Pancreas 5:255–260

15 Chronic Pancreatitis: Pathology

The term chronic pancreatitis implies that clinical manifestation of the disease and anatomical changes of the gland persist or increase, even when the initial cause or factors leading to pancreatitis have been eliminated. Chronic pancreatitis without clinical manifestation may be more frequent than believed. In one postmortem study, mild or moderate chronic inflammation of the gland was found in 13% of the cases [11]. Interstitial fibrosis with a few or no inflammatory cells is common in the elderly, and such findings should not be interpreted as chronic pancreatitis [9].

15.1
Gross Pathology

Chronic calcifying pancreatitis, seen in the majority of patients, is characterized grossly by a pancreas that is nodular, hard and misshaped. It may be either enlarged or atrophic.

15.2
Histopathology

According to the classification of Marseille [14], chronic pancreatitis is morphologically characterized by an irregular sclerosis with destruction and permanent loss of exocrine parenchyma which may be either focal, segmental, or diffuse. These changes may be associated with varying degrees of dilatation of segments of the duct system. Thus, dilatation of the duct of Wirsung and of its small ducts may occur together or independently. No obvious cause of the duct dilatation may be found, but most often it is associated with strictures of the ducts or intraductal protein plugs and calculi (calcification). All types of inflammatory cells may be present in varying degrees as well as edema and focal necrosis. Cysts and pseudocysts are not uncommon. They may be sterile or infected. Some communicate with ducts, while others do not. Compared with the degree of acinar destruction, the islets of Langerhans are relatively well preserved. Based on the predominating structural features, the following descriptive terms can be used [14]:
- Chronic pancreatitis with focal necrosis
- Chronic pancreatitis with segmental or diffuse fibrosis
- Chronic pancreatitis with or without calculi
- Obstructive chronic pancreatitis

15.3
Chronic Pancreatitis With Focal Necrosis

Focal necroses were present in 11.9% and pancreatic pseudocysts in 39.6% in the gland of patients who underwent resection operations for chronic pancreatitis [16]. The incidence was independent of the scarring process.

15.4
Chronic Pancreatitis With Segmental or Diffuse Fibrosis

Chronic pancreatitis may occur with segmental or nonsegmental fibrosis. It is found segmental in 41%–45% of the cases [6, 7, 15]. In keeping with the Marseille classification [14], Stolte [16] has further differentiated fibrosis into 4 classes: grade I = slight scarring, grade II = moderate scarring, grade III = high-grade scarring, and grade IV = complete scarring.

Slight scarring shows a predominantly perilobular arrangement and extends into the lobuli in a moderate degree. In grade IV, considerable scarred reconstruction with almost complete destruction of the exocrine parenchyma has taken place.

The extent and composition of the cellular inflammatory infiltrate is dependent on the degree of fibrosis. In slight scarring, there is also only a slightly developed infiltrate composed of lymphocytes, plasma cells and scattered macrophages. In pronounced scarring, only slight lymphocytic infiltrates can be demonstrated.

In case of protracted fibrosis, reactive fibrosis of the intima of arteries and arterioles develops, the extent of which follows the degree of fibrosis.

The islets of Langerhans exhibit relatively few alterations in light microscopy; in electron microscopy, however, a relative decrease in B-cells and increase in A-cells is found [5]. Only in advanced stages, a more distinct reduction of the islets is found, probably due to perivascular fibrosis of the intrainsular capillaries.

The ductal system is dilated with increasing scarring. Increased convolutions and caliber variations of the duct arise. In the scarring process, folding of the lamina propria ensues from the formation of new fibers, resulting in reduced drainage of the secretions [16]. Depending on the degree of scarring, protein-rich secretion plugs can be demonstrated in the dilated ducts, mainly in the tributaries to the smallest side branches of the main pancreatic duct. Probably as a result of inspissation of the secretions, calcifications can develop in the ducts.

The structural alterations of the ductal system form an essential requirement for the protracted course of the disease. Progressive impairment of drainage of secretion ensuing from fibrosis and epithelial damage in the ducts are responsible for limiting the protective functions of the ductal epithelium, so that pancreatic secretions can continuously erode ductal tissue. A vicious circle ensues, with progressive scarring in chronic pancreatitis [10].

Special forms of segmental fibrosis are chronic pancreatitis associated with pancreas divisum and groove pancreatitis. In the former, which was found in 3.6% of the cases reported by Stolte [15], only one anlage shows chronic pancreatitis, whereas the other is well preserved. Groove pancreatitis, found in 12% of the patients, comprises an inflammatory process in the groove between duodenum, common bile duct, and head of the pancreas without necessarily involving the head of the pancreas [1, 13, 15, 18].

A rare type of chronic pancreatitis seems to be the *shrunken* pancreas, a morphological variant of idiopathic chronic pancreatitis. The gland is irregularily narrowed throughout. Two of the 6 reported patients with this variant also had inflammatory bowel disease [2].

15.5
Obstructive Chronic Pancreatitis

Obstructive chronic pancreatitis is a distinctive form of chronic pancreatitis, which is histologically easily distinguishable from alcoholic and nonalcoholic chronic pancreatitis [3]. It is characterized by uniform dilatation of the ductal system proximal to the occlusion of one of the major ducts (e.g., by tumor or by scars), diffuse atrophy of the acinar parenchyma, and uniform diffuse fibrosis [4, 8, 12, 19].

Calculi are uncommon.

The papilla of Vater shows inflammatory infiltration in 69% and fibrosis in 81% of patients undergoing surgery for chronic pancreatitis, but these minor changes obviously are not enough to induce obstructive chronic pancreatitis, nor do they parallel the degree of chronic pancreatitis [17].

References

1. Becker V, Mischke U (1991) Groove pancreatitis. Int J Pancreatol 10:173–182
2. Bulgim O, Manning A, Lintott D, Axon A (1987) The "shrunken" pancreas: a morphological variant of idiopathic chronic pancreatitis. Br J Radiol 60:543–546
3. De Angelis C, Valente G, Spaccapietra M, Angonese C, Del Favero G, Naccarato R, Andriulli A (1992) Histological study of alcoholic, nonalcoholic, and obstructive chronic pancreatitis. Pancreas 7:193–196
4. Kahrilas PJ, Hogan WJ, Geenen JE, Stewart ET, Dodds WJ, Arndorfer RC (1987) Chronic recurrent pancreatitis secondary to a submucosal ampullary tumor in a patient with neurofibromatosis. Dig Dis Sci 32:102–107
5. Klöppel G, Bommer G, Commandeur G, Heitz P (1978) The endocrine pancreas in chronic pancreatitis. Immunocytochemical and ultrastructural studies. Virchows Arch [Pathol Anat] 377:157–174
6. Klöppel G, Maillet B (1991) Pseudocysts in chronic pancreatitis: a morphological analysis of 57 resection specimens and 9 autopsy pancreata. Pancreas 6:266–274
7. Klöppel G, Maillet B (1991) Chronic pancreatitis: evolution of the disease. Hepatogastroenterology 38:408–412
8. Laugier R, Camatte R, Sarles H (1983) Chronic obstructive pancreatitis after healing of a necrotic pseudocyst. Am J Surg 146:551–557
9. Martin ED (1984) Different pathomorphological aspects of pancreatic fibrosis, correlated with etiology: anatomical study of 300 cases. In: Gyr KE, Singer MV, Sarles H (eds) Pancreatitis – Concepts and Classification. Excerpta Medica, Amsterdam–New York–Oxford, pp 77–82
10. Morgenroth K, Kozuschek W, Hotz J (1991) Pancreatitis. Walter de Gruyter, Berlin–New York
11. Olsen TS (1978) The incidence and clinical relevance of chronic inflammation in the pancreas in autopsy material. Acta Pathol Microbiol Scand A 86:361–365
12. Sarles H, Cambon P, Choux R, Payan MJ, Odaira S, Laugier R, Sahel J (1988) Chronic obstructive pancreatitis due to tiny (0.6 to 8 mm) benign tumors obstructing pancreatic ducts: report of three cases. Pancreas 3:232–237

13. Seitz K, Rettenmaier G, Stolte M (1985) Rinnen-Pankreatitis – pathologische Anatomie und sonographische Befunde. Ultraschall 6:131–133
14. Singer MW, Gyr K, Sarles H (1985) Revised classification of pancreatitis. Report of the Second International Symposium on the Classification of Pancreatitis in Marseille, France, March 28–30, 1984. Gastroenterology 89:683–685
15. Stolte M (1984) Chronische Pankreatitis. Morphologie – Pankreatographie – Differentialdiagnose. perimed Fachbuch-Verlagsgesellschaft, Erlangen
16. Stolte M (1987) Chronische Pankreatitis. Verh Dtsch Ges Pathol 71:175–186
17. Stolte M, Waltschew A (1986) The papilla of Vater and chronic pancreatitis. Hepatogastroenterology 33:163–169
18. Stolte M, Weiß W, Volkholz H, Rösch W (1982) A special form of segmental pancreatitis: "groove pancreatitis". Hepatogastroenterology 29:198–208
19. Stolte M, Zink W, Schaffner O (1983) Duodenalwandzysten und Erkrankungen der Bauchspeicheldrüse. Leber Magen Darm 13:140–149

16 Chronic Pancreatitis: Epidemiology

Data we have on the incidence and prevalence of chronic pancreatitis in various countries is sparse. This deficiency may be explained by several factors:
- The diagnosis of chronic pancreatitis, especially at an early stage, is not easy and requires an experienced doctor, expensive equipment and invasive procedures. An unknown, but probably substantial number of patients with irritable bowel syndrome or other conditions may be incorrectly diagnosed as having *chronic pancreatitis.*
- The generally accepted classifications of pancreatic diseases are not generally known or used. As a result, an interinstitutional data comparison is not possible at present. For example, chronic pancreatitis may be misdiagnosed as acute pancreatitis, and vice versa, and sequelae of acute pancreatitis, e.g., scars seen on endoscopic retrograde cholangiopancreatography (ERCP), may be deemed chronic pancreatitis (see Chap. 4 and Sects. 17.3, 17.4).
- Postmortem examinations do not reflect the true incidence of the disease since in most countries the rate of autopsies is declining. In addition, diagnoses provided on death certificates are not sufficiently accurate for exact statistical analysis.

Nevertheless, the sparse data available on epidemiology of chronic pancreatitis show some similarities among different centers:
- The incidence of chronic pancreatitis per 1000 hospital admissions from Marseille, Cape Town, Sao Paulo and Mexico City varies only very little from 3.1 to 4.9 (Table 16.1) [1, 3, 4, 6].
- Incidence data for chronic pancreatitis collected from the literature appearing between 1946 and 1985 show an overall increase, but not to a level of statistical significance. However, in four areas, where data have been repeatedly published (Minne-

Table 16.1. Overall incidence of chronic pancreatitis in different parts of the world

Authors	Localization	Incidence per 1000 hospital admissions
Durbec et al. [1]	Marseille	3.1
Marks et al. [3]	Cape Town	4.4[a]
– Black patients		4.8
– White patients		3.8
Mott et al. [4]	Sao Paulo	4.9
Roblez-Diaz et al. [6]	Mexico City	4.4

[a] Rate includes acute and chronic pancreatitis

sota, Zurich, Stockholm, and Copenhagen), the incidence increased during the time of investigation. The data show an enormous difference in incidence among the areas investigated for nearly the same period (Fig. 16.1) [8]. Data from a single center, Mexico City, also show a higher incidence, but reveal the problems connected with such statistical evaluations. During the first phase of investigation (1975–1980), the diagnosis of chronic pancreatitis derived from the demonstration of pancreatic calcifications on abdominal plain films, whereas in the second phase (1982–1987), computed tomography, ERCP, and histology were used (Fig. 16.2) [6].

In the only prospective study for evaluation of chronic pancreatitis from Copenhagen, incidence rate was 4 per 100000 inhabitants per year and prevalence rate 13 per 100000 inhabitants [7]. A more recent preliminary evaluation of the Rochester (Minnesota) population suggests the incidence may be increasing, particularly in

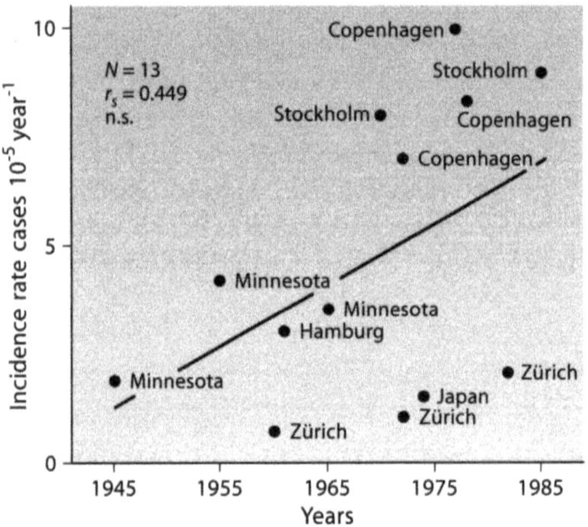

Fig. 16.1. Incidence rate of chronic pancreatitis over the years 1945–1985. (From [8] with permission)

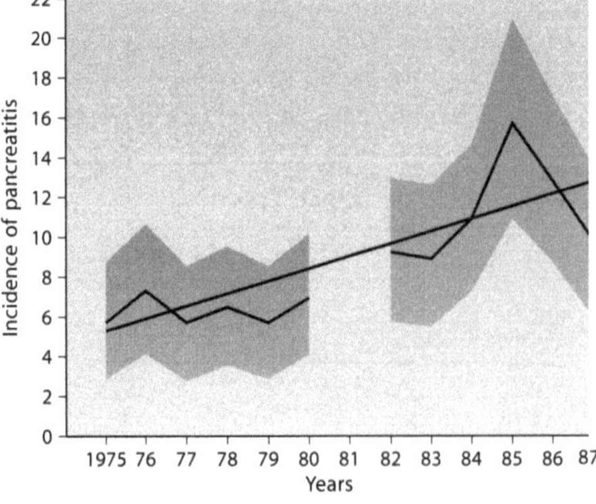

Fig. 16.2. Incidence of pancreatitis in a tertiary care hospital in Mexico City. The *shaded areas* represent 95% confidence limits. (From [6] with permission)

women. The mean age- and sex-adjusted incidence per 100 000 population from 1976 to 1988 was 4.7 (6.7 for men and 3.2 for women) [5].

Further studies from these centers using the same diagnostic criteria would be of great interest as well as other epidemiological studies from other parts of the world using worldwide accepted criteria for the diagnosis of chronic pancreatitis [2]. These studies may perhaps also clarify, whether there are country-to-country differences in susceptibility to alcohol-induced damage of the pancreas. The incidence of chronic pancreatitis is the same in Denmark and Sweden (Fig. 16.1), even though Danes consume more alcohol than Swedes [8].

References

1. Durbec JP, Sarles H (1984) Epidemiology of chronic pancreatitis. Alcohol and dietary habits. In: Gyr KE, Singer MV, Sarles H (eds) Pancreatitis – Concepts and Classification. Elsevier Science Publ., Amsterdam, pp 351–353
2. Lankisch PG, Andrén-Sandberg Å (1993) Standards for the diagnosis of chronic pancreatitis and for the evaluation of treatment. Int J Pancreatol 14:205–212
3. Marks IN, Girdwood AH, Bornman PC, Feretis C (1984) The prevalence and etiology of pancreatitis in Cape Town. In: Gyr KE, Singer MV, Sarles H (eds) Pancreatitis – Concepts and Classification. Excerpta Medica, Amsterdam–New York–Oxford, pp 345–350
4. Mott CB, Guarita DR, Machado MCC, Bettarello A (1984) Epidemiology and etiology of chronic pancreatitis in Sao Paulo (Brasil): a prospective study of 200 cases. In: Gyr KE, Singer MV, Sarles H (eds) Pancreatitis – Concepts and Classification. Excerpta Medica, Amsterdam–New York–Oxford, pp 355–358
5. Riela A, Zinsmeister AR, Melton LJ, DiMagno EP (1990) Trends in the incidence and clinical characteristics of chronic pancreatitis. Pancreas 5:727 (abstr)
6. Robles-Díaz G, Vargas F, Uscanga L, Fernández-del Castillo C (1990) Chronic pancreatitis in Mexico City. Pancreas 5:479–483
7. The Copenhagen Pancreatitis Study Group (1981) Copenhagen Pancreatitis Study. An interim report from a prospective epidemiological multicentre study. Scand J Gastroenterol 16:305–312
8. Worning H (1990) Incidence and prevalence of chronic pancreatitis. In: Beger HG, Büchler M, Ditschuneit H, Malfertheiner P (eds) Chronic Pancreatitis. Springer, Berlin–Heidelberg, pp 8–14

17 Chronic Pancreatitis: Diagnosis

17.1
Clinical Manifestation

17.1.1
Signs and Symptoms

The case history of a patient with chronic pancreatitis has typical characteristics that should alert the physician to pursue further investigations to verify or exclude the suspected diagnosis. Nevertheless, the diagnostic delay is appalling, reaching as long as 30 months in the case of alcoholics and 60 months for patients with other etiologies [13, 144].

Leading symptoms are attacks of severe pain, either focused mostly in the left or middle upper abdomen, sometimes radiating around the abdomen like a girdle, or localized in the back (Fig. 17.1) [160]. The lack of a characteristic site of pancreatic pain may contribute to the late diagnosis of this disease [13, 144].

Pain may occur independently of meals or within 30 min after a meal, thereby resembling the abdominal angina caused by celiac or mesentery artery stenosis [218, 219]. In patients with such symptoms, Otte [202] found a high incidence of isolated duct stenosis and slightly impaired pancreatic function. In this group of patients, weight loss may be an early symptom, indicating an avoidance of food intake in anticipation of subsequent pain. In other patients, weight loss may be a late symptom, reflecting increasing exocrine pancreatic insufficiency and resulting in diarrhea and steatorrhea.

In chronic pancreatitis, pain is often severe and tends to be prolonged, but is less intense than in acute pancreatitis. In some studies, about half of patients described their pain as severe, while the other half described it as moderate or mild [257]. Few studies have been carried out using pain scores and/or quality of life measures [31, 125].

Radiation of pain to other parts of the body is poorly understood. Bliss et al. [30] used electrical stimuli to localize the pain and the direction of its radiation. Stimulation of the tail of the gland, for example, usually induced pain in the left upper abdomen, whereas stimulation of the head usually induced it on the right.

The association between alcohol consumption and pain in chronic pancreatitis is not clear either. Some patients drink alcohol in an effort to relieve the pancreatic pain; others experience a painful attack after having consumed alcohol. In South Africa it has been observed that painful attacks of pancreatitis usually start about 12–48 h after a drinking bout – that is, the "afternoon after the night before" [176].

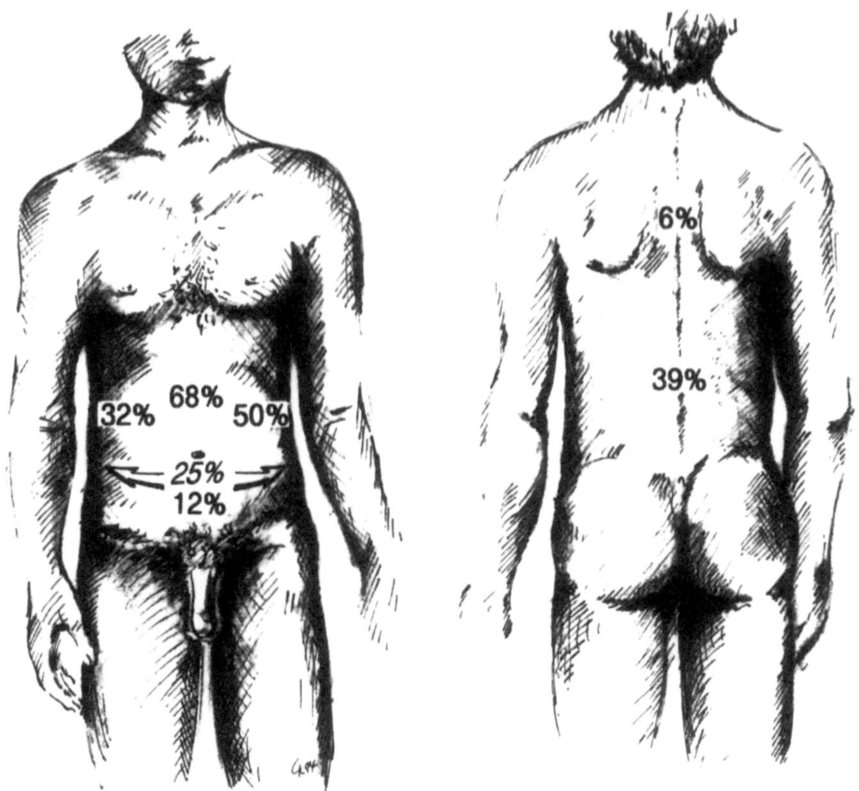

Fig. 17.1. Major sites of pain in 311 patients with painful chronic pancreatitis

Besides pain, other leading symptoms are diarrhea, diabetes-related symptoms, and icterus, the latter as in acute pancreatitis because of the inflammatory swelling of the head of the pancreas or the presence of a pancreatic pseudocyst (Table 17.1). Overall, it is significant that pain is the most frequent initial symptom in both alcohol-induced and idiopathic chronic pancreatitis. Diabetes-related symptoms occur more frequently in idiopathic than in alcoholic pancreatitis (Table 17.1) [160].

Table 17.1. Initial symptoms in chronic pancreatitis [160]

Initial symptom	Alcoholic chronic pancreatitis ($n = 230$)	Idiopathic chronic pancreatitis ($n = 95$)	All ($n = 325$)
Pain	208 (90%)	76 (80%)[a]	284 (87%)
Diarrhea	5 (2%)	6 (6%)	11 (3%)
Diabetes-related symptoms	15 (7%)	13 (14%)[b]	28 (9%)
Icterus	2 (1%)	—	2 (1%)

Fisher's exact test: [a] $p = 0.02$; [b] $p = 0.05$.

Weight loss is a frequent symptom. It may be due either to reduced oral food intake because of fear of postprandial pain, or to severe exocrine pancreatic insufficiency, especially reduction of lipase secretion, leading to diarrhea and steatorrhea.

Loss of body weight does not necessarily occur in chronic pancreatitis. In a study in which normal body weight was defined according to the Broca index (body length in cm minus 100=normal weight in kg), a normal weight was found in 62% of 107 patients with chronic pancreatitis at the beginning of the disease and in 56% of 273 patients after an observation time of 11.3 years [160].

In about 7% of patients with chronic pancreatitis the disease is primarily painless and in about half of the patients with initially painful chronic pancreatitis, pain may disappear after a 10-year follow-up [138]. In the latter patients symptoms of exocrine and endocrine pancreatic insufficiency are dominant.

17.1.2
Physical Examination

When patients present for physical examination during a painful attack of chronic pancreatitis, they frequently, as in the case of acute pancreatitis, try to relieve their pain by flexing the spine, by sitting forward with the knees flexed against the chest, by squatting and clasping the knees to chest, or by lying on one side with the knees flexed (Fig. 17.2).

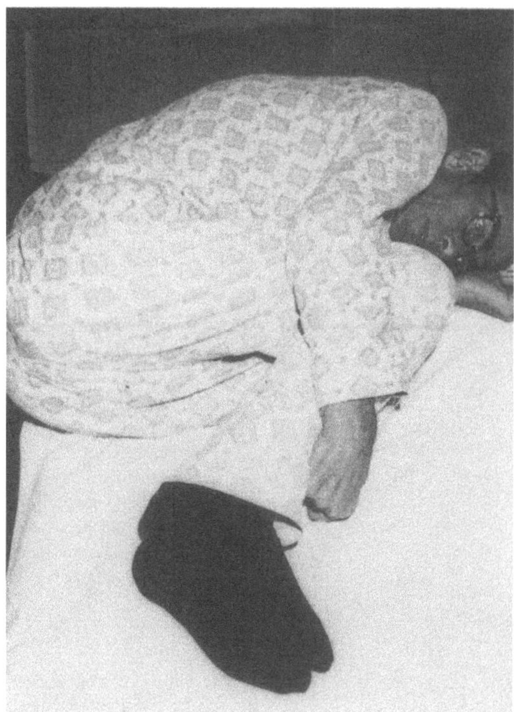

Fig. 17.2. Patient with chronic pancreatitis with knees flexed up against the chest for pain relief

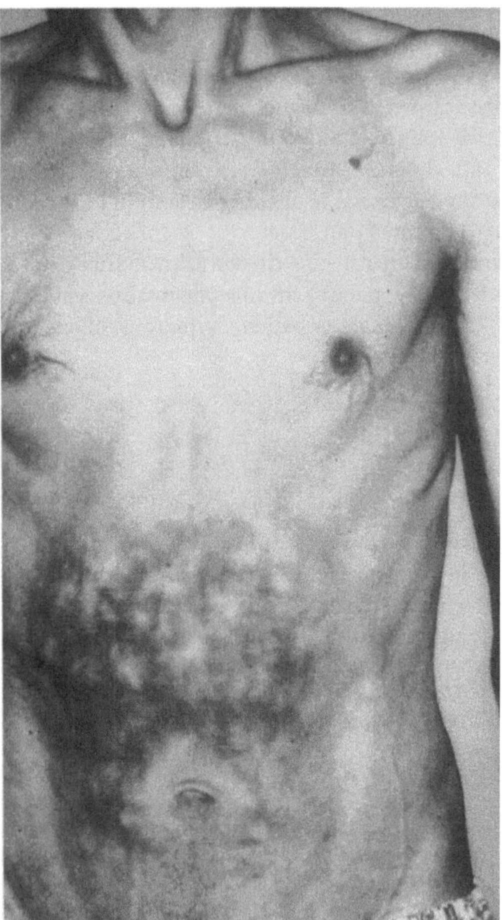

Fig. 17.3. Patient with chronic pancreatitis and an erythema ab igne. (From [130] with permission)

Table 17.2. Causes of exocrine pancreatic insufficiency

- **Overall reduction of enzyme formation or delivery due to**
  Chronic pancreatitis
  Acute pancreatitis (mostly short-term insufficiency)
  Carcinoma obstructing the pancreatic duct
  Major pancreatic resection
  Pancreatic trauma (mostly short-term insufficiency)
  Primary sclerosing cholangitis
  Kwashiorkor
  Hereditary disorder or congenital abnormalities
  Cystic fibrosis
  Shwachman syndrome
- **Isolated deficiency in following enzymes**
  Lipase
  Trypsin
  Amylase
- **Failure of enzyme activation of the small intestine due to**
  Enterokinase insufficiency

During an asymptomatic interval, standard physical examination does not help in establishing the diagnosis [124]. Very rarely, a pancreatic pseudocyst is palpable as an abdominal tumor, or an enlarged spleen is felt as the expression of portal hypertension.

Skin signs are not characteristic [22], but erythema ab igne (redness of the skin caused by application of hot water bottles or electric pads to relieve pain; Fig. 17.3) may be observed on the abdominal wall or on the back. However, this sign is seen both in chronic pancreatitis and pancreatic cancer [49, 130, 186].

17.2
Laboratory Investigations

17.2.1
Basic Laboratory Tests

Pancreatic amylase and lipase activities are elevated only during acute attacks, not during asymptomatic intervals. In later stages of chronic pancreatitis, there is often no elevation of activity of these enzymes, even during acute exacerbations with much pain.

In asymptomatic periods, or periods with few complaints, serum alkaline phosphatase and gamma-glutamyl-transferase activities may be elevated as a result of cholestasis from common bile duct stenosis. β-carotene level in the serum may be decreased because of fat malabsorption [152], and serum calcium may be decreased due to hypoalbuminemia, hypomagnesemia, or possibly malabsorption. If serum calcium levels are elevated, primary hyperparathyroidism should be suspected. Serum glucose levels and glucose tolerance tests may provide evidence of coexistent diabetes mellitus.

17.2.2
Tests of Exocrine Pancreatic Function

17.2.2.1
General Remarks

Exocrine pancreatic insufficiency may be due to an overall reduction of enzymes, to an isolated enzyme deficiency, or to failure of enzyme activation in the small intestine (Table 17.2). The main reason for an overall reduction of enzymes is chronic pancreatitis. Other reasons include a major pancreatic resection and a carcinoma obstructing the pancreatic duct. In addition, transient insufficiency may occur, following acute pancreatitis or pancreatic trauma. In some cases of primary sclerosing cholangitis, exocrine pancreatic insufficiency is present. Finally, overall reduction of enzymes is one of the main features of several congenital or hereditary disorders of the pancreas (see Chaps. 1, 21).

Testing for exocrine pancreatic insufficiency is recommended when chronic pancreatitis is suspected, especially in patients with relapsing abdominal pain, obstructive jaundice, weight loss, fatty stool, and newly detected diabetes mellitus (Table 17.3). Follow-up function tests are also useful after an attack of pancreatitis to retrospectively clarify whether the disease was due to acute pancreatitis or to an acute attack of chronic pancreatitis. Furthermore, repeated function tests during the course of chronic pancreatitis may be indicated to determine whether there has been amelioration or deterioration [138].

There are two different ways of testing exocrine pancreatic function:

- By means of direct tests, in which the parameters of pancreatic secretion are measured in duodenal or pure pancreatic juice following stimulation of the pancreas, or
- By means of indirect tests, in which measurements of enzymes or of enzyme breakdown products in serum, in urine, or feces are used to draw conclusions about exocrine pancreatic function [81]

17.2.2.2
Direct Pancreatic Function Tests

17.2.2.2.1
Determinations in Duodenal Juice

A major technical problem associated with measuring pancreatic volume, bicarbonate and enzyme contents in duodenal juice after stimulation of the pancreas is how to prevent contamination by gastric juice and loss of duodenal contents either into the jejunum or by reflux into the stomach.

For intubation, several double- or multiple-lumen tubes have been recommended, and for calculating loss of duodenal contents, nonabsorbable markers such as polyethylene glycol (PEG) or ^{57}Co-labelled vitamin B_{12} (not allowed in several centers for ethical reasons because of the radiation exposure) have been recommended. The recovery data in investigations using these markers, however, differ considerably, and, unfortunately, are difficult or almost impossible to compare, as methods for intubation, position of patients, markers, their concentration, and infusion rate vary from study to study [122]. With PEG as a marker, recovery was very high or almost complete in some studies [129, 216], but amounted only to 40% in others [245, 249]. This may be due to the left lateral position of the patients [249], thus increasing the difficulties for quan-

---

Table 17.3. Indications for a pancreatic function test

- Suspected chronic pancreatitis because of
  Relapsing upper abdominal pain
  Diarrhea/steatorrhea
  Obstructive jaundice
  Unexplained weight loss
  Calcification in the area of the pancreas
- Follow-up investigations in known chronic pancreatitis
- Follow-up investigations after acute pancreatitis for clarification whether temporary exocrine and endocrine function impairment and morphological changes have returned to normal or whether a transition to chronic pancreatitis has occurred

titative collection of duodenal secretion, or to the advanced distal position of the tube in the small intestine [245]. Furthermore, low recovery rates do not necessarily represent high losses of duodenal contents, since it is almost impossible to control adequate mixing of markers and duodenal juice. A recovery rate of 85% has been said to indicate that the collection technique is probably satisfactory, recovery of less than 85% means that the collection technique needs to be modified [256].

When pancreatic enzymes are measured in duodenal aspirates, either in the secretin-pancreozymin test (SPT) or the Lundh test, salivary isoamylase may contribute to a normal or – compared with the other enzymes – high total amylase output. Salivary isoamylase was found in 75% of the aspirates of the Lundh test [231] and in 18% of patients who underwent an SPT [140]. In the latter, it occurred more often in patients with abnormal pancreatic function than in those with normal function (40.5% vs. 8%) [140].

17.2.2.2.2
Secretin Test

Tests of secretory capacity, such as the secretin test, are based on two assumptions, namely, that a decrease in the capacity to secrete fluid, bicarbonate, and enzymes indicates pancreatic damage, and that the dosage of stimulant which provides submaximal or maximal stimulation to normal glands also exerts the same effect on the diseased pancreas [256].

After the Lagerlöf's [118] evaluation of the secretin test, Dreiling [69], Burton et al. [47], Petersen and Myren [205] and other investigators (for review see [17]) have provided more information on the usefulness of the test. Secretin has been applied by rapid intravenous injection, subcutaneously, and by continuous intravenous infusion [122].

The results of these studies are difficult to compare because the type of secretin preparation, potency, dosage, and the test procedures used differed from study to study [122]. When making comparisons one also has to consider whether syringes containing plastic material has been used for injections and especially for infusions, because plastic surfaces can bind secretin. This binding can be avoided by dissolving secretin in serum albumin [29].

17.2.2.2.3
Secretin-Cholecystokinin-Pancreozymin (Cerulein) Test

Secretin administration allows for a correct evaluation of only the hydrokinetic function of the pancreas, but the enzyme output after the secretin wash-out varies considerably and is even normal in many patients with chronic pancreatitis [57]. Cholecystokinin (CCK) has therefore been added to the test procedure in many European centers in order to assess the pancreatic enzyme output [122].

Like secretin, CCK has also been administered by different methods: as a single intravenous injection before, with, and after secretin, or as a continuous intravenous infusion alone, or in combination with secretin [122].

Some centers have replaced CCK by cerulein (pancreatic secretion-stimulating peptide from frog skin with 7 out of 8 C-terminal amino acids identical with CCK) which is cheaper and, if combined with secretin infusion, provides a similar stimulation of pancreatic enzyme secretion as CCK [52, 88, 209].

The most satisfactory stimulant or combination of stimulants for measuring whether pancreatic secretory capacity is normal or impaired, has not yet been determined. The tests are not yet standardized. Therefore, the test performance differs from center to center, each center having its own levels of normalcy. We (PGL) perform the test as follows: After passage of a duodenal tube, pancreatic secretion is collected over 15 min. This is followed by the injection of secretin (1 CU/kg body weight) and 30 min later by injection of cholecystokinin-pancreozymin (CCK-PZ: 1 Ivy dog unit/kg body weight). Stimulated pancreatic secretion is collected in 15-min periods. Following secretin, bicarbonate concentration and output are measured, whereas after CCK-PZ amylase, lipase, and trypsin are estimated. Pancreatic enzymes are discontinued 3 days prior to the investigation.

There is no widely accepted classification of exocrine pancreatic function test results, but a simple categorization using the results of the SPT and fecal fat analysis has been employed in our studies for many years and prove to be helpful (Table 17.4) [125, 145].

When the SPT is compared with endoscopic retrograde cholangiopancreatography (ERCP), it is found that both test results diverge in 0%–20% of the cases. Seven studies have debated whether pancreatic duct changes detected by ERCP really reflect the state of the gland, or whether the duct changes are only the expression of scarring and healing inflammatory processes [7, 83, 84, 95, 96, 146, 170]. Three of the studies graded the test results for severity in a larger number of patients [146, 170, 201]; 3 used the Cambridge classification for evaluation of ERCP [39, 146, 170]. Otte [201] found corresponding grades of impairment based on results of SPT and ERCP in 53% of all 210 patients investigated, which is in the same range as in another study [146]: 64% in 202 patients. With regard to only patients with abnormal SPT and ERCP results, the following percentages have been reported: 34% by Otte [201], 51% by Malfertheiner et al. [170], and 37% by Lankisch et al. [146]. This indicates that one cannot expect test results of one method to correspond to those of another. This contrasts with a smaller study: Bozkurt et al. [39] reported that all their patients with a Cambridge III classifi-

Table 17.4. Grading of exocrine pancreatic insufficiency according to results of the SPT and fecal fat analysis [145]

Exocrine pancreatic insufficiency[a]	Secretin-pancreozymin test		Fecal fat estimation
	Enzyme output	Bicarbonate concentration	
Mild	Abnormal	Normal	Normal
Moderate	Abnormal	Abnormal	Normal
Severe	Abnormal	Abnormal	Abnormal

[a] Mild to moderate exocrine pancreatic insufficiency means compensated (that is, enzyme substitution not required); severe means decompensated (enzyme substitution required).

cation of ERCP also had global exocrine pancreatic insufficiency. Domínguez-Muñoz et al. [66] compared the results of ERCP, computed tomography (CT) and indirect pancreatic function tests and the serum pancreolauryl test (PLT) and found that the development of exocrine pancreatic functional impairment depended primarily on the degree of ductal changes, where parenchymal abnormalities play a less important role.

In a study grading the SPT results and the ERCP examinations for severity, Lankisch et al. [146] found a significant correlation between both investigations (Fig. 17.4). However, ERCP showed significantly more severe changes. In 30 (15%) of 202 patients, totally nonparallel results were obtained (such as a normal SPT and an abnormal ERCP, or vice versa). Patients with an abnormal ERCP, but normal SPT result, had significantly more frequently a history of acute pancreatitis as compared to the second group with an abnormal SPT and a normal ERCP. In a long-term follow-up of 20 patients with an abnormal ERCP and a normal SPT, only 3 actually developed chronic pancreatitis or were suspected to have chronic pancreatitis, whereas in the remaining cases no symptoms of acute pancreatitis or abdominal pain suggestive of chronic pancreatitis occurred. In the other group (abnormal SPT, normal ERCP), all patients developed chronic pancreatitis in the course of follow-up. This is in accordance with another comparable study [120].

SPT \ ERCP	Normal	Slight changes	Moderate changes	Severe changes
Normal	85	3	15	5
Slight exocrine pancreatic insufficiency	4	2	4	10
Moderate exocrine pancreatic insufficiency	3	3	9	15
Severe exocrine pancreatic insufficiency	0	4	7	33

Fig. 17.4. Comparison of SPT with ERCP results in 200 patients. The correlation between both investigations was significant ($p < 0.001$). However, only 129 (64%) patients had parallel SPT and ERCP results, matching in all four gradings of severity (*medium-shaded areas*); 43 (21%) patients had abnormal results for both SPT and ERCP, but the severity gradings did not parallel (*light-shaded areas*). Finally, 30 (15%) patients showed totally nonparallel results, with a normal SPT and an abnormal ERCP, or vice versa (*dark-shaded areas*). (From [146] with permission)

Comparisons of ERCP with functional and histological changes have shown that the SPT reflects better than the ERCP examination the histological changes in chronic pancreatitis [95, 96].

Following acute pancreatitis, duct changes as demonstrated by ERCP are distinctly more frequent than loss of exocrine pancreatic function [50]. During a longer observation period, exocrine pancreatic insufficiency improves, whereas the duct abnormalities remain unchanged [15, 16].

A long-term follow-up study of patients following acute pancreatitis showed that the majority of patients with duct abnormalities as a result of acute pancreatitis do not develop chronic pancreatitis or symptoms suggestive of the disease [227].

17.2.2.2.4
Lundh Test

In contrast to the exogenous stimulation of the pancreas by the secretin test and the SPT, the Lundh test [162] makes use of an endogenous stimulation of the pancreas by a test meal. The test procedure is simple: after intubation of the duodenum, a test meal (300 ml) is given that contains 6% fat, 5% protein, and 15% carbohydrates. Duodenal contents are aspirated either in 4 consecutive 30-min fractions or, more commonly, in a single 2-h collection. Trypsin is the most frequently measured enzyme, since it is less sensitive to changes of pH and more discriminating than lipase and phospholipase [101]. All enzymes may be reduced in severe exocrine pancreatic insufficiency [260]. It is recommended that at least 2 enzymes should be measured, preferably trypsin and lipase, to improve the reliability of the results [101].

Several research groups have shown that the simple Lundh test is helpful in the diagnosis of chronic pancreatitis, particularly when associated with steatorrhea – that is, severely impaired exocrine pancreatic function [1, 41, 44, 158, 187, 253]. James [103] found that the overall diagnostic rate in chronic pancreatitis was 90% and that of pancreatic carcinoma 79%.

Several investigators have compared the Lundh test with the secretin or the secretin-CCK test (for review see also James [103]). The results showed considerable divergence: in some studies there was a good correlation between both tests [163], especially in severe exocrine pancreatic insufficiency [185], but not in mild cases [92]. Rolny and Jagenburg [212] reported that the Lundh test was much less sensitive than the secretin-CCK test. Braganza and Rao [43] found the opposite, namely, that the indirect test was distinctly superior. This was partly because of the disproportionate reduction in tryptic response to endogenous stimulation of chronic pancreatitis; it was only one-third of the response to exogenous stimulation.

Most investigators who favor the Lundh test stress that it is simple, physiological, and inexpensive, and easily performable in most hospitals. Disadvantages limiting the usefulness of the test, however, are:
- It is based on the endogenous release of secretin and CCK; thus, in case of mucosal damage – for example, in celiac disease – the impaired hormonal release may lead to an abnormal result [62, 258]. Therefore, the test cannot distinguish pancreatic from nonpancreatic disease.

- Hormonal release depends on the integrity of the gastroduodenal anatomy, which makes it difficult to interpret test results after operations, such as Billroth-II gastrectomy [259].
- Volume and bicarbonate secretory capacity cannot be assessed.

17.2.2.3
Indirect Pancreatic Function Tests

17.2.2.3.1
Parotid Saliva Test

In experimental pancreatitis, reduction of amylase content of parotid glands was found in rats [107], and a marked decrease of maximal bicarbonate concentration of parotid saliva in dogs [106]. In humans, the levels were significantly lower than those in patients with nonpancreatic diseases, and it was postulated that this parotid saliva test should be superior to the SPT [108]. Two subsequent studies comparing the parotid saliva test with the SPT showed that the former had a sensitivity which was practically zero or very low [64, 128], so that it cannot be recommended as a screening test.

17.2.2.3.2
Serum Tests

Evocative Tests. As an alternative to duodenal intubation, testing for increased levels of serum amylase, lipase and immunoreactive trypsin after stimulation with secretin and/or pancreozymin, bombesin, morphine and prostigmin has been used as an index for pancreatic function. It has been claimed that in case of a normal pancreas, a negligible rise of all the enzymes is to be expected, but in case of pancreatic insufficiency, particularly in an early stage, the rise would be significant. The validity of the test has been debated for many years. Several groups demonstrated disappointing results [14, 156, 193]. Two large studies correlating the evocative test with the SPT in patients with pancreatic and nonpancreatic disease have shown that this test is neither sensitive nor specific and is not to be recommended [201, 222].

Isoamylase Determination. Total amylase levels in serum and urine are normal in chronic pancreatitis except during acute exacerbation of the disease. Aw et al. [18] showed, by means of electrophoretic separation, that pancreatic isoamylase is lowered in chronic pancreatitis. Since then, serum and urinary amylase have been fractionated by polyacrylamide gel electrophoresis, Sephadex chromatography, electrophoresis, and isoelectric focusing. Later on, a photometric test was developed using an amylase inhibitor isolated from wheat (*Triticum aestivum*) with a 100-fold higher specificity against salivary amylase than pancreatic isoamylase (for review see [197, 198, 230]). Furthermore, a specific isoamylase measurement based on a double monoclonal-antibody technique has been developed [213, 246].

Although isoamylase determinations are helpful in the diagnosis of unexplained hyperamylasemia [159], the above mentioned methods have not widely been applied since they have generally been restricted to specialized centers. Using different methods in patients with chronic pancreatitis, several authors [27,104,165,258] have shown that low isoamylase levels support the diagnosis of chronic pancreatitis, whereas normal levels do not exclude the diagnosis.

Since serum enzyme estimations can serve as a screening test for chronic pancreatitis, both pancreatic isoamylase (inhibitor method) and immunoreactive trypsin estimations were tested in 180 patients who underwent an SPT for diagnostic parameters (Figs. 17.5, 17.6). Eighty-two of these patients suffered exocrine pancreatic insufficiency. Specificity of pancreatic isoamylase and immunoreactive trypsin measurements was high in patients with nonpancreatic diseases (pancreatic isoamylase 98,5%,

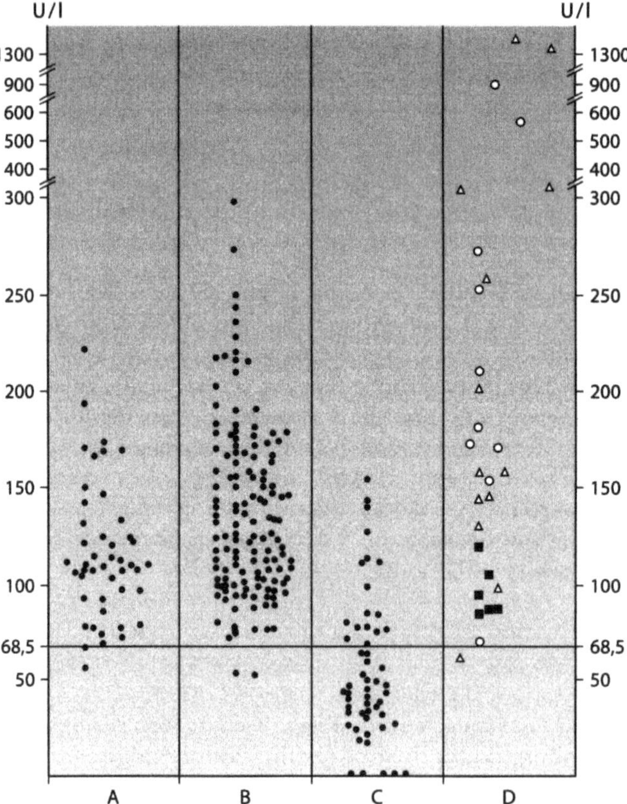

Fig. 17.5. Pancreatic isoamylase estimations in 46 healthy controls (*A*) and 218 patients undergoing an SPT for diagnostic purposes. The SPT was normal in 136 patients (*B*) and abnormal in 82 patients (*C* and *D*). Estimations were performed after an acute attack of the disease in 13 patients (*D; open triangles*), in 10 patients with pancreatic pseudocysts (*open circles*), and in 6 patients older than 60 years (*closed squares*). (From [133] with permission)

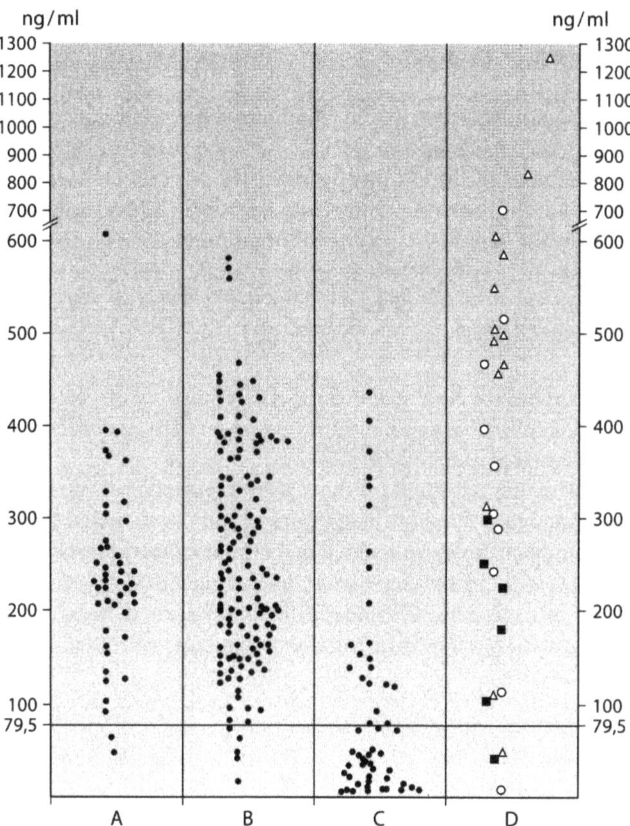

Fig. 17.6. Immunoreactive trypsin estimations in 46 healthy controls (*A*) and 218 patients undergoing an SPT for diagnostic purposes. The SPT was normal in 136 patients (*B*) and abnormal in 82 patients (*C* and *D*). Estimations were performed after an acute attack of the disease in 13 patients (*D; open triangles*), in 10 patients with pancreatic pseudocysts (*open circles*), and in 6 patients older than 60 years (*closed squares*). (From [133] with permission)

immunoreactive trypsin 96.3%). None of the patients with nonpancreatogenic steatorrhea had a low serum enzyme level. Sensitivity, unfortunately, was low in patients with exocrine pancreatic insufficiency (pancreatic isoamylase 45.1%, immunoreactive trypsin 41.5%). Since the low sensitivity might have been due to the still active inflammatory process, i.e., to the acute phase of the disease or the presence of a pseudocyst, such patients were excluded from a second investigation. Furthermore, a small group of patients over 60 years of age were also excluded since both pancreatic isoamylase and immunoreactive trypsin may decrease with age [11, 38, 115, 194]. The end result was increase in sensitivity for pancreatic isoamylase to 67.9% and immunoreactive trypsin to 58.5%. It was concluded that highly specific pancreatic isoamylase measurement is not sensitive enough to be used as a screening test for exocrine pancreatic insufficiency but may be used to determine the etiology of steatorrhea [133]. These findings are in keeping with reports of other groups using different methods [8, 77, 252].

Immunoreactive Serum Trypsin. Radioimmunoreactive trypsin [244] is not detectable after total pancreatectomy [116]. It increases in acute pancreatitis [75], acute exacerbation of chronic pancreatitis [116], and renal failure [117, 119], and may also be raised in the presence of pancreatic cysts with hyperamylasemia [116]. Several studies have shown that the sensitivity of immunoreactive serum trypsin is limited: Although low serum trypsin levels have been said to have an excellent predictive value in diagnosing chronic exocrine pancreatic disease [239], chronic pancreatitis was confirmed by low serum trypsin levels in only 32%–69.2% of patients [38, 75, 116, 119, 238].

The relatively high incidence of falsely normal test results may be explained by the fact that, unlike amylase, serum trypsin tends to stay raised for a longer time after an acute attack of pancreatitis [127].

Low serum trypsin levels have been reported in some patients with diabetes mellitus. Pancreatic function had, however, not been tested in these cases [58]. Furthermore, low serum trypsin and pancreatic isoamylase levels have been reported in some patients with insulin-dependent diabetes mellitus [19, 58, 80, 82, 109, 229, 244]. A comparative study, however, showed that a decrease in serum enzymes did not reflect an impairment of pancreatic function in patients with insulin-dependent diabetes mellitus [139].

17.2.2.3.3
Fecal Tests

Trypsin, Chymotrypsin, and Elastase-1 Estimation. About 0.5% of chymotrypsin and trypsin secreted from the pancreas appear in feces [5]. The development of synthetic low molecular substrates has enabled the specific titrimetric estimation of trypsin and chymotrypsin in stools [12, 94]. Both random samples [12] and 24-h collection of feces [189] have been used. The test is obviously not invasive but is also not popular with laboratory technicians; it requires a titrimeter, which is not available in all hospitals. More recently, with the development of several photometric methods, the use of this test has become more widespread [33, 73, 105, 192, 207].

Falsely normal test results are possible in cases of mild to moderate exocrine pancreatic insufficiency and when pancreatic enzyme therapy has not been discontinued 5 days prior to the test. Falsely abnormal test results can be obtained in patients with diarrhea (low enzyme concentration perhaps due to dilution) and with sprue (decreased liberation of hormones that stimulate pancreatic secretion), after Billroth-II gastrectomy (may be due to postcibal asynchrony), after reduced oral feeding in a cachectic state (decreased pancreatic enzyme synthesis possibly due to protein malnutrition), and in patients with obstructive jaundice (lack of stimulation of bile) (Table 17.5) [171].

Table 17.5. Specificity and sensitivity of indirect pancreatic function tests [171]

Test procedure	Studies (*n*)	Patients (*n*)	Specificity
Fecal chymotrypsin	4	256	84% (73%– 89%)
NBT-PABA test[a]	2	384	87% (87%– 88%)
Pancreolauryl test	11	604	82% (39%–100%)
			Sensitivity
Fecal chymotrypsin	10	361	78% (50%–100%)
NBT-PABA test[a]	3	255	87% (85%– 94%)
Pancreolauryl test	11	371	90% (55%–100%)

[a] 1 g NBT-PABA plus 6-h collection period.

The test has been successfully applied in children with chronic pancreatitis and cystic fibrosis for the detection of pancreatic insufficiency [23, 45, 59, 207].

Recently, an enzyme immunoassay was developed for the measurement of fecal elastase-1. This test has been evaluated against the SPT and found to be an effective, noninvasive, easy-to-perform tubeless pancreatic function test with high sensitivity and specificity. It has been claimed to be more sensitive than fecal chymotrypsin estimation and more specific than the PLT since it is not affected by extrapancreatic diseases or intraluminal degradation and is not influenced by exogenous administration of pancreatic extracts [65, 110, 161, 236]. However, two groups, including one of our own, have shown that in comparison with a direct pancreatic function test, fecal elastase-1 estimations are not sensitive enough to diagnose mild to moderate exocrine pancreatic insufficiency, which is often a clinical problem. Also, the test is not superior to fecal chymotrypsin estimation [4, 137].

Fecal Fat Estimation. Steatorrhea and azotorrhea occur when stimulated lipase and protease output falls below 10% of normal [63]. The estimation of fat in stools collected for 72 h [250] is a safe procedure for the diagnosis of steatorrhea. It may be used as an index for pancreatic function when performed before and after enzyme replacement therapy or as a measure of the effectiveness of the latter therapy. It is also not invasive but, again, is not popular with the laboratory technicians and requires proper laboratory equipment. Nevertheless, this test is recommended as the best investigation available for detecting steatorrhea of pancreatic and nonpancreatic origin.

Recently it has been suggested that patients with gastrointestinal diseases have more severe diarrhea with a given degree of steatorrhea than patients with pancreatic insufficiency. Contributing factors were the underlying gastrointestinal disorders, the osmotic and secretory effects of malabsorbed food, and the probably higher intraluminal concentration of hydrolyzed lipid [32] causing higher fecal losses of water [114]. Unfortunately, further investigations have shown that fecal fat concentration was of no value for a differential diagnosis between pancreatic and nonpancreatic steatorrhea [153, 210].

It has been suggested that fecal fat estimation could be replaced by fecal weight measurements. In a large series of 1269 measurements, comparing fecal weight with fecal fat, Lembcke [150] found in 26.3% of the patients no correlation between both methods: 12.8% had steatorrhea in the presence of normal fecal weight; 13.5% had normal fecal fat content with elevated fecal weight. Thus it is not possible to diagnose steatorrhea just by measuring fecal weight. It has frequently been recommended to inspect stools of patients suspected to suffer from steatorrhea. This has recently been prospectively evaluated. It was found that the visual diagnosis of steatorrhea is dependent on the clinical experience of observers (i.e., experienced gastroenterologists or medical technicians, but not young doctors), and the amount of fecal fat excretion. The specificity of visual diagnosis was good: about 80% of stools with a fat content of more than 15 g/day were correctly diagnosed. However, the sensitivity of the visual diagnosis in moderate steatorrhea (7–15 g/day) was poor. Thus, at least in these cases, the unpopular smellier van de Kamer method will (unfortunately) still be required [131].

A nuclear magnetic resonance (NMR) spectrometry estimation of total stool fat was shown to correlate very well with the fecal fat estimation of van de Kamer and coworkers [225]. However, use of this method is restricted to highly specialized centers.

More recently, a new method, the near-infrared reflectance analysis, has been developed which enables the qualitative measurement of fecal fat and nitrogen concentrations and fecal water content as well as carbohydrate content [25, 26, 151, 237]. This method is very attractive due to the clean measurement and the short analysis time of < 1 min, but the high costs of the instrument presently limit its wider use.

17.2.2.3.4
Urine Tests

Bentiromide and Pancreolauryl Test. For the bentiromide test (in Europe known as the NBT-PABA test; no longer available in several countries of the world including the United States of America and Germany), the patient receives, together with the test meal, N-benzoyl-L-tyrosyl-para-aminobenzoic acid, which is split in the duodenum by the pancreas-specific chymotrypsin. Para-aminobenzoic acid (PABA) is absorbed in the gut, conjugated in the liver, and excreted in the urine. The amount excreted serves as a measure of exocrine pancreatic function.

The test may be falsely abnormal because of disturbances of absorption or conjugation, or renal insufficiency. It has recently been shown that the bentiromide test is not affected by small bowel or liver disease [180]. But it is generally agreed that the specificity of the test may be improved by repetition with the split product (pure PABA) for individual absorption, conjugation and excretion [182]. By means of radioactively marked PABA, the control test may be performed together with the general test on the same day [42, 181, 242]. To avoid possible interference with the test results, all medication except digitalis should be discontinued 2 days prior to the test, especially sulfonamides, sulfonylurea, laxatives, diuretics, vitamins, and pancreatic enzymes. 48 h prior to and during the test no food conserved by benzoic acid should be given, as benzoic acid may influence the test results. Bacterial overgrowth of the gut can lead to falsely normal test results, since some bacteria split the NBT-PABA peptide [93].

In the second type of oral pancreatic function tests, the PLT, the patient receives, together with the test meal, fluorescein-dilauric acid, which is split by the pancreas-specific cholinesterase. One part of the substance (fluorescein) is absorbed and excreted with the urine. Two days later the test is repeated with fluorescein to exclude individual defect of absorption, or metabolic disorder of the liver, or renal insufficiency. The T/C ratio is determined from the excretion result of the test day (T) and control day (C).

Intake of vitamin B_2 and sulfasalazine preparations interfere with the test. These as well as pancreatic enzymes must be discontinued 5 days prior to the test. Falsely abnormal test results have been reported for patients with biliary dyskinesia (insufficient hydrolysis of the ester), or after a Billroth-II operation (possibly because of postcibal asynchrony), but also in patients with inflammatory bowel disease [79, 111, 172].

Both oral tests, or their modifications, have been used successfully for diagnosing pancreatic insufficiency due to chronic pancreatitis or cystic fibrosis in children [99, 173, 196, 217, 226].

Since correct urine collection may be difficult in elderly, severely ill, and out-patients, a shortening of the test procedure would be desirable. Several research groups have developed serum tests for the measurement of paraaminobenzoic acid and fluorescein in serum [36, 53, 60, 121, 126]. Modifications of such tests use metoclopramide and secretin to stimulate the pancreas [168, 169].

17.2.2.3.5
Value of Indirect Pancreatic Function Tests to Confirm
or to Exclude Exocrine Pancreatic Insufficiency

All indirect pancreatic function tests are easily performed (exception: fecal fat analysis), and none has any risks or side effects. The results depend more on competent laboratory performance than on the experience of the examining doctor, in contrast to morphological procedures, such as ultrasound, CT, and ERCP, which require an experienced investigator.

The results of indirect pancreatic function tests depend to a high degree on:
- *Selection of the patients*
  When patients are selected on the basis of accurate case histories, a higher prevalence of chronic pancreatitis is to be expected, thus enhancing the predictive value of the function test [79].
- *Instructions given to the patients*
  When, for example, in the bentiromide test or PLT, the patient takes the test pills before or after breakfast, instead of in the middle of the test meal, this can lead to false-positive results because of postcibal asynchrony.
- *Severity of exocrine pancreatic insufficiency*
  In cases of mild exocrine insufficiency, all indirect pancreatic function tests may yield normal results.

Sensitivity of fecal chymotrypsin test results is high in patients with severe exocrine pancreatic insufficiency [5, 71, 132, 145, 240]. False-negative results occur if exocrine pancreatic insufficiency is mild to moderate or if pancreatic enzyme substitution is not discontinued 3–5 days prior to the test. False-positive results may occur in cases of diarrhea, celiac disease, cachectic state due to chronic inflammatory diseases or tumors, anorexia nervosa, Billroth-II resection, and extrahepatic biliary obstruction.

The PLT and the bentiromide test are very reliable detectors of severe exocrine pancreatic insufficiency, but not mild or moderate insufficiency [145, 172, 240]. In comparative investigations of patients with pancreatic steatorrhea, the sensitivity of all 3 tests was 92%–100%. In patients with mild to moderate exocrine pancreatic insufficiency, tubeless pancreatic function tests are more reliable than fecal chymotrypsin measurements [145].

Serum tests in a report by Lankisch et al. [126] have yielded the same sensitivity and specificity as urine tests. Other investigators have had more reliable results from serum tests [168, 169, 243], or have found that metabolic measurements of the products of PABA, viz. the arylamines, were of higher value than serum estimation [76]. The optimal cutoff point for separating normal from abnormal pancreatic function was after 210 min in the PLT, and after 150 min in the bentiromide test. The latter test was slightly less sensitive and specific than the PLT [126] (Figs. 17.7, 17.8).

The results of direct and indirect pancreatic function tests may show whether exocrine pancreatic insufficiency is decompensated, i.e., whether steatorrhea is likely to be present, thus avoiding the unpopular van de Kamer method for fecal fat estimation [250]. DiMagno et al. [63] found that steatorrhea usually does not occur before stimulated lipase secretion fell below 10% of normal (Fig. 17.9), which was confirmed in a subsequent study [135]. Lankisch et al. [141] showed that the PLT, but not the bentiromide test, yields a similar correlation (Fig. 17.10).

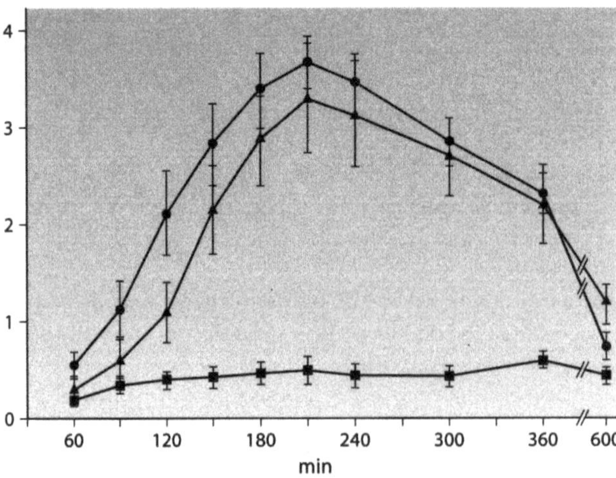

Fig. 17.7. Fluorescein concentration in the serum (micrograms per milliliter; ± SEM) on the test day in 22 healthy controls (*closed circles*), 17 patients with nonpancreatic diseases and normal pancreatic function (*closed triangles*), and 31 patients with exocrine pancreatic insufficiency (*closed squares*). (From [126] with permission)

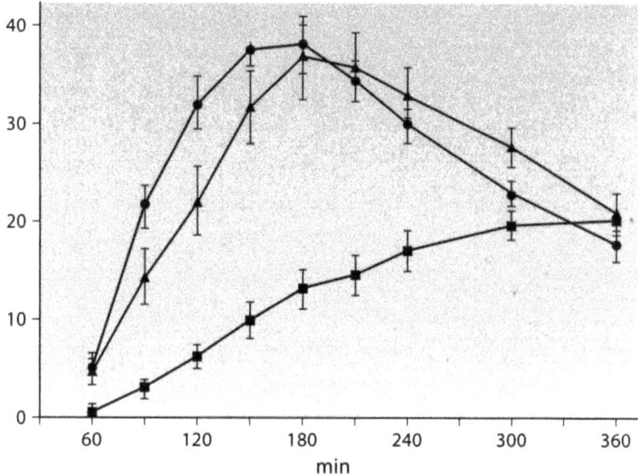

Fig. 17.8. *p*-Aminobenzoic acid concentration in the serum (nanomoles per milliliter; mean ± SEM) in 22 healthy controls (*closed circles*), 17 patients with nonpancreatic diseases and normal pancreatic function (*closed triangles*), and 31 patients with exocrine pancreatic insufficiency (*closed squares*). (From [126] with permission)

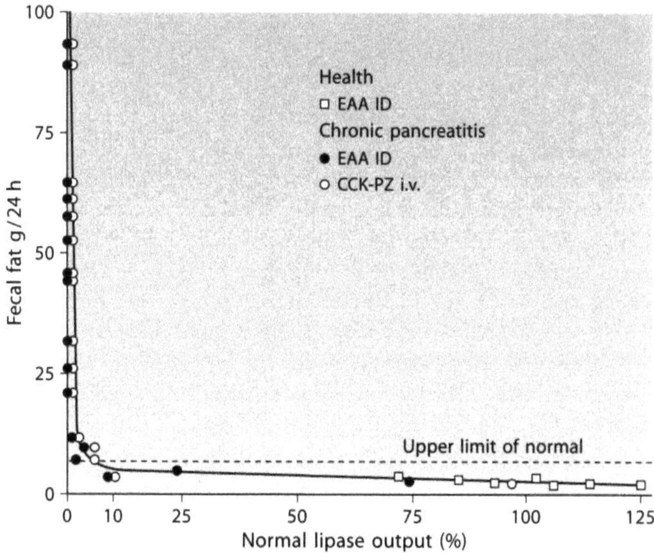

Fig. 17.9. Relation of lipase outputs per hour to 24-h fecal fat excretion in healthy subjects and patients with chronic pancreatitis. Values above the *horizontal dashed line* denote steatorrhea (>7 g of fat/24 h). *EAA ID* = essential amino acids introaduodenally. (From [63] with permission)

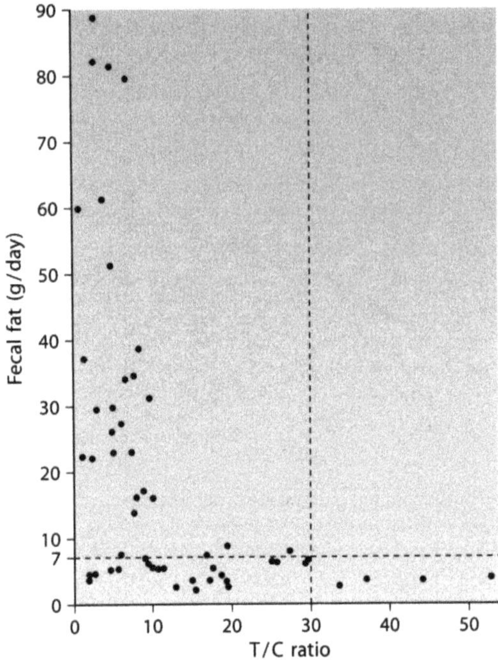

Fig. 17.10. Comparison of daily fecal fat excretion with the results of the urine PLT in 54 patients with exocrine pancreatic insufficiency proven by the SPT. The T/C ratio is determined from the excretion result of the test day (T) and control day (C). Similar to Fig. 17.9, steatorrhea usually does not occur before the T/C ratio falls below 10. (From [141] with permission)

17.2.2.3.6
Plasma Amino Acid Consumption Test

A new interesting exocrine pancreatic function test measures amino acid levels in plasma following stimulation of the exocrine pancreas with secretin and pancreozymin. All patients with normal exocrine pancreatic function showed > 12% decrease in amino acids; in patients with moderate to severe pancreatic insufficiency, this decrease was < 12% [67, 98]. Furthermore, the plasma amino acid consumption test is unaffected by anatomic alterations following gastrectomy [97]. This would give it an advantage over the PLT and fecal chymotrypsin estimation.

Unfortunately, subsequent studies led to almost totally different results [2, 37, 90, 91, 112, 154, 175]. Further clarification is necessary before this test can be recommended as a screening test for exocrine pancreatic insufficiency.

17.2.2.3.7
Breath Analysis Tests

Repeated efforts to use breath analysis as a substitute for direct pancreatic function tests have been unsuccessful [134]. One more recently developed rice flour breath hydrogen test [113] has been shown to be of the same value as the bentiromide test [204]. Another more recently developed breath analysis test seems to be diagnostically valuable only in cases of severe exocrine pancreatic insufficiency [56]. It has been also used in animal experiments [191] and for monitoring enzyme replacement treatment [190].

Here again, further attempts to use breath analysis tests for detecting mild exocrine pancreatic insufficiency would be of great interest.

17.2.2.3.8
Dual-Label Schilling Test

Brugge et al. [46] suggested that insufficient degradation of R-protein (nonintrinsic factor cobalamin-binding proteins present in the saliva, gastric juice, and other body fluids) was responsible for cobalamin malabsorption in pancreatic insufficiency. They performed a modified dual-label Schilling test (pancreatic dual-label Schilling test) to evaluate pancreatic exocrine function. It was found that the cobalamin is not absorbed in the ileum unless the R-protein is cleaved by pancreatic enzymes.

Two subsequent studies based on this test in patients with exocrine pancreatic insufficiency led to varying results. Whereas Leung et al. [157] found a sensitivity of only 50%, Chen et al. [54] reported that they were able to detect patients with both severe and relatively mild pancreatitis. They found a good correlation between the test results and ERCP examinations. Further investigations are required.

Since vitamin B_{12} levels are usually normal [155], vitamin B_{12} absorption does not appear to be a major problem in chronic pancreatitis patients. In the presence of a large variety of pancreatic function tests, the addition of a radioactive pancreatic function test seems outdated.

This is also true for a similar test, the in vitro test of degradation of haptocorrin, a cobalamin-binding glycoprotein that requires the collection of duodenal juice during endoscopy after stimulation with secretin [87, 174].

17.2.2.3.9
Pancreatic Polypeptide

Pancreatic polypeptide is a peptide hormone which is localized both in the islets and between the acinar cells of the exocrine pancreas, especially in the head of the pancreas. The expectation that there may be a close correlation between pancreatic polypeptide release and exocrine pancreatic function was only partly met, since mild to moderate exocrine pancreatic insufficiency could not be diagnosed with sufficient sensitivity [55].

17.2.3
Tests of Endocrine Pancreatic Function

In chronic pancreatitis, a glucose tolerance test may give evidence of diabetes mellitus. Serum insulin levels may reflect a deficiency of insulin secretion as a result of destroyed islet cells. Serum glucagon levels may also be reduced for the same reason. Reduced glucagon secretion renders the diabetes of chronic pancreatitis extremely brittle [68].

17.3
Imaging Procedures

17.3.1
Conventional Radiology

Pancreatic calcifications may be visualized on plain films of the abdomen (Fig. 17.11). Calcifications may appear in diffuse patterns throughout the gland either as relatively large concretions or small scattered stones. It is important to ascertain whether calcifications reside within the pancreas itself and not in an adjacent structure. An oblique or lateral projection can be of great help in confirming whether the calcification is situated in the retroperitoneum behind the stomach. The precise site of calcification within the pancreas can vary. At times, stones are visible at first in the head of the pancreas to the right of the spine and then, as time goes on, more diffusely throughout the gland. Less often is calcification initially visible in the tail of the pancreas.

Incidence data for pancreatic calcifications vary considerably. Pancreatic calcifications were once considered as a late complication and indicative of severe exocrine pancreatic insufficiency [248]. Pancreatic calcification has also been found in the early stage of the disease prior to the development of steatorrhea [142] and may also occur in association with inflammatory scars following acute pancreatitis [143].

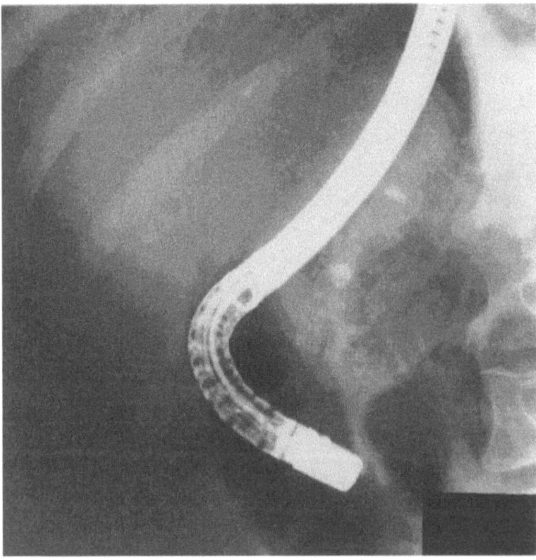

Fig. 17.11. Chronic calcific pancreatitis. Prior to instillation of contrast material into the pancreatic duct at the time of ERCP, survey film reveals multiple intraductal stones throughout pancreatic ducts in a 35-year-old man with chronic calcific pancreatitis who was receiving large amounts of narcotic agents for intractable abdominal pain. The large size of the pancreatic calculi suggests that the main pancreatic duct is considerably dilated. ERCP confirmed marked dilatation of the pancreatic duct. The patient underwent a lateral pancreaticojejunostomy, and at the time of discharge 1 week later was experiencing only residual pancreatic pain. Approximately 80% of patients experienced relief of pain following lateral pancreaticojejunostomy. However, only 40%–50% of patients remain relatively pain-free (see Chap. 19)

Studies of Ammann et al. [6, 9] have shown that pancreatic calcifications may vanish in late stages of the disease [10]. Thus, pancreatic calcifications are a sign that something has happened to the pancreas – in most cases probably chronic pancreatitis –, but their presence is not a parameter for the staging of the disease. Therefore, in light of the latest research, the prognostic importance of pancreatic calcifications is questionable (see Sects. 18.2.1, 20.2.5).

During a suspected flare-up of chronic pancreatitis, just as in primary acute pancreatitis, a chest X-ray and plain films of the abdomen, one in a standing position, should be performed to detect pleural effusions, free air in the abdomen, or evidence of an ileus.

If pain is localized on the left side of the abdomen, or if there is rectal bleeding, a barium enema or colonoscopy may be necessary to detect complete or incomplete colonic stenosis due to involvement of the colon by spread of the pancreatic inflammatory process; the splenic flexure is the portion of the colon usually involved [136]. If common bile duct stenosis is suspected, ERCP or percutaneous transhepatic cholangiography may be necessary.

Should the spleen be enlarged, and especially, if esophageal varices are also present, a dynamic contrast-enhanced CT scan or a magnetic resonance imaging (MRI) should be performed to determine whether there is splenic vein thrombosis [123].

17.3.2
Ultrasound and Computed Tomography

Diagnostic ultrasound (Fig. 17.12a, b) and CT have decisively facilitated the clinical investigations of patients with chronic pancreatitis. Without discomfort to the patient, these studies enable the detection of gallstones and pancreatic calcifications (Fig. 17.13), the evaluation of pancreatic pseudocysts and abscesses, the enlargement of the whole organ or parts of the pancreas [21], and the detection of segmental pancreatitis [241]. Both imaging procedures appear to be of similar value in detecting abnormalities of the pancreas itself. CT has the advantage of detecting pancreatitis-induced changes in surrounding structures. Ultrasound is less invasive, less expensive, and more readily available than CT.

The sensitivity of ultrasound in chronic pancreatitis is 80%–90%, the specificity about 90%. Abnormalities include a dilated pancreatic duct (20%–77%), an irregular outline of the organ (23%–60%), an irregular echo pattern (50%–92%), and a diffuse or partial enlargement of the organ (12%–57%) (Fig. 17.12a, b) [147]. Only one study has investigated the correlation of ultrasonographically detected morphological findings with pancreatic function test results. A distinct, but not very close correlation between the severity of functional impairment and the morphological picture of the parenchymal destruction was found [34]. Especially in the early stage of chronic pancreatitis, functional impairment precedes morphological abnormalities. Ultrasound may fail to distinguish chronic pancreatitis from pancreatic carcinoma. In cases of suspected pancreatic carcinoma, ultrasound-guided pancreatic biopsy may be helpful in the differential diagnosis [183]. While advanced stages of chronic pancreatitis can very well be detected by means of ultrasound, in the early stage the detection of the

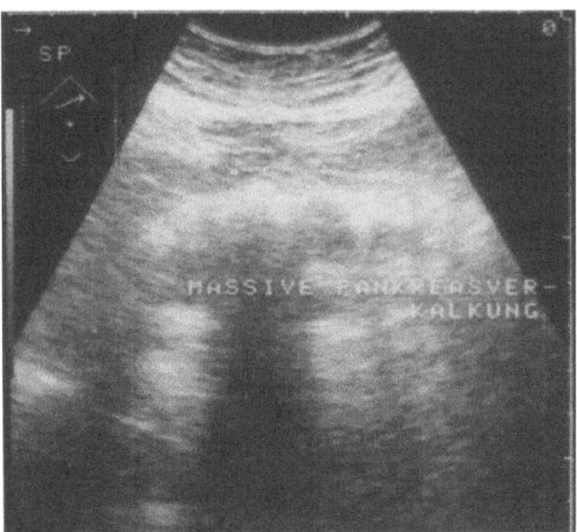
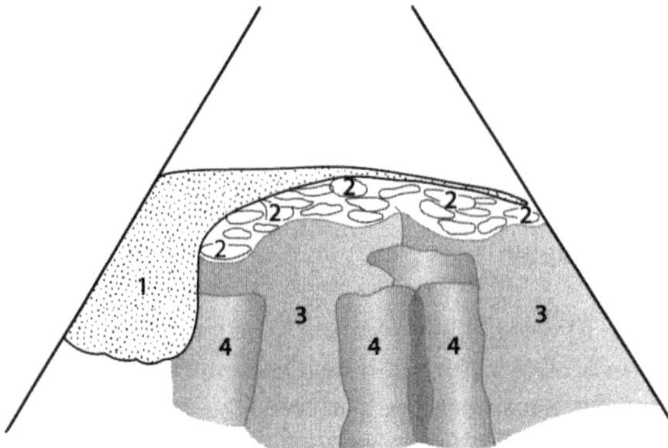

Fig. 17.12 a. 84-year-old male patient with chronic pancreatitis of unknown etiology. *1* head of the pancreas, *2* multiple pancreatic calcifications (massive Pankreasverkalkung), *3* acoustic shadow, *4* repetitive echoes

disease by ultrasound mostly depends on the skill and the experience of the investigator and may be impossible (Table 17.6) [78].

In cases where ERCP fails or proves nondiagnostic, it may be possible to perform ultrasound-guided percutaneous pancreatography for further clarification. This technique has been performed without significant complications [149, 178].

The development of specialized techniques has enabled measurements of the diameter of the pancreatic duct. Secretin stimulation in healthy persons can induce a distinct dilatation of the pancreatic duct within minutes after injection [35, 85, 86, 177]. After secretin stimulation, normal individuals show a distinct pancreatic duct dilatation of more than 90% of basal duct diameter; in comparison, most patients with chronic pancreatitis show no distinct secretin-induced duct enlargement, presumably because of periductal fibrosis [86]. This diagnostic procedure is certainly dependent on the ultrasound equipment and the experience of the investigator.

CT is particularly useful when ultrasound examination fails because of severe meteorism. After oral contrast to visualize stomach and small intestine, the pancreas can be well demonstrated by CT. An intravenous contrast bolus injection is necessary in

Fig. 17.12 b. The 42-year-old male patient with alcohol-induced chronic pancreatitis showed a dilated pancreatic duct *(5)* behind a stone (Stein) *(3)* located between head and body of the gland *(2)*. *1* liver, *4* acoustic shadow

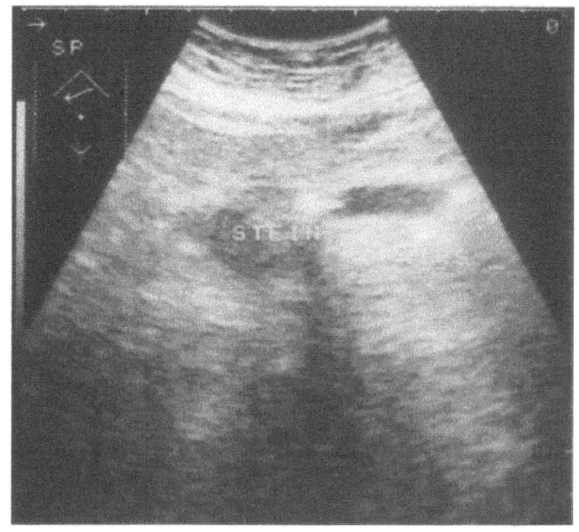

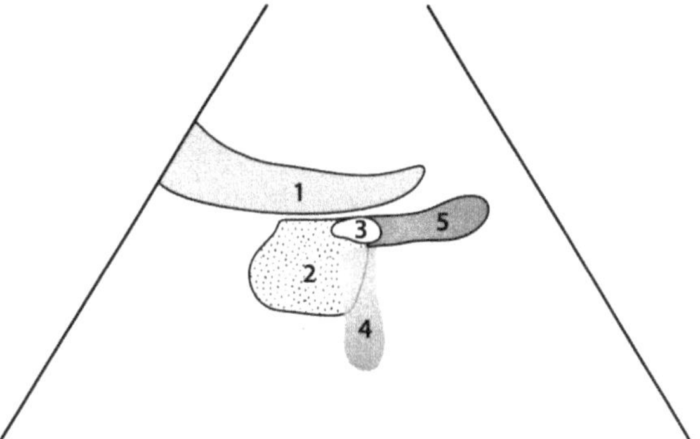

Table 17.6. The sonographic image of the early and late stage of chronic pancreatitis [78, 147]

Early stage
- Homogenous diffuse elevation of the echo-amplitude, pattern of structure retained
- Cobblestone-like pattern of echoes of medium size
- Medium to large size echoes, nonhomogenously dispersed on normal background

Late stage
- Nonhomogenous-heterogenous pattern of echoes with changing appearances of dense and cystic areas
  Exceptional variability of echo-amplitudes and extension of echoes
- Changes in organ size. Sometimes only partial enlargement (caput >3 cm, corpus >2.5 cm, cauda >3 cm, anterior-posterior measurement)
- Tissue calcifications
- Stones in the pancreatic duct
- Cysts
- Dilatation of the pancreatic duct (>2.5 mm)
- Deformation of the organ (outer contour)
- Increase in consistency of pancreatic tissue
- Decreased mobility of pancreas during diaphragmatic excursions
- Enlargement of the common bile duct concomitant with an enlarged head of the pancreas

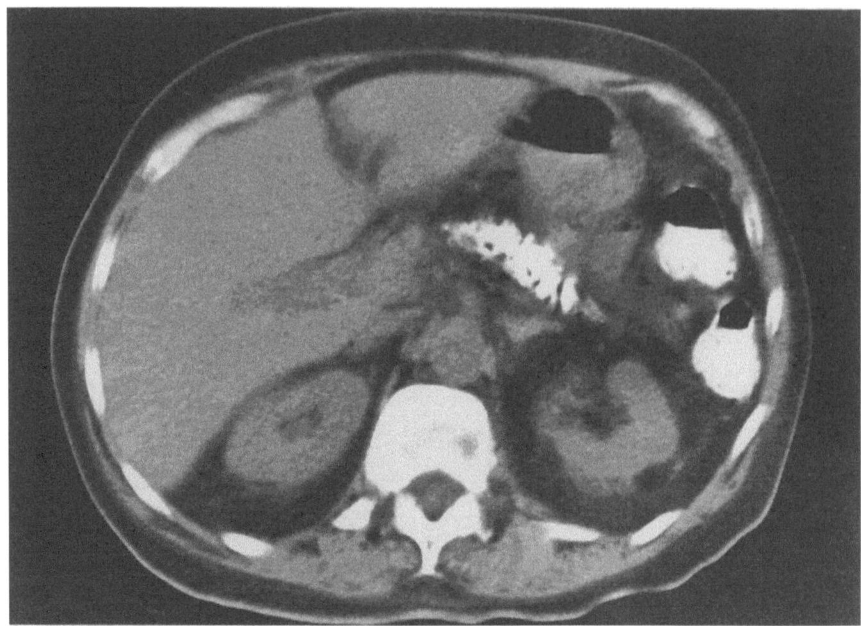

Fig. 17.13. Chronic calcific pancreatitis. Unenhanced CT scan reveals numerous large pancreatic stones in the main pancreatic duct with possible extension into side branches as well. This 50-year-old man with alcoholic chronic pancreatitis had experienced only three prior brief episodes of abdominal pain and had never been hospitalized for pancreatitis. He was not diabetic and was not experiencing steatorrhea. This case illustrates that extensive calcification can occur in a patient without significant abdominal pain and without steatorrhea or diabetes mellitus

acute inflammatory attacks of chronic pancreatitis for the detection of necrotic areas and is helpful to delineate splenic vein thrombosis and associated varices.

The sensitivity and specificity of ultrasonography and CT in patients with chronic pancreatitis are in the same range of about 80%–90% (Table 17.7) [3, 34, 61, 147, 148,

Table 17.7. Computed tomography pictures of chronic pancreatitis [147]

Organ size	Usually enlargement of parts or of the whole organ, rarely also shrinkage of the pancreas
Density of tissue	Nonhomogenous pattern, sometimes with cysts or calcification. Generally slightly increased density
Contour	Irregular form
Pancreatic duct	Dilated (this can be determined by CT only, if diameter is >5 mm)
Bile ducts	Dilated, with enlargement of the head of the pancreas
Duodenum	Compressed, with enlargement of the head of the pancreas
Splenic vein	Occasionally thrombosed, sometimes with spleen enlargement
Other signs	Thickening of peritoneum and renal fascia next to the pancreas; involution of retroperitoneal adipose tissue

Table 17.8. Cambridge classification of pancreatic morphology in chronic pancreatitis as evaluated by computed tomography and ultrasound [148, 220]

Changes	Computed tomography and ultrasound
Normal	Main pancreatic duct <2 mm Normal gland size and shape Homogenous parenchyma
Equivocal	One only of the following signs: Main pancreatic duct between 2 and 4 mm Slight enlargement ($<2 \times$ normal) Heterogenous parenchyma
Mild	Two or more signs needed for diagnosis: Main pancreatic duct between 2 and 4 mm Slight enlargement Heterogenous parenchyma
Moderate	Small cavities <10 mm Duct irregularity Focal acute pancreatitis Increased echogenicity of the duct wall Contour irregularity
Marked	As above with one or more of: Large cavities (>10 mm) Gross gland enlargement ($>2 \times$ normal) Intraductal filling defects or calculi Duct obstruction, structure or gross irregularity Contiguous organ invasion

203]. There is no good correlation between functional impairment and the severity of parenchymal destruction as seen by CT. In minimal functional impairment, morphological abnormalities are rarely seen by CT [167, 170].

A classification for CT and ultrasound, similar to that for ERCP findings (Table 17.8) [20, 148] at the Cambridge Classification Meeting in 1983, has been devised, but is not widely used in clinical practice at the present time.

17.3.3
Magnetic Resonance Imaging

MRI has been used in a variety of pancreatic diseases. Alterations in the signal intensity of the pancreatic parenchyma are well seen. In addition, alterations in the size of the pancreatic duct are also well demonstrated (Figs. 17.14a–d, 17.15a, b). With a specialized technique termed magnetic resonance cholangiopancreatography (MR-CP), the pancreatic duct shows abnormalities that are visible by the technique of ERCP (Figs. 17.15a, b, 17.16a, b). Additional studies are required to determine whether MRI is more accurate than CT or ERCP in demonstrating changes of chronic pancreatitis.

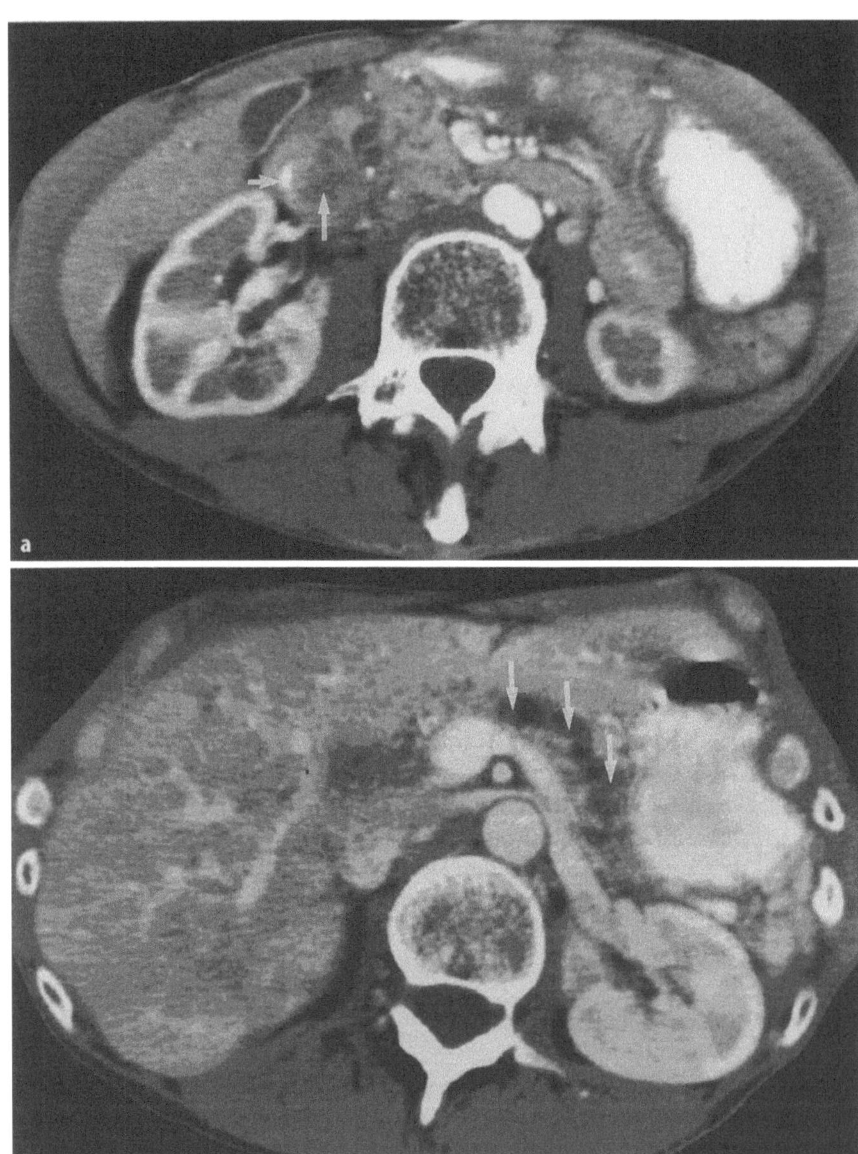

Fig. 17.14a, b. Chronic pancreatitis with dilated pancreatic duct. **a** Dynamic contrast-enhanced CT scan at the level of the pancreatic head in a 45-year-old woman with intractable abdominal pain for 1 year shows an enlarged pancreatic head which enhances heterogenously (*vertical arrow*) and contains punctate calcifications. Contrast is seen within the descending duodenum (*horizontal arrow*). The appearance is consistent with chronic pancreatitis, but carcinoma in the head of the pancreas cannot be excluded. **b** CT scan image obtained through the body and tail shows an irregularly dilated pancreatic duct (*arrows*)

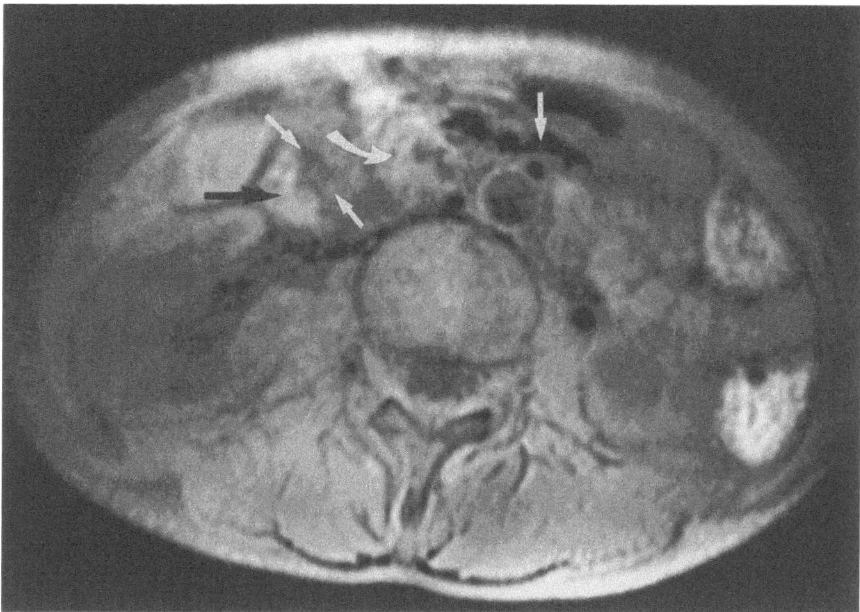

Fig. 17.14c. Chronic pancreatitis with dilated pancreatic duct. T1-weighted fat-suppressed spin echo MR image through the head of the pancreas demonstrates an area of focal increased signal intensity (*oblique arrows*) in the head of the pancreas adjacent to the duodenum (*black arrow*) compatible with pancreatitis or tumor. In an adjacent portion of the pancreatic head, there is increased signal intensity (*curved arrow*) indicating a relatively normal pancreatic parenchyma. The dilated main pancreatic duct is seen in the body of the pancreas (*vertical arrow*)

17.3.4
Endoscopic Retrograde Cholangiopancreatography

ERCP demonstrates better than any other imaging procedure changes of the pancreatic duct system and the common bile duct. An accurate diagnosis of chronic pancreatitis is facilitated by meticulous performance of pancreatography according to the recommendations of Axon et al. [20] given at the International Workshop on the Classification of Pancreatitis at Cambridge. Optimal radiographs are obtained when endoscopists collaborate with experienced radiologists using modern equipment. The series should include a pre-ERCP control film (Fig. 17.11). The main duct should be filled to the tail (or sufficiently to clearly define any obstruction), and the branches should be filled to the second generation (Fig. 17.17a, b). Movement blur and injection of air bubbles must be avoided. Films should be taken during the filling phase to detect small filling defects, and also during emptying, in the supine position.

Serving as a basis for uniformity and comparative studies, the Cambridge classification [20] grades pancreatogram results from normal or equivocal chronic pancreatitis to marked or severe chronic pancreatitis (Table 17.9) [20]. Its use is strongly recommended (Figs. 17.15a, b, 17.17a, b, 17.18, 17.19a, b; see also Figs. 18.2, 18.4) [125].

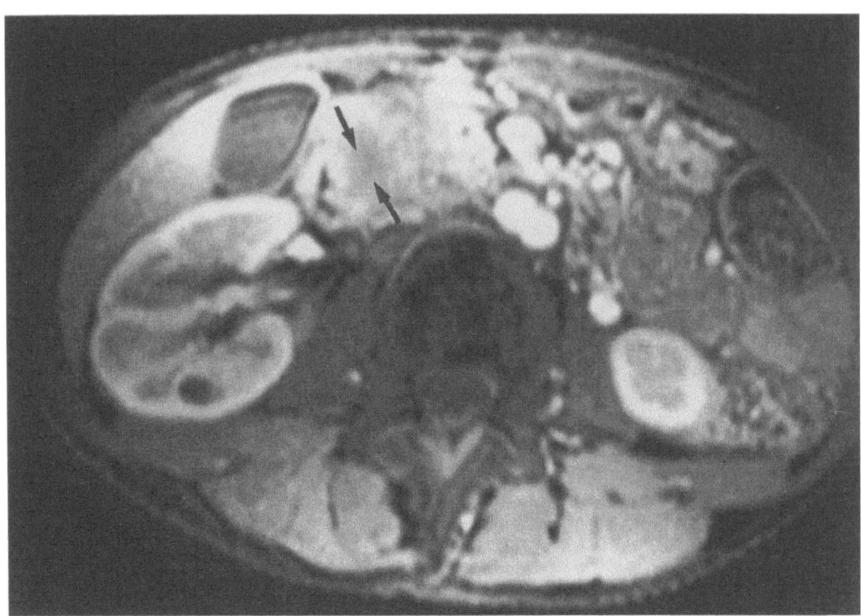

Fig. 17.14d. Chronic pancreatitis with dilated pancreatic duct. Dynamic contrast-enhanced MR image through the head of the pancreas demonstrates an area of focal diminished enhancement corresponding to the area of diminished signal intensity on Fig. 17.14c (*oblique arrows*). This focal abnormality raises the suspicion of a mass lesion. Despite this concern, she underwent a lateral pancreaticojejunostomy, and 1.5 years later remains symptom-free. When the head of the pancreas is considerably enlarged and the remainder of the pancreas is relatively normal aside from ductal dilatation, chronic pain usually originates from the diseased head of the gland. Under these circumstances, and especially when carcinoma is suspected, a Whipple operation should be performed. In this case, the signal abnormalities seen in the head of the pancreas on Figs. 17.14c–d presumably represent fibrosis within an area of chronic pancreatitis rather than tumor

Table 17.9. Cambridge classification of pancreatograms in chronic pancreatitis [20]

Terminology	Main duct	Abnormal side branches	Additional features
Normal	Normal	None	
Equivocal	Normal	Fewer than 3	
Mild changes of chronic pancreatitis	Normal	3 or more	
Moderate changes of chronic pancreatitis	Abnormal	More than 3	
Marked changes of chronic pancreatitis	Abnormal	More than 3	One or more: large cavity, obstruction, filling defects, severe dilatation or irregularity

An abnormal ERCP does not definitely establish the diagnosis of chronic pancreatitis. Pancreatic duct abnormalities may be age-dependent [223, 224], or may represent persistent damage of acute necrotizing pancreatitis [15, 16, 146, 227].

Fig. 17.15a,b. Chronic pancreatitis with dilated pancreatic duct. **a** ERCP reveals a massively dilated pancreatic duct with considerably dilated secondary branches. The duct in the head was narrow and could not be well seen. On this delayed film, the duct has not drained, consistent with obstructive pancreatitis. The endoscope has been withdrawn into the stomach. **b** The corresponding MR-CP image (magnetic resonance cholangiopancreatography) demonstrates similar findings with a markedly dilated main pancreatic duct and dilated side branches. The duct is not visible in the head of the pancreas. Fluid is seen in the duodenal sweep (*arrows*). The gallbladder and biliary tree are well seen and are normal

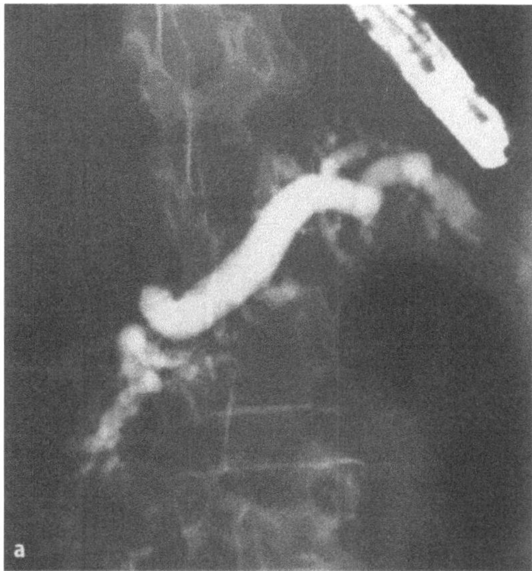

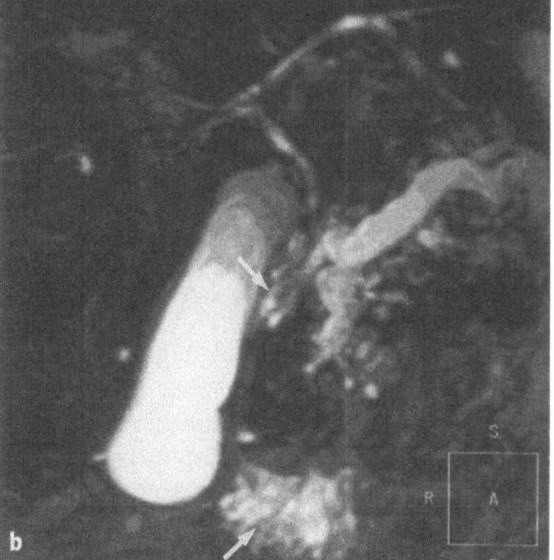

The presence of a normal pancreatic duct system does not definitely exclude chronic pancreatitis.

However, in chronic pancreatitis the severity of duct abnormalities has been found to increase with the duration of the disease [51].

Pancreatic duct abnormalities including pancreas divisum (Figs. 17.16a,b, 17.19a, b, 17.20), which has been found in 5% of a series of chronic pancreatitis patients (see Sect. 1.2.2), are demonstrable by ERCP. This investigation not only detects pancreatic and common bile duct changes, but offers also the possibility of duodenoscopy, aspiration of pure pancreatic juice for cytology and the determination of albumin, immunoglobulins, enzymes, and tumor markers. First studies comparing results of MR-CP

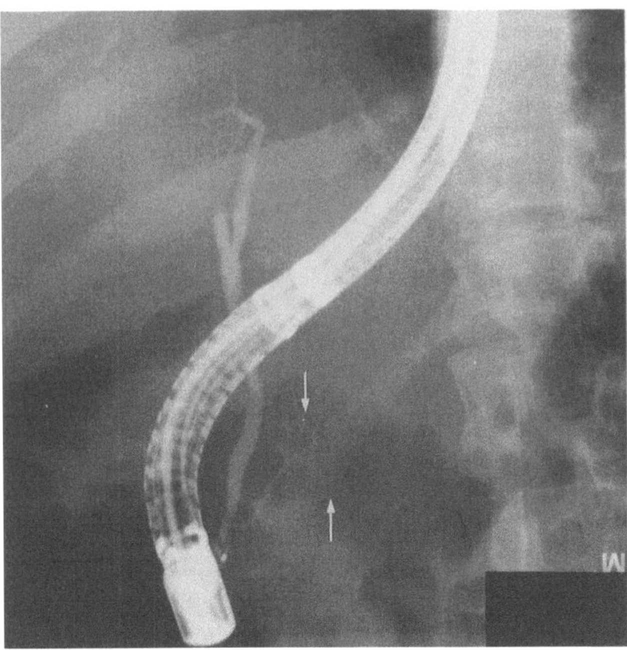

Fig. 17.16a. Pancreas divisum. ERCP shows filling of the common bile duct and the ventral pancreatic duct. There was no opacification of the duct in the body and tail. The pancreatic duct is narrow and exhibits multiple side branches near and at its termination (*arrows*). Differential diagnosis includes pancreas divisum, obstruction to the pancreatic duct, and previous resection of the pancreas. Confirmation of pancreas divisum requires opacification of the dorsal duct. This was not possible in this case for technical reasons

with ERCP show that both imaging procedures can see the pancreatic duct and common bile duct reasonably well [232].

Two decades ago, the complication rate of ERCP was reported to be about 3% and the death rate 0.3% [28]. More recently, post-ERCP pancreatitis was reported in 5.1% in more than 25 000 patients undergoing ERCP [228]. Nevertheless, even recent reports indicate that pancreatitis after ERCP is an underreported event which induces severe and even lethal outcomes with a mortality as high as 13% in seriously ill patients [234].

False-negative and false-positive results are clinically important, particularly the failure to distinguish changes of chronic pancreatitis and the failure to distinguish pancreatic tumor from chronic pancreatitis. These errors can be explained, as follows:
- Duct abnormalities that can be recognized on ERCP develop only in the late stages of pancreatitis.
- Similarities between chronic pancreatitis and pancreatic carcinoma may lead to an erroneous interpretation of the X-ray findings. There is no secure ductal abnormality to establish either the presence or absence of a pancreatic carcinoma, not even the presence of pancreatic calcifications. Carcinoma may be very difficult to distinguish from chronic pancreatitis on ERCP. Chronic calcifying pancreatitis may predispose to pancreatic carcinoma.

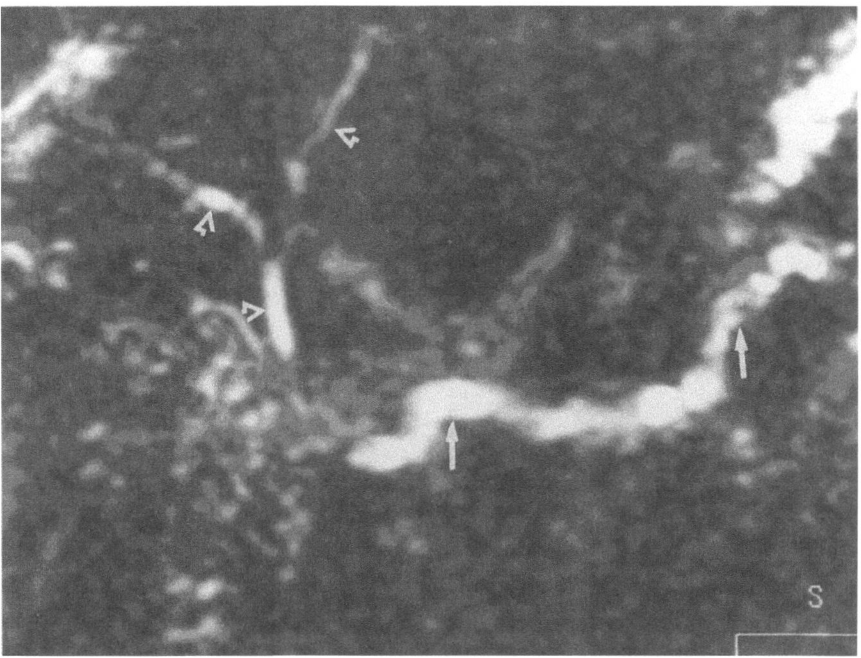

Fig. 17.16b. Pancreas divisum. MR-CP (magnetic resonance cholangiopancreatography) demonstrates a dilated and beaded pancreatic duct in the body and tail of the pancreas consistent with the dorsal duct (*arrows*). This is an example of chronic pancreatitis involving the dorsal ductal system sparing the ventral duct. The biliary tree is visualized (*arrowheads*)

In summary, indications for the use of an ERCP are the following:
- ERCP should be performed in suspected chronic pancreatitis to prove or exclude abnormalities of the pancreatic duct, common bile duct system, and the papilla of Vater and its surroundings. Pancreatic abnormalities include distortion of the ductal system with ductal stricture or obstruction, intraductal calcification, ductal dilatation, and pseudocysts; biliary abnormalities include common bile duct stricture, biliary tract gravel, choledochal cyst, and structural abnormalities of the sphincter of Oddi.
- In cases of known chronic pancreatitis and relapsing pain episodes, ERCP can detect abnormalities of the common bile duct or the pancreatic duct which are responsible for the pain and require surgery.
  The presence of significant pancreatic ductal dilatation allows for consideration of a lateral pancreaticojejunostomy (Figs. 17.14a–d, 17.15a, b). Marked isolated stenosis of the pancreatic duct with obstructive pancreatitis allows for distal pancreatic resection. Diffuse ductal pathology raises the important question as to whether any operative manipulation would yield a favorable clinical result.
- In abdominal trauma associated with recurrent abdominal discomfort of uncertain etiology, ERCP may identify a traumatic stricture of the pancreatic duct, ductal disruption, or a pseudocyst.

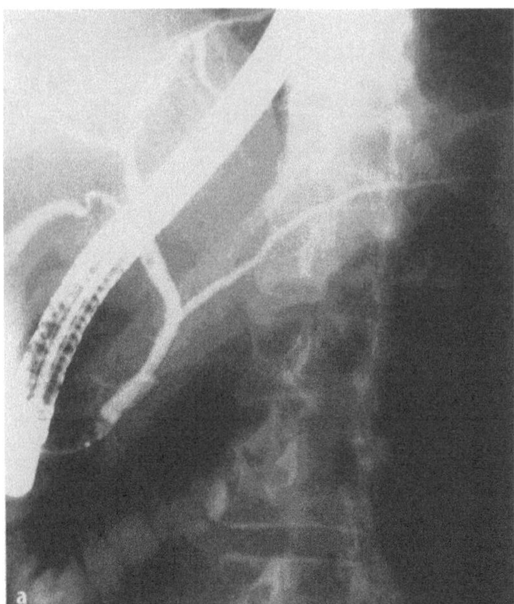

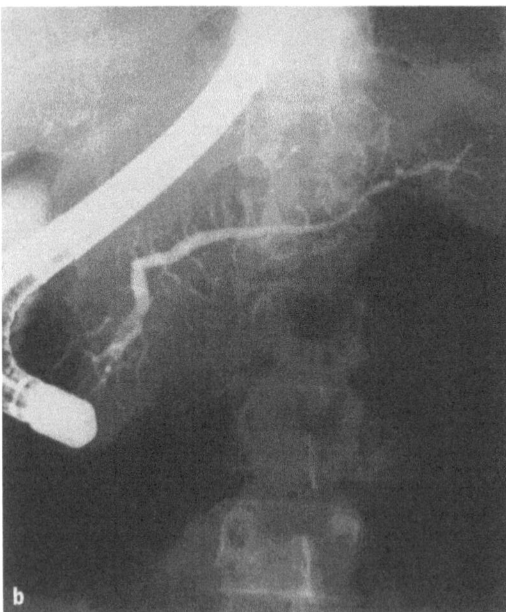

Fig. 17.17 a, b. Normal ERCP. **a** ERCP reveals a normal pancreatic duct with very slender normal side branches. There is an air bubble in the common bile duct just below the endoscope. **b** ERCP reveals a normal main pancreatic duct with completely filled side branches, some of which may be slightly dilated. The side branch changes were considered to be minimal and not diagnostic of chronic pancreatitis

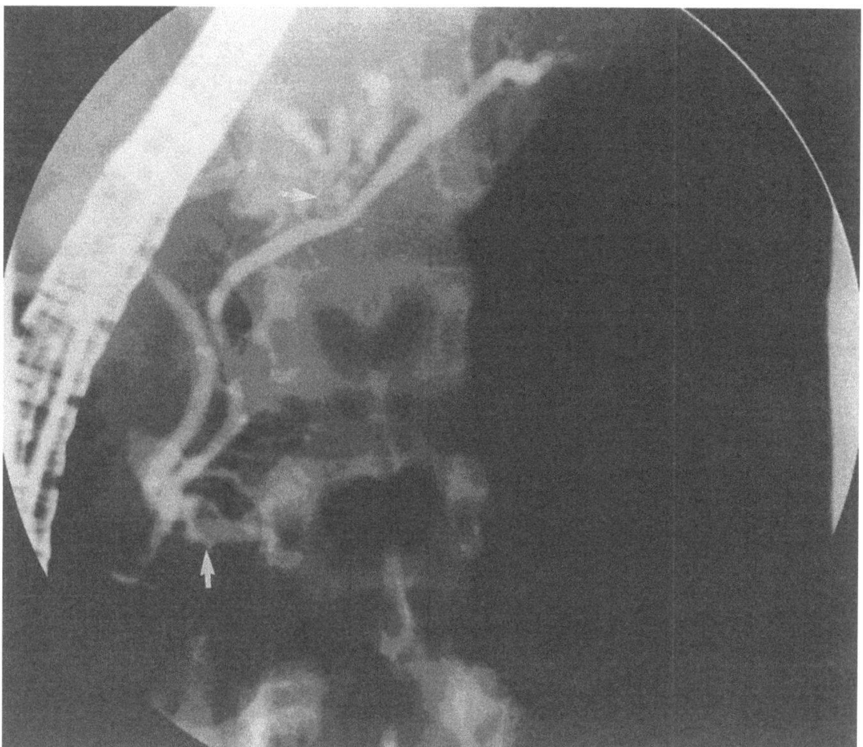

Fig. 17.18. Chronic calcific pancreatitis. ERCP reveals slight dilatation and contour irregularities of the main pancreatic duct and considerable dilatation of side branches. Calculi are visible in several side branches (*arrows*). The 22-year-old man with idiopathic pancreatitis experienced episodes of mild abdominal pain for several years and has subsequently become pain-free during the past 3 years. This case illustrates the unpredictability of the clinical course in chronic pancreatitis. In some series, patients with idiopathic chronic pancreatitis have experienced a more benign course than those with alcoholic pancreatitis

- In pleural effusion and pancreatic ascites, ERCP may demonstrate leakage from a pseudocyst or from a ductal disruption (Fig. 17.21 a, b). This information is, therefore, of great usefulness for surgical or endoscopic treatment [100, 102, 179].
- Occasionally, after surgery for pancreatic pseudocyst, the patient continues to experience episodes of abdominal pain. ERCP may reveal persisting pancreatic ductal stenosis and, at times, the development of a second pseudocyst related to this stenosis.
- ERCP is very helpful in the postoperative assessment of patency of ductal anastomosis to jejunum.
- Accuracy in interpretation of ERCP is enhanced by an indepth knowledge of the case history of the patient [208].

Fig. 17.19a, b. Pancreas divisum. ERCP performed on a 38-year-old woman with 10 years of idiopathic recurrent pancreatitis. **a** Cannulation of the ventral duct shows a short segment of dilated irregular duct with clubbed side branches. **b** Cannulation of the dorsal duct shows subtle contour changes with dilated side branches (*arrows*). This is an example of idiopathic chronic pancreatitis involving both the dorsal and ventral ducts in a patient with pancreas divisum

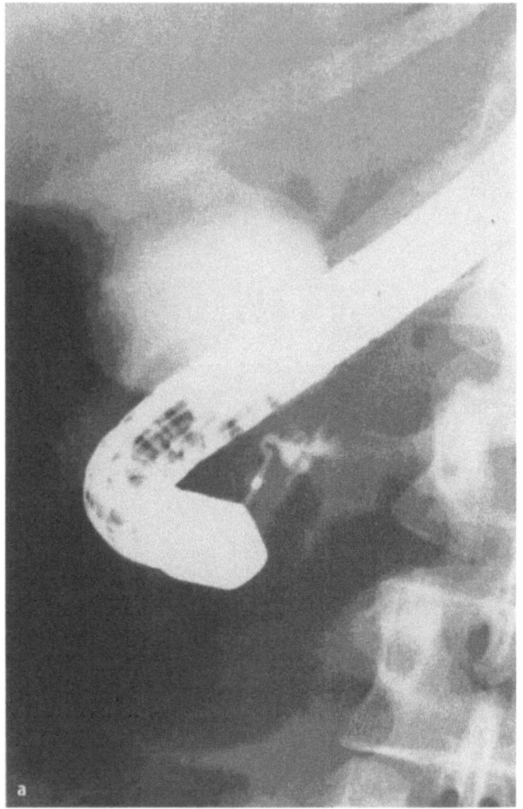

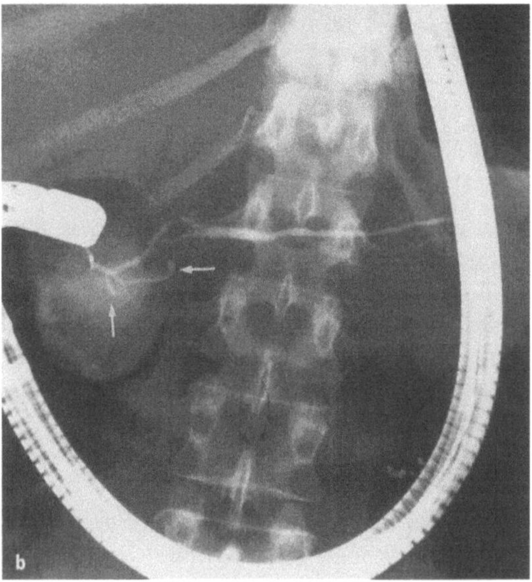

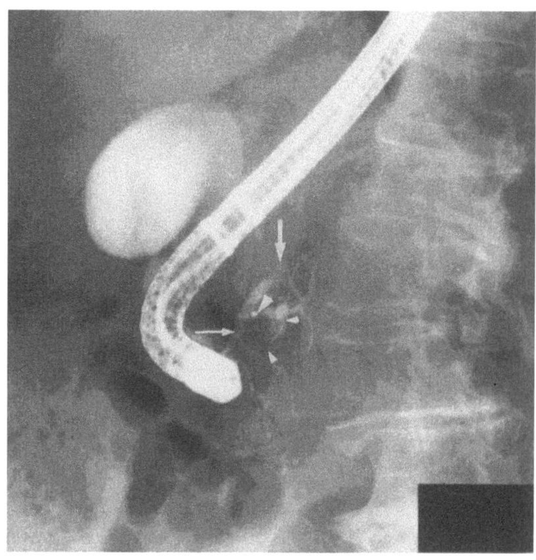

Fig. 17.20. Obstruction of main pancreatic duct. ERCP in an 80-year-old woman with persistent epigastric pain shows complete obstruction of the pancreatic duct in the head of the gland. The pancreatic duct is mildly dilated and has a blunt termination (*vertical arrow*). The catheter has been inserted several centimeters into the main pancreatic duct (*arrowheads*). The accessory duct has been filled in retrograde fashion (*horizontal arrow*). At surgery, a carcinoma of the body of the pancreas was found, and a distal pancreatectomy was performed

17.3.5
Endoscopic Ultrasound

Whereas a unique role has been established for endoscopic ultrasound (EUS) in the detection of pancreatic malignancy [214], the role of this relatively new imaging procedure in the detection of chronic pancreatitis has still to be clarified (Figs. 17.22, 17.23).

In a prospective study, Nattermann et al. [195] compared EUS and ERCP in 114 patients with either chronic pancreatitis or after acute interstitial pancreatitis. When patients were staged according to the Cambridge classification for ERCP results in chronic pancreatitis [20] into groups with normal pancreatic duct (0), minimal, moderate, and severe changes (I, II and III), sensitivity of EUS was 63%, 88%, 100%, and 100% in these groups. In another prospective study, Wiersema et al. [255] investigated 69 patients with chronic abdominal pain of suspected pancreatic origin with EUS and ERCP. All of the 19 patients with abnormal pancreatogram results had also abnormal EUS findings. In addition, in the group of patients in an early stage of chronic pancreatitis (no or minimal changes on ERCP), the sensitivity of EUS was 86% versus 50% with ERCP. In another prospective study, Rösch et al. [215] investigated the role of EUS in the evaluation of patients with suspected pancreatic disease (Table 17.10). The

Table 17.10. Role of EUS in evaluation of 57 patients with suspected pancreatic disease [215]

Final diagnosis	n	Clinical evaluation (%)	EUS (%)	ERCP (%)	CT (%)
Normal pancreas	19	53	95	63	84
Chronic pancreatitis	24	67	79	67	79
Ampullopancreatic malignancy	14	36	64	43	71

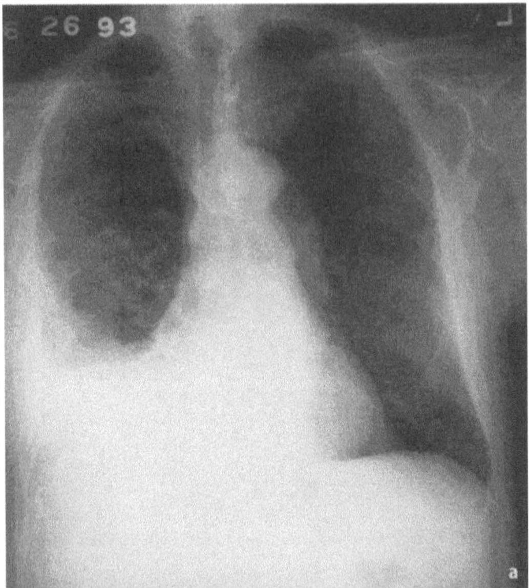

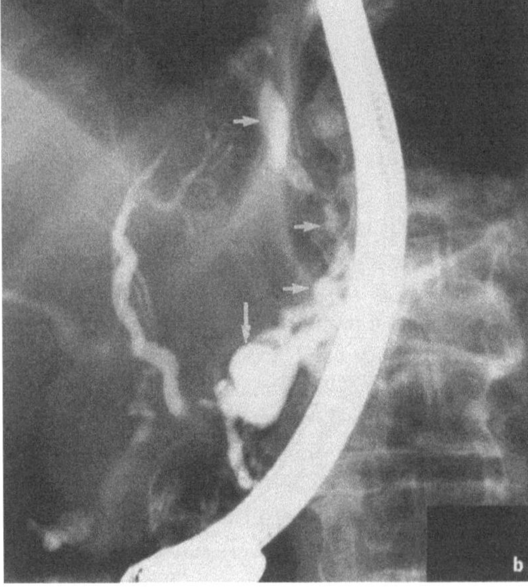

Fig. 17.21 a,b. Chronic pancreatitis with ductal disruption and pleural effusion. **a** Chest X-ray in this 74-year-old man with alcoholic chronic pancreatitis reveals opacification of the right lung base consistent with a moderate-sized right pleural effusion. At thoracentesis, amylase-rich fluid was aspirated. **b** ERCP reveals a normal common bile duct. Opacification of the main pancreatic duct reveals an amorphous collection at the genu consistent with a pseudocyst that is in communication with the main pancreatic duct (*vertical arrow*). The remainder of the pancreatic duct is dilated. In the vicinity of the pseudocyst, there is a disruption of the pancreatic duct with extravasation of contrast material (*horizontal arrows*) extending into the right pleural space. Attempts at passing a pancreatic stent to the level of the extravasation failed. The patient underwent a Roux-en-Y lateral pancreaticojejunostomy. A right chest tube eliminated the pleural effusion. This case demonstrates the role of decompression of a pseudocyst and dilated pancreatic duct in closing a pancreatic fistula

ultrasound method was superior to clinical evaluation and ERCP, and ranked similarly with CT. At present, EUS limitations seem to be in the diagnosis of early pancreatitis and in the correct differentiation of pancreatic masses, especially in differentiating focal inflammation from malignancy. However, we can now do fine-needle aspiration with this procedure through the posterior wall of the stomach for cytology and K-ras. Further limitations of EUS are certainly that this method requires special experience and expensive equipment. Further studies are necessary.

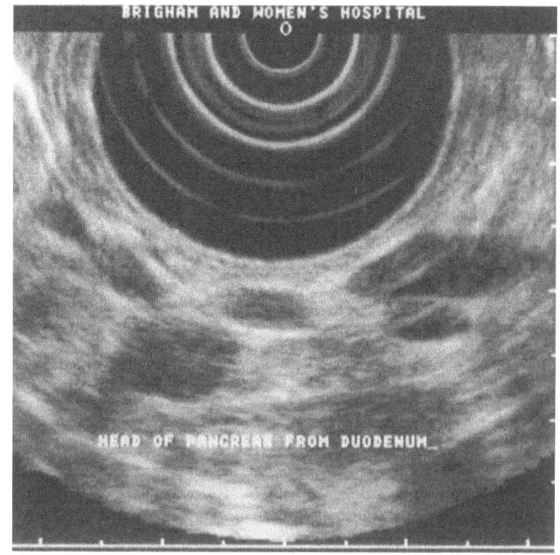

Fig. 17.22. Chronic pancreatitis. Endoscopic ultrasound shows the head of the pancreas as imaged from the duodenum. There are small hypoechoic areas strongly suggestive of chronic pancreatitis. The hypoechoic areas are thought to represent tiny cystic areas

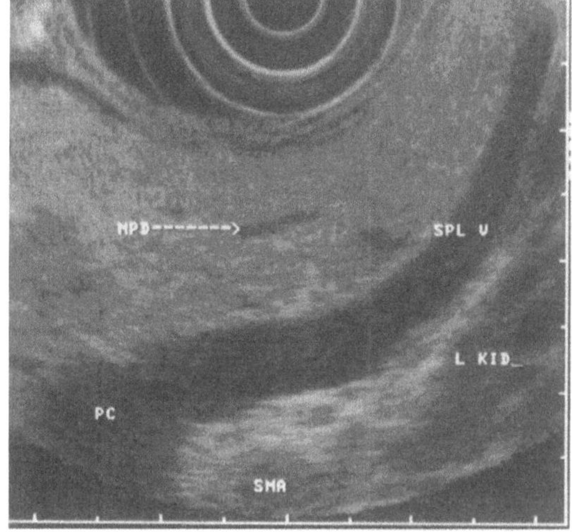

Fig. 17.23. Normal pancreas. Endoscopic ultrasound shows the body and tail of the pancreas as imaged from the posterior wall of the stomach. The pancreatic parenchyma is relatively homogenous in appearance. The main pancreatic duct (*MPD*), splenic vein (*SPL v*), and portal confluence (*PC*), left kidney (*L KID*), and superior mesenteric artery (*SMA*) are well shown

Finally, Buscail et al. [48] investigated prospectively 81 patients with suspected pancreatic disease. Sensitivity of EUS for diagnosis of chronic pancreatitis was 88%, of ERCP 74%, and of CT scan 75%.

A preliminary report [247] shows that EUS is valuable in detecting groove pancreatitis, which is a special form of chronic pancreatitis [24, 241].

At present, among imaging procedures for diagnosing chronic pancreatitis, ERCP remains the gold standard. EUS may be as good as ERCP. However, we need more data in terms of following individuals whose EUS is positive but ERCP thus far is negative. We also need correlation with direct pancreatic function tests, such as the secretin test or the SPT.

17.3.6
Angiography

Angiography is occasionally helpful in the diagnosis of chronic pancreatitis. The demonstration of pseudoaneurysms in peripancreatic arteries in pancreatitis, and their absence in carcinoma of the pancreas, has been reported to be a helpful differential feature [254]. Angiography is sometimes combined with CT to search for a pancreatic pseudoaneurysm as a cause of hemorrhage into a pancreatic pseudocyst [74, 81, 166, 206, 233]. This method can also be used for arterial embolization to stop bleeding [221].

17.3.7
Pancreatic Duct Manometry

Measurements of intraductal pressure have been made in patients without pancreatic disease and those with ductal abnormalities. Thus far, among patients without pancreatic disease, intraductal pressure has been found to be 7 mm Hg by direct puncture at surgery in one patient [72] and 10–16 mm Hg by ERCP among 33 patients without pancreatic disease [40, 199, 235]. By comparison, in three studies of intraductal pressure measured by puncture at surgery in 59 patients with a dilated duct, intraductal pressure ranged from 18–48 mm Hg [40, 72, 164], whereas in studies from two other groups endoscopically measured manometric pressure of the pancreatic duct was 16.2 or 18 mm Hg in patients without pancreatitis [199, 200, 211].

Further studies are necessary to evaluate the role of pancreatic duct manometry in diagnosis and treatment of chronic pancreatitis.

17.4
Synopsis of Diagnostic Procedures

17.4.1
General

At present, there is no generally accepted standardized procedure available to diagnose chronic pancreatitis and evaluate the severity of the disease. This makes it difficult to compare reports on chronic pancreatitis throughout the world and also contributes to long delays in diagnosing the disease [13, 144].

The following is a suggested synopsis of standards for the diagnosis of the disease [125].

Case history, physical examination, basic laboratory tests, and some basic imaging procedures must be performed in each patient. The timing of morphological and functional procedures should be guided by the nature of the presenting complaint (pain or weight loss and/or diarrhea and/or steatorrhea) (Fig. 17.24).

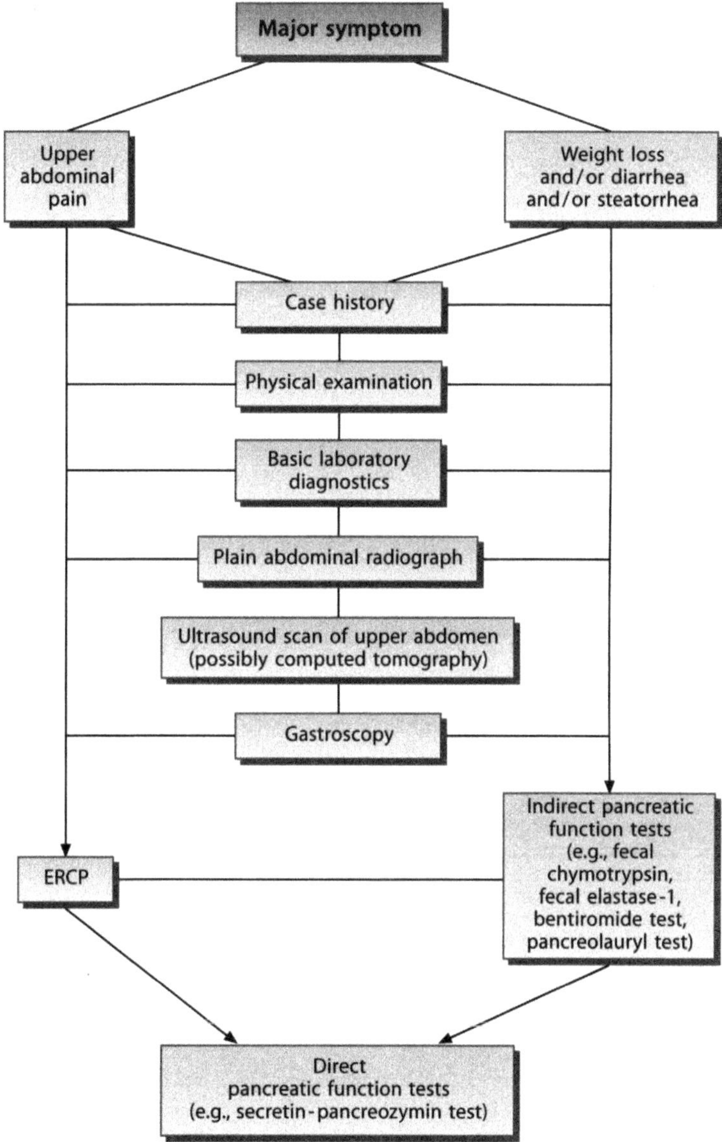

Fig. 17.24. Diagnostic procedure according to major symptoms when chronic pancreatitis is suspected. If epigastric complaints dominate, ERCP should be performed in addition to (possibly even before) indirect pancreatic function tests. If weight loss, diarrhea, or steatorrhea dominate, indirect pancreatic function tests should be performed before ERCP. If ERCP and indirect pancreatic function tests are inconclusive but chronic pancreatitis still suspected, a direct pancreatic function test is indicated to confirm or refute this suspicion

17.4.2
Case History

Relapsing and otherwise unexplained attacks of pain are frequently misdiagnosed as chronic pancreatitis. Thus, other explanations for pain, such as gallstone disease, peptic ulcer, and inflammatory bowel disease must be excluded [124].

Pain should be classified in order to assess the course of the disease and treatment. One could use a visual analogue scale, for example from 0–10, or a shorter scale, for example "no pain", "mild", "moderate severe", and "severe pain" (Table 17.11). It is important to note frequency of pain attacks: whether the pain is continuous, or, if not, the number of pain attacks per week, month, or year.

Table 17.11. Recommended staging of chronic pancreatitis

A **Symptoms**
  - Pain (for example visual analogue scale 0–10)
  - Weight loss, nausea, vomiting, diarrhea (absence/presence, frequency, amount)

B **Morphology**
  - Ultrasound
  - Computed tomography
  - ERCP (according to the Cambridge classification)

C **Exocrine pancreatic function**
  - SPT plus fecal fat analysis
    Mild exocrine pancreatic insufficiency:
    Enzyme secretion reduced, bicarbonate concentration and fecal fat excretion normal
    Moderate exocrine pancreatic insufficiency:
    Enzyme secretion and bicarbonate concentration reduced, fecal fat excretion normal
    Severe exocrine pancreatic insufficiency:
    Enzyme secretion and bicarbonate concentration reduced, steatorrhea

D **Endocrine pancreatic insufficiency (diabetes mellitus)**
  - Absent (no treatment)
  - Moderate (diet plus/minus oral medication)
  - Severe (insulin treatment)

Finally, it should be established whether pain affects the quality of life of the patient (e.g., whether or not the patient is restricted in her or his activities). If analgesics are used, their type and dosage should be registered.

Weight loss, nausea, vomiting, and diarrhea, in contrast to pain, are of less importance for the patient's life. An evaluation should include the presence or absence of these symptoms, whether they are caused by dietary habits, and if nausea, vomiting, and diarrhea are present, their frequency and impact on the patient's lifestyle should be mentioned.

17.4.3
Physical Examination

Other than during an acute attack of chronic pancreatitis, standard physical examination will not be useful for diagnosis, since palpable masses and skin signs are rare.

17.4.4
Basic Laboratory Tests

Pancreatic enzyme elevations can be detected only during acute attacks. *It is, however, of outmost importance to know that even if amylase and lipase levels are normal, this does not exclude an acute attack of chronic pancreatitis.* In the advanced stage of the disease, acute inflammation may produce pain without enzyme elevations.

17.4.5
Basic Imaging Procedures

A plain abdominal film for locating pancreatic calcifications, ultrasound examination of the abdomen, and – if these are inconclusive – a CT are advisable to assess size and texture of the pancreas and the existence of any masses or cystic alterations.

If calcifications in the area of the pancreas are demonstrated by any of these imaging procedures, this means "chronic pancreatitis". Only in a few cases can pancreatic calcifications be detected after an attack of acute pancreatitis [143].

17.4.6
Gastroscopy

An endoscopy of the upper gastrointestinal tract should be performed to exclude other causes of abdominal pain [124]. *It should be noted that peptic ulcers have been observed in up to 37.5% in some series of chronic pancreatitis* (see Sect. 18.3.3) [70, 89, 160, 184, 188, 251]. Thus, even in a patient with proven chronic pancreatitis, an endoscopy may be indicated to evaluate pain.

17.4.7
ERCP or Function Test: Which Step Next?

Diagnosis of chronic pancreatitis may require both functional and morphological tests. Together, these tests allow for more accurate results. To borrow an analogy from daily life, nobody would pronounce judgment on a beautiful car before she/he has tested its function, in this case, its engine. And, morphologically speaking, a beat-up car, nevertheless, may function because of its excellent motor [125].

Several studies have shown that ERCP and the SPT, both gold standards for morphological and functional examinations of the pancreas, do not lead to corresponding results. There may be totally nonparallel results in up to 15%–23%, i.e., the SPT result may be abnormal and the ERCP result normal, or vice versa (see Sect. 17.2.2.2.3) [146, 201].

An abnormal ERCP or an abnormal SPT result does not necessarily establish the diagnosis of chronic pancreatitis. An abnormal SPT does not distinguish between chronic pancreatitis, pancreatic carcinoma, or resolving acute pancreatitis. Similarly, an abnormal ERCP may be due to a severe attack of previous acute pancreatitis leaving scars rather than being a sign of chronic pancreatitis. Such scars may persist long after the acute inflammation has returned to normal [227]. Only when both clinical symptoms of chronic pancreatitis and an abnormal SPT, or ERCP, or both, coexist, can one make the diagnosis of chronic pancreatitis.

The results of an exocrine pancreatic function test depend to a great extent on the accuracy of the examination procedure, instructions to the patient, and the patient's compliance. The gold standard test, the SPT, is time-consuming and, therefore, not too popular. Morphological examinations, on the other hand, depend on the investigator's experience with ultrasound, CT, and especially ERCP. Since these imaging procedures are not time-consuming and, with the exception of ERCP which is usually done under conscious sedation, not invasive, they are much more popular than the function tests. Accuracy of both the function tests and the imaging procedures depends on the severity of the disease, that is, they may be normal in mild chronic pancreatitis. It is believed that a combination of function tests and morphological examinations is necessary to diagnose chronic pancreatitis as well as to stage severity and to establish prognosis of complications [125].

Therefore, it is recommended
- *To perform an ERCP in symptomatic patients* to detect the source of the patient's pain in the pancreatic duct or elsewhere.
- *To perform a function test*
  in a referral center, an SPT and fecal fat analysis to prove exocrine pancreatic insufficiency, to stage its severity, and to find out whether pancreatic enzyme substitution is necessary (Table 17.4).
  in a nonreferral center, an indirect pancreatic function test such as the urinary PLT or the bentiromide test (see Sect. 17.2.2.3.4), or fecal enzyme estimation (chymotrypsin or elastase-1; see Sect. 17.2.2.3.3) may be sufficient. In a number of patients with mild to moderate exocrine pancreatic insufficiency, these tests may remain normal. But for practical purposes, it is important that such normal *indirect test results exclude chronic pancreatitis as the cause of steatorrhea.*
  The staging of ERCP results and of other imaging procedures, such as ultrasound and CT, should be performed according to the Cambridge classification (Tables 17.8, 17.9) [20, 148].
- *To test endocrine pancreatic function, an oral glucose tolerance test* and, possibly, 2-h fasting postprandial blood glucose as well as hemoglobin A_{1c} estimation. Endocrine pancreatic insufficiency may be simply classified as *absent, moderate* (diabetes mellitus treated only with diet plus/minus oral medication), and *severe* (requiring insulin treatment) [125, 138].

References

1. Aenishänslin WH, Kayasseh L, Stalder GA (1973) Die Pankreasfunktionsprüfung mit dem Lundh-Test. Resultatübersicht anhand von 246 Tests. Dtsch Med Wochenschr 98:2192–2196
2. Allen AM, Oates PS (1992) Measuring total plasma amino acid concentrations as a test of exocrine pancreatic function. Gut 33:392–396
3. Alpern MB, Sandler MA, Kellman GM, Madrazo BL (1985) Chronic pancreatitis: ultrasonic features. Radiology 155:215–219
4. Amann ST, Bishop M, Toskes PP (1995) Fecal pancreatic elastase 1: is it the test we have been looking for? Gastroenterology 108:A341 (abstr)
5. Ammann R (1967) Fortschritte in der Pankreasfunktionsdiagnostik. Experimentelle Medizin, Pathologie und Klinik, Band 22. Springer, Berlin–Heidelberg–New York
6. Ammann RW, Akovbiantz A, Largiadèr F, Schueler G (1984) Course and outcome of chronic pancreatitis. Longitudinal study of a mixed medical-surgical series of 245 patients. Gastroenterology 86:820–828
7. Ammann RW, Buehler H, Bruehlmann W, Kehl O, Muench R, Stamm B (1986) Acute (nonprogressive) alcoholic pancreatitis: prospective longitudinal study of 144 patients with recurrent alcoholic pancreatitis. Pancreas 1:195–203
8. Ammann RW, Bühler H, Pei P (1982) Comparative diagnostic accuracy of four tubeless pancreatic function tests in chronic pancreatitis. Scand J Gastroenterol 17:997–1002
9. Ammann RW, Largiadèr F, Akovbiantz A (1979) Pain relief by surgery in chronic pancreatitis? Relationship between pain relief, pancreatic dysfunction, and alcohol withdrawal. Scand J Gastroenterol 14:209–215
10. Ammann RW, Muench R, Otto R, Buehler H, Freiburghaus AU, Siegenthaler W (1988) Evolution and regression of pancreatic calcification in chronic pancreatitis. A prospective long-term study of 107 patients. Gastroenterology 95:1018–1028
11. Ammann RW, Pei P, Satz N, Woodtli W (1982) Variations with age of immunoreactive serum trypsin: higher reference ranges in "healthy" elderly people. Klin Wochenschr 60:243–246
12. Ammann RW, Tagwercher E, Kashiwagi H, Rosenmund H (1968) Diagnostic value of fecal chymotrypsin and trypsin assessment for detection of pancreatic disease. A comparative study. Am J Dig Dis 13:123–146
13. Andersen BN, Thorsgaard Pedersen N, Scheel J, Worning H (1982) Incidence of alcoholic chronic pancreatitis in Copenhagen. Scand J Gastroenterol 17:247–252
14. Andriulli A, Masoero G, Fico D, Zago P, Marchetto M (1986) Evocative test of serum pancreatic enzymes to bombesin in chronic pancreatitis. Am J Gastroenterol 81:562–565
15. Angelini G, Cavallini G, Pederzoli P, Bovo P, Bassi C, Di Francesco V, Frulloni L, Sgarbi D, Talamini G, Castagnini A (1993) Long-term outcome of acute pancreatitis: a prospective study with 118 patients. Digestion 54:143–147
16. Angelini G, Pederzoli P, Caliari S, Fratton S, Brocco G, Marzoli G, Bovo P, Cavallini G, Scuro LA (1984) Long-term outcome of acute necrohemorrhagic pancreatitis. A 4-year follow-up. Digestion 30:131–137
17. Arvanitakis C, Cooke AR (1978) Diagnostic tests of exocrine pancreatic function and disease. Gastroenterology 74:932–948
18. Aw SE, Hobbs JR, Wootton IDP (1967) Urinary isoamylases in the diagnosis of chronic pancreatitis. Gut 8:402–407
19. Axon ATR, Ashton MG, Lintott DJ (1979) Chronic pancreatitis and inflammatory bowel disease. Clin Radiol 30:179–182
20. Axon ATR, Classen M, Cotton PB, Cremer M, Freeny PC, Lees WR (1984) Pancreatography in chronic pancreatitis: international definitions. Gut 25:1107–1112
21. Baert AL, Delorme G (eds) (1994) Radiology of the Pancreas. Springer, Berlin–Heidelberg–New York
22. Barba A, Piubello W, Vantini I, Cocchetto R, Caliari S, Vallaperta P, Scuro LA, Sapuppo A, Cavallini G (1982) Skin lesions in chronic alcoholic pancreatitis. Dermatologica 164:322–326
23. Barbero GJ, Sibinga MS, Marino JM, Seibel R (1966) Stool trypsin and chymotrypsin. Value in the diagnosis of pancreatic insufficiency in cystic fibrosis. Am J Dis Child 112:536–540
24. Becker V, Mischke U (1991) Groove pancreatitis. Int J Pancreatol 10:173–182

25. Benini L, Caliari S, Bonfante F, Guidi GC, Brentegani MT, Castellani G, Sembenini C, Bardelli E, Vantini I (1992) Near infrared reflectance measurement of nitrogen faecal losses. Gut 33: 749–752
26. Benini L, Caliari S, Guidi GC, Vaona B, Talamini G, Vantini I, Scuro LA (1989) Near infrared spectrometry for faecal fat measurement: comparison with conventional gravimetric and titrimetric methods. Gut 30:1344–1347
27. Berk JE, Ayulo JA, Fridhandler L (1979) Value of pancreatic-type isoamylase assay as an index of pancreatic insufficiency. Dig Dis Sci 24:6–10
28. Bilbao MK, Dotter CT, Lee TG, Katon RM (1976) Complications of endoscopic retrograde cholangiopancreatography (ERCP). A study of 10 000 cases. Gastroenterology 70:314–320
29. Bitar KN, Zfass AM, Makhlouf GM (1978) Binding of secretin to plastic surfaces. Gastroenterology 75:1080–1082
30. Bliss WR, Burch B, Martin MM, Zollinger RM (1950) Localization of referred pancreatic pain induced by electric stimulation. Gastroenterology 16:317–323
31. Bloechle C, Izbicki JR, Knoefel WT, Kuechler T, Broelsch CE (1995) Quality of life in chronic pancreatitis – Results after duodenum-preserving resection of the head of the pancreas. Pancreas 11:77–85
32. Bo-Linn GW, Fordtran JS (1984) Fecal fat concentration in patients with steatorrhea. Gastroenterology 87:319–322
33. Bode C, Bode JC (1986) Usefulness of a simple photometric determination of chymotrypsin activity in stools – results of a multicentre study. Clin Biochem 19:333–337
34. Bolondi L, Gaiani S, Casanova P, Santi V, Labò G (1986) Critical evaluation and controversial points of ultrasound findings in chronic pancreatitis. In: Malfertheiner P, Ditschuneit H (eds) Diagnostic Procedures in Pancreatic Disease. Springer, Berlin–Heidelberg–New York, pp 149–154
35. Bolondi L, Gaiani S, Gullo L, Labò G (1984) Secretin administration induces a dilatation of main pancreatic duct. Dig Dis Sci 29:802–808
36. Bornschein W (1981) Der PABA-Peptid-Serum-Test. Untersuchungen zur methodischen Verbesserung eines indirekten Pankreasfunktionstests. Dtsch Med Wochenschr 106:1676–1677
37. Borovicka J, Schwizer W, Remy B, Fried M (1995) Cerulein-induced changes in plasma amino acid concentrations are not a valid test for pancreatic insufficiency. Am J Gastroenterol 90: 1111–1115
38. Bossuyt PJ, Van den Bogaert R, Scharpé SL, Van Maercke Y (1981) Relation of age to isoenzyme pattern and total activity of amylase in serum. Clin Chem 27:451–454
39. Bozkurt T, Braun U, Leferink S, Gilly G, Lux G (1994) Comparison of pancreatic morphology and exocrine functional impairment in patients with chronic pancreatitis. Gut 35:1132–1136
40. Bradley III EL (1982) Pancreatic duct pressure in chronic pancreatitis. Am J Surg 144:313–316
41. Braganza JM, Herman K, Hine P, Kay G, Sandle GI (1978) Pancreatic enzymes in human duodenal juice – a comparison of responses in secretin pancreozymin and Lundh Borgström tests. Gut 19:358–366
42. Braganza JM, Kay GH, Tetlow VA, Herman KJ (1983) Observations on the BT PABA/^{14}C-PABA tubeless test of pancreatic function. Clin Chim Acta 130:339–347
43. Braganza JM, Rao JJ (1978) Disproportionate reduction in tryptic response to endogenous compared with exogenous stimulation in chronic pancreatitis. Br Med J 2:392–394
44. Bramwell Cook H, Lennard-Jones JE, Sherif SM, Wiggins HS (1967) Measurement of tryptic activity in intestinal juice as a diagnostic test of pancreatic disease. Gut 8:408–414
45. Brown GA, Sule D, Williams J, Puntis JWL, Booth IW, McNeish AS (1988) Faecal chymotrypsin: a reliable index of exocrine pancreatic function. Arch Dis Child 63:785–789
46. Brugge WR, Goff JS, Allen NC, Podell ER, Allen RH (1980) Development of a dual label Schilling test for pancreatic exocrine function based on the differential absorption of cobalamin bound to intrinsic factor and R protein. Gastroenterology 78:937–949
47. Burton P, Evans DG, Harper AA, Howat HT, Oleesky S, Scott JE, Varley H (1960) A test of pancreatic function in man based on the analysis of duodenal contents after administration of secretin and pancreozymin. Gut 1:111–124
48. Buscail L, Escourrou J, Moreau J, Delvaux M, Louvel D, Lapeyre F, Tregant P, Frexinos J (1995) Endoscopic ultrasonography in chronic pancreatitis: a comparative prospective study with conventional ultrasonography, computed tomography, and ERCP. Pancreas 10:251–257

49. Butler ML (1977) Erythema ab igne, a sign of pancreatic disease. Am J Gastroenterol 67:77–79
50. Büchler M, Malfertheiner P, Block S, Maier W, Beger HG (1985) Morphologische und funktionelle Veränderungen des Pankreas nach akuter nekrotisierender Pankreatitis. Z Gastroenterol 23:79–83
51. Caletti G, Brocchi E, Agostini D, Balduzzi A, Bolondi L, Labò G (1982) Sensitivity of endoscopic retrograde pancreatography in chronic pancreatitis. Br J Surg 69:507–509
52. Cavallini G, Mirachian R, Angelini G, Vantini I, Vaona B, Bovo P, Gelpi F, Ederle A, Dobrilla G, Scuro LA (1978) The role of caerulein in tests of exocrine pancreatic function. Scand J Gastroenterol 13:3–15
53. Cavallini G, Piubello W, Brocco G, Micciolo R, Chech G, Angelini G, Benini L, Riela A, Dalle Molle L, Vantini I, Scuro LA (1985) Serum PABA and fluorescein in the course of Bz-Ty-PABA and pancreolauryl test as an index of exocrine pancreatic insufficiency. Dig Dis Sci 30:655–663
54. Chen W-L, Morishita R, Eguchi T, Kawai T, Sakai M, Tateishi H, Uchino H (1989) Clinical usefulness of dual-label Schilling test for pancreatic exocrine function. Gastroenterology 96: 1337–1345
55. Cichy W, Lankisch PG, Arnold R, Creutzfeldt W (1984) Evaluation of serum pancreatic polypeptide estimations following hormonal stimulation for the diagnosis of exocrine pancreatic insufficiency. Digestion 30:218–223
56. Cole SG, Rossi S, Stern A, Hofmann AF (1987) Cholesteryl octanoate breath test. Preliminary studies on a new noninvasive test of human pancreatic exocrine function. Gastroenterology 93: 1372–1380
57. Creutzfeldt W (1964) Funktionsdiagnostik bei Erkrankungen des exokrinen Pankreas. Verh Dtsch Ges Inn Med 70:781–801
58. Dandona P, Elias E, Beckett AG (1978) Serum trypsin concentrations in diabetes mellitus. Br Med J II:1125
59. de Pedro C, Codoceo R, Vazquez P, Hernanz A (1986) Fecal chymotrypsin levels in children with pancreatic insufficiency. Clin Biochem 19:338–340
60. Delchier J-C, Soule J-C (1983) BT-PABA test with plasma PABA measurements: evaluation of sensitivity and specificity. Gut 24:318–325
61. DiMagno EP (1986) Ultrasound, computed tomography and endoscopic retrograde pancreatography in the diagnosis of chronic pancreatitis: a comparative evaluation. In: Malfertheiner P, Ditschuneit H (eds) Diagnostic Procedures in Pancreatic Disease. Springer, Berlin–Heidelberg–New York–Tokyo, pp 185–191
62. DiMagno EP, Go VLW, Summerskill WHJ (1972) Impaired cholecystokinin-pancreozymin secretion, intraluminal dilution, and maldigestion of fat in sprue. Gastroenterology 63:25–32
63. DiMagno EP, Go VLW, Summerskill WHJ (1973) Relations between pancreatic enzyme outputs and malabsorption in severe pancreatic insufficiency. N Engl J Med 288:813–815
64. Dobrilla G, Valentini M, Filippini M, Bonoldi MC, Felder M, Moroder E, Schnabl D, Gaspa U (1979) Study of parotid and mixed saliva in the diagnosis of chronic pancreatitis. Digestion 19: 180–185
65. Domínguez-Muñoz JE, Hieronymus C, Sauerbruch T, Malfertheiner P (1995) Fecal elastase test: evaluation of a new noninvasive pancreatic function test. Am J Gastroenterol 90:1834–1837
66. Domínguez-Muñoz JE, Manes G, Pieramico O, Büchler M, Malfertheiner P (1995) Effect of pancreatic ductal and parenchymal changes on exocrine function in chronic pancreatitis. Pancreas 10:31–35
67. Domschke S, Heptner G, Kolb S, Sailer D, Schneider MU, Domschke W (1986) Decrease in plasma amino acid level after secretin and pancreozymin as an indicator of exocrine pancreatic function. Gastroenterology 90:1031–1038
68. Donowitz M, Hendler R, Spiro HM, Binder HJ, Felig P (1975) Glucagon secretion in acute and chronic pancreatitis. Ann Intern Med 83:778–781
69. Dreiling DA, Janowitz HD (1962) The measurement of pancreatic secretory function. In: Ciba Foundation Symposium on the Exocrine Pancreas. Churchill, London, pp 225–252
70. Dreiling DA, Naqvi MA (1969) Peptic ulcer diathesis in patients with chronic pancreatitis. Am J Gastroenterol 51:503–510
71. Dürr HK, Otte M, Forell MM, Bode JC (1978) Fecal chymotrypsin: a study on its diagnostic value by comparison with the secretin-cholecystokinin test. Digestion 17:404–409

72. Ebbehøj N, Borly L, Madsen P, Svendsen LB (1986) Pancreatic tissue pressure and pain in chronic pancreatitis. Pancreas 1:556–558
73. Ehrhardt-Schmelzer S, Otto J, Schlaeger R, Lankisch PG (1984) Faecal chymotrypsin for investigation of exocrine pancreatic function: a comparison of two newly developed tests with the titrimetric method. Z Gastroenterol 22:647–651
74. El Hamel A, Parc R, Adda G, Bouteloup PY, Huguet C, Malafosse M (1991) Bleeding pseudocysts and pseudoaneurysms in chronic pancreatitis. Br J Surg 78:1059–1063
75. Elias E, Redshaw M, Wood T (1977) Diagnostic importance of changes in circulating concentrations of immunoreactive trypsin. Lancet 2:66–68
76. Ertan A, Degertekin H, Akdamar K, Godiwala T, Mather F (1986) A new criterion in the assessment of bentiromide as a test of exocrine pancreatic function in alcoholics. Pancreas 1:176–179
77. Fahrenkrug J, Magid E (1980) Concentration of immunoreactive trypsin and activity of pancreatic isoamylase in serum compared in pancreatic diseases. Clin Chem 26:1573–1576
78. Freise J, Gebel M, Wellmann W, Huchzermeyer H (1981) Sonographie und endoskopische retrograde Pankreatikographie – Alternative oder komplementäre Untersuchungsverfahren in der Diagnostik der chronischen Pankreatitis und des Pankreaskarzinoms? Ultraschall 2:65–69
79. Freise J, Ranft U, Fricke K, Schmidt FW (1984) Chronische Pankreatitis: Sensitivität, Spezifität und prädiktiver Wert des Pankreolauryltests. Z Gastroenterol 22:705–712
80. Frier BM, Saunders JHB, Wormsley KG, Bouchier IAD (1976) Exocrine pancreatic function in juvenile-onset diabetes mellitus. Gut 17:685–691
81. Funnell IC, Bornman PC, Krige JEJ, Beningfield SJ, Terblanche J (1994) Endoscopic drainage of traumatic pancreatic pseudocyst. Br J Surg 81:879–881
82. Gamble DR, Moffatt A, Marks V (1979) Serum immunoreactive trypsin concentrations in infectious and non-infectious illnesses and in juvenile diabetes. J Clin Pathol 32:897–901
83. García-Pugés AM, Navarro S, Ros E, Elena M, Ballesta A, Aused R, Vilar-Bonet J (1986) Reversibility of exocrine pancreatic failure in chronic pancreatitis. Gastroenterology 91:17–24
84. Girdwood AH, Hatfield ARW, Bornman PC, Denyer ME, Kottler RE, Marks IN (1984) Structure and function in noncalcific pancreatitis. Dig Dis Sci 29:721–726
85. Glaser J, Högemann B, Krummenerl T, Schneider M, Hultsch E, van Husen N, Gerlach U (1987) Sonographic imaging of the pancreatic duct. New diagnostic possibilities using secretin stimulation. Dig Dis Sci 32:1075–1081
86. Glaser J, Högemann B, Schneider M, Hultsch E, van Husen N, Gerlach U (1989) Significance of a sonographic secretin test in the diagnosis of pancreatic disease. Results of a prospective study. Scand J Gastroenterol 24:179–185
87. Guéant JL, Champigneulle B, Djalali M, Bigard MA, Gaucher P, Hassouni A, Nicolas JP (1986) In-vitro test of haptocorrin degradation for biological diagnosis of exocrine pancreatic dysfunction using duodenal juice collected during endoscopy. Lancet 2:709–712
88. Gullo L, Costa PL, Fontana G, Labò G (1976) Investigation of exocrine pancreatic function by continuous infusion of caerulein and secretin in normal subjects and in chronic pancreatitis. Digestion 14:97–107
89. Gullo L, Costa PL, Labò G (1977) Chronic pancreatitis in Italy. Aetiological, clinical and histological observations based on 253 cases. Rendic Gastroenterol 9:97–104
90. Gullo L, Pezzilli R, Ventrucci M (1996) Diagnostic value of the amino acid consumption test in pancreatic diseases. Pancreas 12:64–67
91. Gullo L, Pezzilli R, Ventrucci M, Barbara L (1990) Caerulein induced plasma amino acid decrease: a simple, sensitive, and specific test of pancreatic function. Gut 31:926–929
92. Gyr K, Agrawal NM, Felsenfeld O, Font RG (1975) Comparative study of secretin and Lundh tests. Am J Dig Dis 20:506–512
93. Gyr K, Felsenfeld O, Imondi AR (1978) Chymotrypsinlike activity of some intestinal bacteria. Am J Dig Dis 23:413–416
94. Haverback BJ, Dyce BJ, Gutentag PJ, Montgomery DW (1963) Measurement of trypsin and chymotrypsin in stool. A diagnostic test for pancreatic exocrine insufficiency. Gastroenterology 44:588–597
95. Heij HA, Obertop H, van Blankenstein M, Nix GAJJ, Westbroek DL (1987) Comparison of endoscopic retrograde pancreatography with functional and histologic changes in chronic pancreatitis. Acta Radiol 28:289–293

96. Heij HA, Obertop H, van Blankenstein M, ten Kate FW, Westbroek DL (1986) Relationship between functional and histological changes in chronic pancreatitis. Dig Dis Sci 31:1009–1013
97. Heptner G, Domschke S, Domschke W (1989) Exocrine pancreatic function after gastrectomy. Specificity of indirect tests. Gastroenterology 97:147–153
98. Heptner G, Domschke S, Schneider MU, Kolb S, Domschke W (1987) Aminosäurespiegel im Plasma – dargestellt als α-Amino-Stickstoff – reagieren auf Stimulation des exokrinen Pankreas: Ansätze für einen Pankreasfunktionstest. Klin Wochenschr 65:1054–1061
99. Hoek FJ, van den Bergh FAJTM, Klein Elhorst JT, Meijer JL, Timmer E, Tytgat GNJ (1987) Improved specificity of the PABA test with p-aminosalicylic acid (PAS). Gut 28:468–473
100. Hotz J, Goebell H, Herfarth C, Probst M (1977) Massive pancreatic ascites without carcinoma. Report of three cases. Digestion 15:200–216
101. Ihse I, Arnesjö B, Kugelberg C, Lilja P (1977) Intestinal activities of trypsin, lipase, and phospholipase after a test meal. An evaluation of 474 examinations. Scand J Gastroenterol 12:663–668
102. Ihse I, Lindström E, Evander A, Lundstedt C (1987) The value of preoperative imaging techniques in patients with chronic pancreatic pleural effusions. Int J Pancreatol 2:269–276
103. James O (1973) The Lundh test. Gut 14:582–591
104. Johnson SG, Levitt MD (1978) Relation between serum pancreatic isoamylase concentration and pancreatic exocrine function. Dig Dis Sci 23:914–918
105. Junge W (1986) Assessment of titrimetric and photometric methods for the determination of chymotrypsin catalytic activity in stool. Clin Biochem 19:323–328
106. Kakizaki G, Noto N, Fujiwara Y, Oizumi T, Soeno T, Saito T (1972) Histologic findings and amylase contents of the pancreas and parotid gland of rats with experimental peritonitis or ileus. Tohoku J Exp Med 108:155–164
107. Kakizaki G, Noto N, Onuma T, Saito T, Izumi S (1971) Experimental study on the correlation between the pancreas and parotid gland. Tohoku J Exp Med 105:223–231
108. Kakizaki G, Saito T, Soeno T, Sasahara M, Fujiwara Y (1976) A new diagnostic test for pancreatic disorders by examination of parotid saliva. Am J Gastroenterol 65:437–445
109. Kamaryt J, Stejskal J, Osicková L (1978) Urinary isoamylases in juvenile diabetics. J Clin Chem Clin Biochem 16:539–541
110. Katschinski M, Schirra J, Bross A, Arnold R, Göke B (1994) Fecal concentration of pancreatic elastase-1 accurately indicates exocrine pancreatic insufficiency. Gastroenterology 106:A300 (abstr)
111. Kay G, Hine P, Braganza J (1982) The pancreolauryl test. A method of assessing the combined functional efficacy of pancreatic esterase and bile salts in vivo? Digestion 24:241–245
112. Kemmer TP, Malfertheiner P, Häberle H, Pohlandt F, Friess H, Büchler M, Ditschuneit H (1992) Die diagnostische Wertigkeit des Aminosäurenabsorptionstests beim Nachweis einer exokrinen Pankreasfunktionsstörung. Z Gastroenterol 30:391–396
113. Kerlin P, Wong L, Harris B, Capra S (1984) Rice flour, breath hydrogen, and malabsorption. Gastroenterology 87:578–585
114. Kim YS, Spritz N (1968) Hydroxy acid excretion in steatorrhea of pancreatic and nonpancreatic origin. N Engl J Med 279:1424–1426
115. Koehn HD, Mostbeck A (1981) Age-dependence of immunoreactive trypsin concentrations in serum. Clin Chem 27:502
116. Koop H, Lankisch PG, Stöckmann F, Arnold R (1980) Trypsin radioimmunoassay in the diagnosis of chronic pancreatitis. Digestion 20:151–156
117. Koop H, Rumpf KW, Lankisch PG, Bothe E, Stöckmann F, Arnold R (1980) Plasma-immunoreactive trypsin in chronic renal failure. Digestion 20:334–335
118. Lagerlöf HO (1942) Pancreatic function and pancreatic disease. Studied by means of secretin. Acta Med Scand Suppl. 128:1–289
119. Lake-Bakaar G, McKavanagh S, Gatus B, Summerfield JA (1980) The relative values of serum immuno-reactive trypsin concentration and total amylase activity in the diagnosis of mumps, chronic renal failure, and pancreatic disease. Scand J Gastroenterol 15:97–101
120. Lambiase L, Forsmark CE, Albert C, Toskes PP (1993) Secretin test diagnoses chronic pancreatitis earlier than ERCP. Gastroenterology 104:A315 (abstr)
121. Lang C, Gyr K, Tonko I, Conen D, Stalder GA (1984) Value of serum PABA as a pancreatic function test. Gut 25:508–512

122. Lankisch PG (1984) Secretin test or secretin-CCK test – gold standard in pancreatic function testing? In: Gyr KE, Singer MV, Sarles H (eds) Pancreatitis – Concepts and classification. Excerpta Medica, ICS 642, Amsterdam–New York, pp 247–259

123. Lankisch PG (1990) The spleen in inflammatory pancreatic disease. Gastroenterology 98:509–516

124. Lankisch PG (1990) Diagnosis of abdominal pain. How to distinguish between pancreatic and extrapancreatic causes. Acta Chir Scand 156:273–278

125. Lankisch PG, Andrén-Sandberg Å (1993) Standards for the diagnosis of chronic pancreatitis and for the evaluation of treatment. Int J Pancreatol 14:205–212

126. Lankisch PG, Brauneis J, Otto J, Göke B (1986) Pancreolauryl and NBT-PABA tests. Are serum tests more practicable alternatives to urine tests in the diagnosis of exocrine pancreatic insufficiency? Gastroenterology 90:350–354

127. Lankisch PG, Buschmann-Kaspari H, Otto J, Schröder K, Koop H (1990) Correlation of pancreatic enzyme levels with the patient's recovery from acute edematous pancreatitis. Klin Wochenschr 68:565–569

128. Lankisch PG, Chilla R, Luerssen K, Koop H, Arglebe C, Creutzfeldt W (1979) Parotid saliva test in the diagnosis of chronic pancreatitis. Digestion 19:52–55

129. Lankisch PG, Creutzfeldt W (1981) Effect of synthetic and natural secretin on the function of the exocrine pancreas in man. Digestion 22:61–65

130. Lankisch PG, Creutzfeldt W (1986) Erythema ab igne (Livedo reticularis e calore): ein Hautzeichen für chronische Pankreaserkrankungen. Z Gastroenterol 24:119–120

131. Lankisch PG, Dröge M, Hofses S, König H, Lembcke B (1996) Steatorrhoea: You cannot trust your eyes when it comes to diagnosis. Lancet 347:1620–1621

132. Lankisch PG, Ehrhardt-Schmelzer S, Koop H, Caspary WF (1980) Der NBT-PABA-Test in der Diagnostik der exokrinen Pankreasinsuffizienz. Dtsch Med Wochenschr 105:1418–1423

133. Lankisch PG, Koop H, Otto J (1986) Estimation of serum pancreatic isoamylase: its role in the diagnosis of exocrine pancreatic insufficiency. Am J Gastroenterol 81:365–368

134. Lankisch PG, Lembcke B (1984) Indirect pancreatic function tests: chemical and radioisotope methods. Clin Gastroenterol 13:717–737

135. Lankisch PG, Lembcke B, Wemken G, Creutzfeldt W (1986) Functional reserve capacity of the exocrine pancreas. Digestion 35:175–181

136. Lankisch PG, Lopez E, Winckler K, Schuster R (1976) Kolonstenosen nach Pankreatitis. Schweiz Med Wochenschr 106:1243–1247

137. Lankisch PG, Löhr M, König H, Schmidt I, Knollmann R, Liebe S (1995) Fecal elastase-1: not helpful in diagnosing slight to moderate exocrine pancreatic insufficiency. Pancreas 11:436 (abstr)

138. Lankisch PG, Löhr-Happe A, Otto J, Creutzfeldt W (1993) Natural course in chronic pancreatitis. Pain, exocrine and endocrine pancreatic insufficiency and prognosis of the disease. Digestion 54:148–155

139. Lankisch PG, Manthey G, Otto J, Koop H, Talaulicar M, Willms B, Creutzfeldt W (1982) Exocrine pancreatic function in insulin-dependent diabetes mellitus. Digestion 25:211–216

140. Lankisch PG, Otto J (1986) Salivary isoamylase in duodenal aspirates. Dig Dis Sci 31:1299–1302

141. Lankisch PG, Otto J, Brauneis J, Hilgers R, Lembcke B (1988) Detection of pancreatic steatorrhea by oral pancreatic function tests. Dig Dis Sci 33:1233–1236

142. Lankisch PG, Otto J, Erkelenz I, Lembcke B (1986) Pancreatic calcifications: no indicator of severe exocrine pancreatic insufficiency. Gastroenterology 90:617–621

143. Lankisch PG, Otto J, Löhr A, Schirren C-A, Schuster R (1989) Pancreatic calcifications in patients with normal pancreatic function. Int J Pancreatol 5:281–293

144. Lankisch PG, Peiper M, Löhr-Happe A, Otto J, Seidensticker F, Stöckmann F (1993) Delay in diagnosing chronic pancreatitis. Eur J Gastroenterol Hepatol 5:713–714

145. Lankisch PG, Schreiber A, Otto J (1983) Pancreolauryl test. Evaluation of a tubeless pancreatic function test in comparison with other indirect and direct tests for exocrine pancreatic function. Dig Dis Sci 28:490–493

146. Lankisch PG, Seidensticker F, Otto J, Lübbers H, Mahlke R, Stöckmann F, Fölsch UR, Creutzfeldt W (1996) Secretin-pancreozymin test (SPT) and endoscopic retrograde cholangiopancreatography (ERCP): both are necessary for diagnosing or excluding chronic pancreatitis. Pancreas 12:149–152

147. Lankisch PG, Staritz M, Freise J (1990) Sicherheit bei der Diagnostik der chronischen Pankreatitis. Z Gastroenterol 28:253–258
148. Lees WR (1986) Critical evaluation and controversial points of computed tomography findings in chronic pancreatitis. In: Malfertheiner P, Ditschuneit H (eds) Diagnostic Procedures in Pancreatic Disease. Springer, Berlin–Heidelberg, pp 161–168
149. Lees WR, Heron CW (1987) US-guided percutaneous pancreatography: experience in 75 patients. Radiology 165:809–813
150. Lembcke B (1984) Malassimilationsdiagnostik. In: Caspary WF (ed) Maldigestion – Malabsorption. Klinik – Differentialdiagnose – Therapie. Gastroenterologische Reihe, Bd. 21. Kali-Chemie Pharma GmbH, Hannover, pp 47–86
151. Lembcke B, Braden B, Stein J (1994) Diagnostik der Steatorrhoe. Z Gastroenterol 32:256–261
152. Lembcke B, Geibel K, Kirchhoff S, Lankisch PG (1989) Serum-β-Carotin: ein einfacher statischer Laborparameter für die Diagnostik der Steatorrhoe. Dtsch Med Wochenschr 114:243–247
153. Lembcke B, Grimm K, Lankisch PG (1987) Raised fecal fat concentration is not a valid indicator of pancreatic steatorrhea. Am J Gastroenterol 82:526–531
154. Lembcke B, Konle O, Duan LP, Caspary WF (1994) Lack of accuracy of plasma α-amino nitrogen profiles as an indicator of exocrine pancreatic function both after continuous and bolus stimulation of the pancreas with secretin and cholecystokinin-pancreozymin. Z Gastroenterol 32: 679–683
155. Lembcke B, Kraus B, Lankisch PG (1985) Small intestinal function in chronic relapsing pancreatitis. Hepatogastroenterology 32:149–151
156. Lesi C, Scandellari A, Cucci AM, Franceschi F, Matacena C, Malaguti P (1985) Changes in serum pancreatic enzymes after hormonal stimulation in chronic pancreatitis. Dig Dis Sci 30:552–557
157. Leung JWC, Frost RA, Burgess R, Braganza JM, Slater DM, Cotton PB (1988) Modified dual label Schilling test for pancreatic exocrine function. Clin Chim Acta 174:93–100
158. Levin GE, Youngs GR, Bouchier IAD (1972) Evaluation of the Lundh test in the diagnosis of pancreatic disease. J Clin Pathol 25:129–132
159. Levitt MD, Ellis CJ, Meier PB (1980) Extrapancreatic origin of chronic unexplained hyperamylasemia. N Engl J Med 302:670–671
160. Löhr A (1990) Der natürliche Verlauf der chronischen Pankreatitis. Die Entwicklung der Leitsymptome Schmerzen, exokrine und endokrine Pankreasinsuffizienz und die Prognose der Erkrankung. Med Diss Göttingen
161. Löser C, Mölgaard A, Fölsch UR (1995) Elastase 1 in faeces: a novel highly sensitive and specific pancreatic function test for easy and inexpensive routine application. Digestion 56:301 (abstr)
162. Lundh G (1962) Pancreatic exocrine function in neoplastic and inflammatory disease; a simple and reliable new test. Gastroenterology 42:275–280
163. Lurie B, Brom B, Bank S, Novis B, Marks IN (1973) Comparative response of exocrine pancreatic secretion following a test meal and secretin-pancreozymin stimulation. Scand J Gastroenterol 8:27–32
164. Madsen P, Winkler K (1982) The intraductal pancreatic pressure in chronic obstructive pancreatitis. Scand J Gastroenterol 17:553–554
165. Magid E, Horsing M, Rune SJ (1977) On the quantitation of iso-amylases in serum and the diagnostic value of serum pancreatic type amylase in chronic pancreatitis. Scand J Gastroenterol 12: 621–627
166. Mahlke R, Elbrechtz F, Petersen M, Schafmayer A, Lankisch PG (1995) Acute abdominal pain in chronic pancreatitis: hemorrhage from a pseudoaneurysm? Z Gastroenterol 33:404–407
167. Malfertheiner P, Büchler M (1989) Correlation of imaging and function in chronic pancreatitis. Radiol Clin North Am 27:51–64
168. Malfertheiner P, Büchler M, Müller A, Ditschuneit H (1987) Fluoresceindilaurat-Serumtest nach Metoclopramid- und Sekretinstimulation zur Pankreasfunktionsprüfung. Beitrag zur Diagnose der chronischen Pankreatitis. Z Gastroenterol 25:225–232
169. Malfertheiner P, Büchler M, Müller A, Ditschuneit H (1987) Fluorescein dilaurate serum test: a rapid tubeless pancreatic function test. Pancreas 2:53–60
170. Malfertheiner P, Büchler M, Stanescu A, Ditschuneit H (1986) Exocrine pancreatic function in correlation to ductal and parenchymal morphology in chronic pancreatitis. Hepatogastroenterology 33:110–114

171. Malfertheiner P, Ditschuneit H (Eds) (1986) Prognostic Procedures in Pancreatic Disease. Springer, Berlin–Heidelberg–New York–Tokyo

172. Malfertheiner P, Peter M, Junge U, Ditschuneit H (1983) Der orale Pankreasfunktionstest mit FDL in der Diagnose der chronischen Pankreatitis. Klin Wochenschr 61:193–198

173. Malis F, Fric P, Kasafírek E, Jodl J, Vávrová V, Slaby J (1979) A peroral test of pancreatic insufficiency with 4-(N-acetyl-L-tyrosyl)aminobenzoic acid in children with cystic fibrosis. J Pediatr 94:942–944

174. Marcoullis G, Gueant J-L, Nicolas J-P (1986) Radioimmunoassay for assessing exocrine pancreatic insufficiency, based on the differential enzymatic degradation of cobalamin-binding proteins. Clin Chem 32:453–460

175. Maringhini A, Nelson DK, Jones JD, DiMagno EP (1994) Is the plasma amino acid consumption test an accurate test of exocrine pancreatic insufficiency? Gastroenterology 106:488–493

176. Marks IN, Bank S (1985) Chronic pancreatitis. Etiology, clinical aspects, and medical management. In: Berk JE (ed) Bockus Gastroentrology, Vol. 5, 4th edn. W.B. Saunders, Philadelphia, pp 4020–4040

177. Masoero G, Bianco A, Rossanino A, Colaferro S, Marchetto M, Cavaliere R (1987) Ultrasonic monitoring of Wirsung duct following secretin in controls and in chronic pancreatitis patients. Pancreas 2:344–349

178. Matter D, Bret PM, Bretagnolle M, Valette PJ, Fond A (1987) Pancreatic duct: US-guided percutaneous opacification. Radiology 163:635–636

179. McLatchie GR, Meek D, Imrie CW (1985) The use of endoscopic retrograde choledocho-pancreatography (ERCP) in the diagnosis of internal fistulae complicating severe acute pancreatitis. Br J Radiol 58:395–397

180. Meyer BM, Campbell DR, Curington CW, Toskes PP (1987) Bentiromide test is not affected in patients with small bowel disease or liver disease. Pancreas 2:44–47

181. Mitchell CJ, Field HP, Simpson FG, Parkin A, Kelleher J, Losowsky MS (1981) Preliminary evaluation of a single-day tubeless test of pancreatic function. Br Med J 282:1751–1753

182. Mitchell CJ, Humphrey CS, Bullen AW, Kelleher J, Losowsky MS (1979) Improved diagnostic accuracy of a modified oral pancreatic function test. Scand J Gastroenterol 14:737–741

183. Mitchell CJ, Wai D, Jackson AM, MacFie J (1989) Ultrasound guided percutaneous pancreatic biopsy. Br J Surg 76:706–707

184. Miyake H, Harada H, Kunichika K, Ochi K, Kimura I (1987) Clinical course and prognosis of chronic pancreatitis. Pancreas 2:378–385

185. Moeller DD, Dunn GD, Klotz AP (1972) Comparison of the pancreozymin-secretin test and the Lundh test meal. Am J Dig Dis 17:799–805

186. Mok DWH, Blumgart LH (1984) Erythema ab igne in chronic pancreatic pain: a diagnostic sign. J R Soc Med 77:299–301

187. Mottaleb A, Kapp F, Noguera ECA, Kellock TD, Wiggins HS, Waller SL (1973) The Lundh test in the diagnosis of pancreatic disease: A review of five years' experience. Gut 14:835–841

188. Mörl M, Piechulek H (1987) Leberschäden bei chronisch-kalzifizierter, alkoholinduzierter Pankreatitis. Z Gastroenterol 25:325–330

189. Muller L, Wisniewski ZS, Hansky J (1970) The measurement of faecal chymotrypsin: a screening test for pancreatic exocrine insufficiency. Aust Ann Med 1:47–49

190. Mundlos S, Kühnelt P, Adler G (1990) Monitoring enzyme replacement treatment in exocrine pancreatic insufficiency using the cholesteryl octanoate breath test. Gut 31:1324–1328

191. Mundlos S, Rhodes JB, Hofmann AF (1987) The cholesteryl octanoate breath test: a new procedure for detection of pancreatic insufficiency in the rat. Pediatr Res 22:257–261

192. Münch R, Bühler H, Ammann R (1983) Chymotrypsinaktivität im Stuhl: Vergleich eines neuen photometrischen Verfahrens mit der titrimetrischen Standardmethode. Schweiz Med Wochenschr 113:1794–1797

193. Myhre J, Nesbitt S, Hurly JT (1949) Response of serum amylase and lipase to pancreatic stimulation as a test of pancreatic function. The mecholyl-secretin and the morphine-secretin tests. Gastroenterology 13:127–134

194. Møller-Petersen J, Pedersen S (1982) Cathodic trypsin-like immunoreactivity in serum: influence of sex, age, renal function, food and diurnal variation. Clin Chim Acta 124:31–37

195. Nattermann C, Goldschmidt AJW, Dancygier H (1993) Endosonography in chronic pancreatitis – a comparison between endoscopic retrograde pancreatography and endoscopic ultrasonography. Endoscopy 25:565–570
196. Nousia-Arvanitakis S, Arvanitakis C, Desai N, Greenberger NJ (1978) Diagnosis of exocrine pancreatic insufficiency in cystic fibrosis by the synthetic peptide N-benzoyl-L-tyrosyl-p-aminobenzoic acid. J Pediatr 92:734–737
197. O'Donnell MD, FitzGerald O, McGeeney KF (1977) Differential serum amylase determination by use of an inhibitor, and design of a routine procedure. Clin Chem 23:560–566
198. O'Donnell MD, McGeeney KF (1976) Purification and properties of an α-amylase inhibitor from wheat. Biochim Biophys Acta 422:159–169
199. Okazaki K, Yamamoto Y, Kagiyama S, Tamura S, Sakamoto Y, Morita M (1988) Pressure of papillary sphincter zone and pancreatic main duct in patients with alcoholic and idiopathic chronic pancreatitis. Int J Pancreatol 3:457–468
200. Okazaki K, Yamamoto Y, Nishimori I, Nishioka T, Kagiyama S, Tamura S, Sakamoto Y, Nakazawa Y, Morita M, Yamamoto Y (1988) Motility of the sphincter of Oddi and pancreatic main ductal pressure in patients with alcoholic, gallstone-associated, and idiopathic chronic pancreatitis. Am J Gastroenterol 83:820–826
201. Otte M (1979) Pankreasfunktionsdiagnostik. Internist 20:331–340
202. Otte M (1979) Klinik der chronischen Pankreatitis. In: Forell MM (ed) Chronische Pankreatitis und Pankreaskarzinom. Klinik, Diagnostik, Therapie. Georg Thieme, Stuttgart, pp 4–12
203. Otte M (1986) Ultrasound in chronic pancreatitis. In: Malfertheiner P, Ditschuneit H (eds) Diagnostic Procedures in Pancreatic Disease. Springer, Berlin–Heidelberg–New York, pp 143–148
204. Patel VP, Jain NK, Agarwal N, Varghese PJG, Pitchumoni CS (1986) Comparison of bentiromide test and rice flour breath hydrogen test in the detection of exocrine pancreatic insufficiency. Pancreas 1:172–175
205. Petersen H, Myren J (1975) Secretin dose-response in health and chronic pancreatic inflammatory disease. Scand J Gastroenterol 10:851–861
206. Pitkäranta P, Haapiainen R, Kivisaari L, Schröder T (1991) Diagnostic evaluation and aggressive surgical approach in bleeding pseudoaneurysms associated with pancreatic pseudocysts. Scand J Gastroenterol 26:58–64
207. Remtulla MA, Durie PR, Goldberg DM (1986) Stool chymotrypsin activity measured by a spectrophotometric procedure to identify pancreatic disease in infants. Clin Biochem 19:341–347
208. Reuben A, Johnson AL, Cotton PB (1978) Is pancreatogram interpretation reliable? – a study of observer variation and error. Br J Radiol 51:956–962
209. Ribet A, Tournut R, Duffaut M, Vaysse N (1976) Use of caerulein with submaximal doses of secretin as a test of pancreatic function in man. Gut 17:431–434
210. Roberts IM, Poturich C, Wald A (1986) Utility of fecal fat concentrations as screening test in pancreatic insufficiency. Dig Dis Sci 31:1021–1024
211. Rolny P, Ärlebäck A, Järnerot G, Andersson T (1986) Endoscopic manometry of the sphincter of Oddi and pancreatic duct in chronic pancreatitis. Scand J Gastroenterol 21:415–420
212. Rolny P, Jagenburg R (1978) The secretin-CCK test and a modified Lundh test. A comparative study. Scand J Gastroenterol 13:927–931
213. Rosenblum JL (1988) Direct, rapid assay of pancreatic isoamylase activity by use of monoclonal antibodies with low affinity for macroamylasemic complexes. Clin Chem 34:2463–2468
214. Rösch T, Braig C, Gain T, Feuerbach S, Siewert JR, Schusdziarra V, Classen M (1992) Staging of pancreatic and ampullary carcinoma by endoscopic ultrasonography. Comparison with conventional sonography, computed tomography, and angiography. Gastroenterology 102:188–199
215. Rösch T, Neuhaus H, Gmeinwieser J, Zapilko R, Siewert JR, Classen M (1993) Role of endoscopic ultrasonography in the evaluation of patients with suspected pancreatic disease. Gastroenterology 104 (Suppl.):A21 (abstr)
216. Rune SJ, Worning H (1985) Evaluation of the marker technique for measurement of exocrine pancreatic secretion rate. Scand J Gastroenterol 20:525–529
217. Sacher M, Kobsa A, Shmerling DH (1978) PABA screening test for exocrine pancreatic function in infants and children. Arch Dis Child 53:639–641
218. Sarles H, Gerolami-Santandrea A (1972) Chronic pancreatitis. Clin Gastroenterol 1:167–193

219. Sarles H, Sahel J, Staub JL, Bourry J, Laugier R (1979) Chronic pancreatitis. In: Howat HT, Sarles H (eds) The Exocrine Pancreas. W.B. Saunders, London–Philadelphia–Toronto, pp 402–439
220. Sarner M, Cotton PB (1984) Classification of pancreatitis. Gut 25:756–759
221. Savastano S, Feltrin GP, Antonio T, Miotto D, Chiesura-Corona M, Castellan L (1993) Arterial complications of pancreatitis: diagnostic and therapeutic role of radiology. Pancreas 8:687–692
222. Schmidt H, Witthöft C (1976) Wert des Provokations(Evokations)-Tests für die Pankreasdiagnostik. Leber Magen Darm 6:227–234
223. Schmitz-Moormann P, Hein J (1976) Altersveränderungen des Pankreasgangsystems und ihre Rückwirkungen auf das Parenchym. Virchows Arch [Pathol Anat] 371:145–152
224. Schmitz-Moormann P, Himmelmann GW, Brandes J-W, Fölsch UR, Lorenz-Meyer H, Malchow H, Soehendra LN, Wienbeck M (1985) Comparative radiological and morphological study of human pancreas. Pancreatitis like changes in postmortem ductograms and their morphological pattern. Possible implication for ERCP. Gut 26:406–414
225. Schneider MU, Demling L, Jones SA, Barker PJ, Domschke S, Heptner G, Domschke W (1987) NMR spectrometry. A new method for total stool fat quantification in chronic pancreatitis. Dig Dis Sci 32:494–499
226. Schönberger W, Weitzel D (1980) Diagnose der exokrinen Pankreasinsuffizienz mit Fluorescein-Dilaurat bei Patienten mit cystischer Fibrose. Monatsschr Kinderheilkd 128:195–198
227. Seidensticker F, Otto J, Lankisch PG (1995) Recovery of the pancreas after acute pancreatitis is not necessarily complete. Int J Pancreatol 17:225–229
228. Sherman S, Lehman GA (1991) ERCP- and endoscopic sphincterotomy-induced pancreatitis. Pancreas 6:350–367
229. Skrha J, Stepán J, Havránek T, Skrha F, Herfort K, Srámková J, Páv J (1981) Isoamylases in diabetes mellitus. Diabetologia 20:129–133
230. Skude G (1977) On human amylase isoenzymes. Scand J Gastroenterol 12, Suppl. 44:1–37
231. Skude G, Ihse I (1976) Salivary amylase in duodenal aspirates. Scand J Gastroenterol 11:17–20
232. Soto JA, Barish MA, Yucel EK, Siegenberg D, Ferrucci JT, Chuttani R (1996) Magnetic resonance cholangiography: comparison with endoscopic retrograde cholangiopancreatography. Gastroenterology 110:589–597
233. Stabile BE, Wilson SE, Debas HT (1983) Reduced mortality from bleeding pseudocysts and pseudoaneurysms caused by pancreatitis. Arch Surg 118:45–51
234. Stanten R, Frey CF (1990) Pancreatitis after endoscopic retrograde cholangiopancreatography. An underreported disease whose severity is often unappreciated. Arch Surg 125:1032–1035
235. Staritz M, Meyer zum Büschenfelde KH (1988) Elevated pressure in the dorsal part of pancreas divisum: the cause of chronic pancreatitis? Pancreas 3:108–110
236. Stein J, Jung M, Sziegoleit A, Zeuzem S, Caspary WF, Lembcke B (1996) Immunoreactive elastase I: clinical evaluation of a new noninvasive test of pancreatic function. Clin Chem 42:222–226
237. Stein J, Purschian B, Bieniek U, Caspary WF, Lembcke B (1994) Near-infrared reflectance analysis: a new dimension in the investigation of malabsorption syndromes. Eur J Gastroenterol Hepatol 6:889–894
238. Steinberg WM, Anderson KK (1984) Serum trypsinogen in diagnosis of chronic pancreatitis. Dig Dis Sci 29:988–993
239. Steinberg WM, Goldstein SS, Davis ND, Anderson KK, Shamma'a JM (1985) Predictive value of low serum trypsinogen. Dig Dis Sci 30:547–551
240. Stock K-P, Schenk J, Schmack B, Domschke W (1981) Funktions-"Screening" des exokrinen Pankreas. FDL-, N-BT-PABA-Test, Stuhl-Chymotrypsinbestimmung im Vergleich mit dem Sekretin-Pankreozymin-Test. Dtsch Med Wochenschr 106:983–987
241. Stolte M, Weiß W, Volkholz H, Rösch W (1982) A special form of segmental pancreatitis: "groove pancreatitis". Hepatogastroenterology 29:198–208
242. Tanner AR, Fisher D, Ward C, Smith CL (1984) An evaluation of the one-day NBT-PABA/^{14}C-PABA in the assessment of pancreatic exocrine insufficiency. Digestion 29:42–46
243. Tanner AR, Robinson DP (1988) Pancreatic function testing: serum PABA measurement is a reliable and accurate measurement of exocrine function. Gut 29:1736–1740
244. Temler RS, Felber J-P (1976) Radioimmunoassay of human plasma trypsin. Biochim Biophys Acta 445:720–728

245. Thomas FB, Sinar D, Caldwell JH, Mekhjian HS, Falko JM (1977) Stimulation of pancreatic secretion of water and electrolytes by furosemide. Gastroenterology 73:221–225
246. Tietz NW, Burlina A, Gerhardt W, Junge W, Malfertheiner P, Murai T, Otte M, Stein W, Gerber M, Klein G, Poppe WA (1988) Multicenter evaluation of a specific pancreatic isoamylase assay based on a double monoclonal-antibody technique. Clin Chem 34:2096–2102
247. Tio TL, Luiken GJHM, Tytgat GNJ (1991) Endosonography of groove pancreatitis. Endoscopy 23:291–293
248. Toskes PP, Greenberger NJ (1983) Acute and chronic pancreatitis. Disease-a-Month 29:1–81
249. Tympner F, Domschke S, Domschke W, Classen M, Demling L (1974) Reproducibility of the response to secretin and secretin plus pancreozymin in man. Scand J Gastroenterol 9:377–381
250. Van de Kamer JH, ten Bokkel Huinink H, Weyers HA (1949) Rapid method for the determination of fat in feces. J Biol Chem 177:347–355
251. Vantini I, Piubello W, Scuro LA, Benini P, Talamini G, Benini L, Micciolo R, Cavallini G (1982) Duodenal ulcer in chronic relapsing pancreatitis. Digestion 24:23–28
252. Ventrucci M, Gullo L, Daniele C, Bartolucci C, Priori P, Platé L, Bonora G, Labò G (1983) Comparative study of serum pancreatic isoamylase, lipase, and trypsin-like immunoreactivity in pancreatic disease. Digestion 28:114–121
253. Waller SL (1975) The Lundh test in the diagnosis of pancreatic disease: A comment from the moderator. Gut 16:657–658
254. White AF, Baum S, Buranasiri S (1976) Aneurysms secondary to pancreatitis. Am J Roentgenol 127:393–396
255. Wiersema MJ, Hawes RH, Lehman GA, Kochman ML, Sherman S, Kopecky KK (1993) Prospective evaluation of endoscopic ultrasonography and endoscopic retrograde cholangiopancreatography in patients with chronic abdominal pain of suspected pancreatic origin. Endoscopy 25:555–564
256. Wormsley KG (1978) Tests of pancreatic secretion. Clin Gastroenterol 7:529–544
257. Worning H (1984) Chronic pancreatitis: pathogenesis, natural history and conservative treatment. Clin Gastroenterol 13:871–894
258. Worning H, Müllertz S, Hess Thaysen E, Bang HO (1967) pH and concentration of pancreatic enzymes in aspirates from the human duodenum during digestion of a standard meal in patients with intestinal disorders. Scand J Gastroenterol 2:81–89
259. Worning H, Müllertz S, Hess Thaysen E, Bang HO (1967) pH and concentration of pancreatic enzymes in aspirates from the human duodenum during digestion of a standard meal in patients with duodenal ulcer and in patients subjected to different gastric resections. Scand J Gastroenterol 2:23–38
260. Worning H, Müllertz S, Hess Thaysen E, Bang HO (1968) pH and concentration of pancreatic enzymes in aspirates from the human duodenum during digestion of a standard meal in patients with pancreatic diseases. Scand J Gastroenterol 3:83–90

18 Chronic Pancreatitis: Complications

18.1
General

The complications of acute pancreatitis are well known and have a decisive influence on the prognosis of the disease, whereas the influence of complications of chronic pancreatitis (Table 18.1) on the natural history of chronic pancreatitis is not fully established.

Complications may be divided into intrapancreatic and extrapancreatic types.

18.2
Intrapancreatic Complications

18.2.1
Pancreatic Calcifications

About 70 years ago, pancreatic calculi were demonstrated for the first time by abdominal X-ray examination in a living patient. This examination has subsequently become routine for diagnosing chronic pancreatitis [99]. It is, however, still not clear, whether pancreatic calcifications are merely a manifestation of the underlying disease or really a complication.

Table 18.1. Complications of chronic pancreatitis

Intrapancreatic complications	Extrapancreatic complications
● Intrapancreatic complications	● Extrapancreatic complications
Calcifications	Stenosis of adjacent viscera
Pseudocyst(s)	– Duodenal stenosis
Abscess(es)	– Colonic stenosis
Acute necrotizing pancreatitis	– Common bile duct stenosis
Carcinoma	Peptic ulcer
	Gastrointestinal bleeding
	Pleural effusion
	Ascites
	Splenic changes
	Osseous lesions
	Metabolic consequences
	Associated diseases
	Extrapancreatic carcinoma

The frequency of pancreatic calcifications in patients with chronic pancreatitis varies [50, 82, 134]. In our own series, 55% of all patients with chronic pancreatitis showed pancreatic calcifications on plain abdominal film [64, 71]. Pancreatic calcifications are even more frequent in painless chronic pancreatitis, occurring in 70%–80% of the patients [18, 64, 82].

Data correlating pancreatic calcifications with chronic pancreatitis have to be viewed with caution. The rate of calcifications detected by plain abdominal films can be falsely high or low:

- Abdominal calcifications in the vicinity of the pancreas do not necessarily indicate chronic pancreatitis. Additional X-ray series including oblique and lateral views may be indicated to discover whether calcifications are within the pancreas or in a nearby structure. Pancreatic calcifications may also occur in a variety of other pancreatic diseases, including cysts, hemangioma, lymphangioma, cystadenoma, cystadenocarcinoma, and islet tumors [99] and may also occur in patients with normal exocrine pancreatic function following acute pancreatitis [65].
- Pancreatic calcifications may be overlooked. Ferrucci et al. [37] showed that they are detected twice as frequently by computed tomography (CT) scans as by plain abdominal films.

Pancreatic calcifications, in addition to steatorrhea and diabetes mellitus, have long been thought to occur only in the advanced stages of chronic pancreatitis [6, 9, 30, 57, 76, 90], when the residual function of the pancreas is reduced to 20% of normal [121]. Although pancreatic calcifications increase in frequency with increasing severity of exocrine pancreatic insufficiency, pancreatic calcifications are by no means an indicator of severe exocrine pancreatic insufficiency. They may occur even in patients with mild to moderate exocrine pancreatic insufficiency, and are independent of endoscopic retrograde cholangiopancreatography (ERCP) findings and of deterioration in endocrine pancreatic function [65].

Remarkably, Ammann et al. [11] have shown a regression of pancreatic calcifications in the late stages of chronic pancreatitis or following drainage procedures.

18.2.1.1
Treatment

Routine eradication of pancreatic calcifications is not possible and seems unnecessary since prognostic importance of pancreatic calcifications in the course of the disease is unknown.

18.2.2
Pancreatic Pseudocysts

In a personal series (P.G.L.), pancreatic pseudocysts occurred in every fourth patient with chronic pancreatitis, significantly more frequent than in acute pancreatitis (Table 18.2).

Table 18.2. Incidence of pancreatic pseudocysts in acute (1980–1994) and chronic (1965–1987) pancreatitis in patients from Göttingen and Lüneburg

Type of pancreatitis	n	Pseudocysts
Acute pancreatitis	602	85 (14%)
Chronic pancreatitis	335	86 (26%)[a]

[a] $p < 0.001$

Table 18.3. Incidence of pancreatic pseudocysts in chronic pancreatitis according to etiology in patients from Göttingen 1965–1987

Etiology	n	Pseudocysts
Alcohol	230	71 (31%)
Nonalcohol	105	15 (14%)[a]

[a] $p < 0.001$

Similar to acute pancreatitis (see Sect. 10.1.3) [61], pancreatic pseudocysts occur more frequently in alcoholics than in nonalcoholics (Table 18.3).

The natural history of pancreatic pseudocysts following acute pancreatitis is well known: 40% show a spontaneous resolution within 6 weeks [21]. In contrast, the natural history of pancreatic pseudocysts in chronic pancreatitis is less well known. Spontaneous resolution is rare [29, 81] and has not been observed when pancreatic calcifications or other evidence of chronic pancreatitis were observed [12].

Pancreatic pseudocysts may contribute considerably to pain and account for about two-thirds of all operations in chronic pancreatitis (Figs. 18.1 a, b, 18.2 a, b) [71]. While 96% of these operated patients are free of pain immediately after operation, median follow-up for 11 years had shown that this figure fell to 53% subsequently. Alcohol abstinence did not significantly reduce pain. Endocrine pancreatic deterioration was significantly more frequent than exocrine. In contrast to previous belief [81], the prognosis for patients with chronic pancreatitis complicated by pancreatic pseudocysts is serious: in the course of follow-up, unemployment increased from 2% to 41%, retirement rose from 0% to 33%, mainly as a result of pancreatitis, and 38% of patients died. In 14% of the latter, deaths were due to pancreatitis [72].

The differential diagnosis of a cystic structure within the pancreas may be difficult. It includes pancreatic pseudocysts, cystic neoplasm [47, 67, 126, 129, 130], hematoma, hydadid cyst [80], von Hippel-Lindau syndrome [116], urinoma [112], metastatic tumor, and true cyst [113]. Cystic neoplasms include serous cystadenomas, mucinous cystadenomas, mucinous cystadenocarcinoma [68], and rarely cystic islet-cell tumors [130]. For details see Sect. 10.1.3.

18.2.2.1
Treatment

Therapy of pancreatic pseudocysts obviously contributing to pain in chronic pancreatitis is surgical or endoscopic. Usually drainage procedures are utilized. Treatment of asymptomatic pseudocysts is conservative, at least in small and medium-sized cysts.

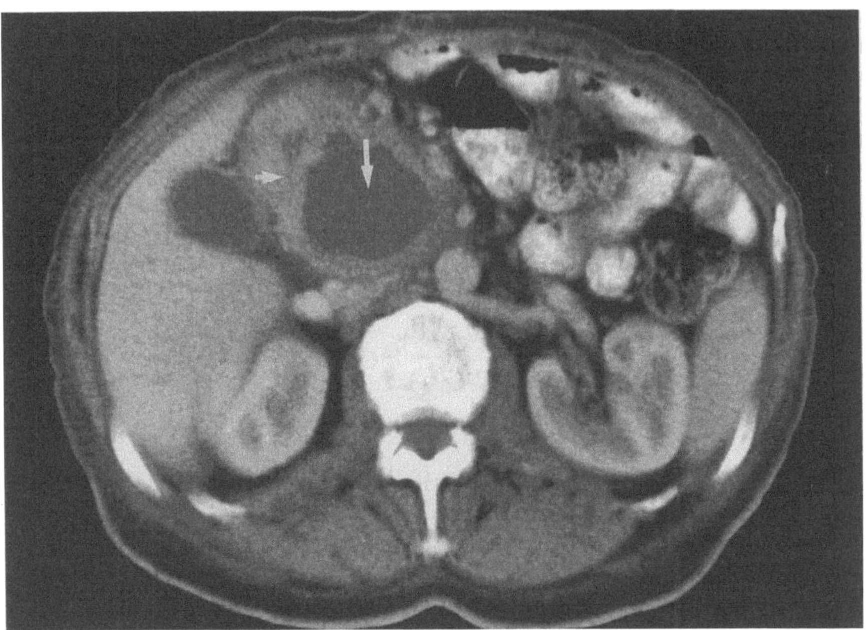

Fig. 18.1 a. Chronic pancreatitis with pseudocyst of the head of the pancreas. Dynamic contrast-enhanced CT scan shows a large, slightly irregular low-attenuation area in the head of the pancreas consistent with an intrapancreatic pseudocyst (*vertical arrow*). There is mass effect on the adjacent duodenum (*horizontal arrow*) which was confirmed by barium enema examination and endoscopy. This 43-year-old man with alcoholic chronic pancreatitis was experiencing intractable mid-abdominal pain. ERCP did not show a communication between the main pancreatic duct and the pseudocyst. Hence, the pseudocyst could not be drained by inserting a stent into the main pancreatic duct. He underwent a Roux-en-Y cystojejunostomy

In patients with asymptomatic large pseudocysts, some surgeons fear rupture due to abdominal trauma and recommend a drainage procedure.

Several recent reports have shown that cystogastrostomy or cystoduodenostomy are very efficient in treating pancreatic pseudocysts [17, 19, 26, 111].

18.2.3
Abscess

This lesion occurs rarely in chronic pancreatitis. Following surgical or endoscopical intervention, or an exacerbation of chronic pancreatitis severe enough to cause necrosis of tissue complicated by secondary infection, an abscess could conceivably develop as in acute pancreatitis (see Sect. 10.1.4).

Recently, *spontaneous* abscess formation in the pancreas and the liver was reported in 1.8% and 1.2% of 336 patients with chronic pancreatitis in a prospective follow-up study. Almost all of them had had pancreaticojejunostomy up to 12 years previously [5].

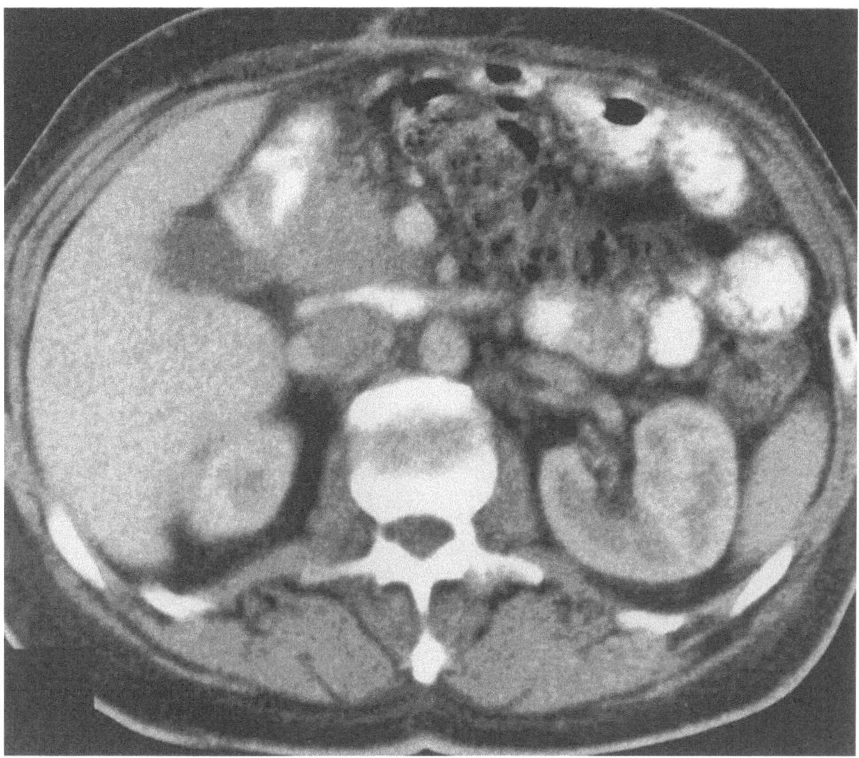

Fig. 18.1 b. Chronic pancreatitis with pseudocyst of the head of the pancreas. Dynamic contrast-enhanced CT scan 2 months later reveals total resolution of the low-attenuation area and reduction in size of the head of the pancreas. He has remained asymptomatic

18.2.3.1
Treatment

Similar to acute pancreatitis, abscess formation in chronic pancreatitis requires surgical drainage or radiologic catheter drainage.

18.2.4
Acute Necrotizing Pancreatitis

Acute pancreatic necrosis has been reported in two prospective studies in 11%–12% of patients with chronic pancreatitis who underwent surgical treatment shortly after an acute attack [73, 87].

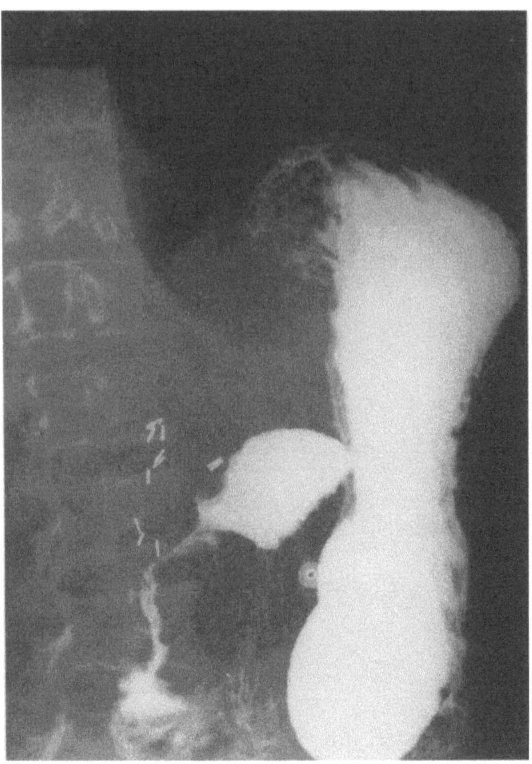

Fig. 18.2 a. Chronic pancreatitis with duodenal stenosis. Barium meal examination reveals marked narrowing and irregularity of the duodenum extending from the apex of the bulb to the third portion of the duodenum. Cholecystectomy clips are visible. The 48-year-old man with chronic pancreatitis secondary to alcohol was experiencing intractable abdominal pain. Duodenal stenosis in chronic pancreatitis is usually attributed to either chronic pancreatitis involving the wall of the duodenum or a pseudocyst in the head of the pancreas

18.2.4.1
Treatment

Necrosectomy has usually been recommended. There are no studies at present of conservative treatment of pancreatic necrosis in chronic pancreatitis. If it is asymptomatic, our recommendation is to treat pancreatic necrosis medically. Surgery is reserved for patients with intractable pain, or some other complication.

18.2.5
Pancreatic Carcinoma

Clinical studies report varying figures concerning the incidence of pancreatic carcinoma in patients with chronic pancreatitis, reaching from 1.4% to 2.7% [7, 10, 64, 84, 117]. Recently, a multicenter historical cohort study of 2015 subjects with chronic pancreatitis was carried out in clinical centers in 6 countries [70]. The cumulative risk of pancreatic carcinoma in patients who were followed for at least 2 years increased distinctly, and 10 and 20 years after the diagnosis of pancreatitis it was 1.8% and 4%, respectively (Fig. 18.3). Thus, the risk of pancreatic carcinoma was significantly elevat-

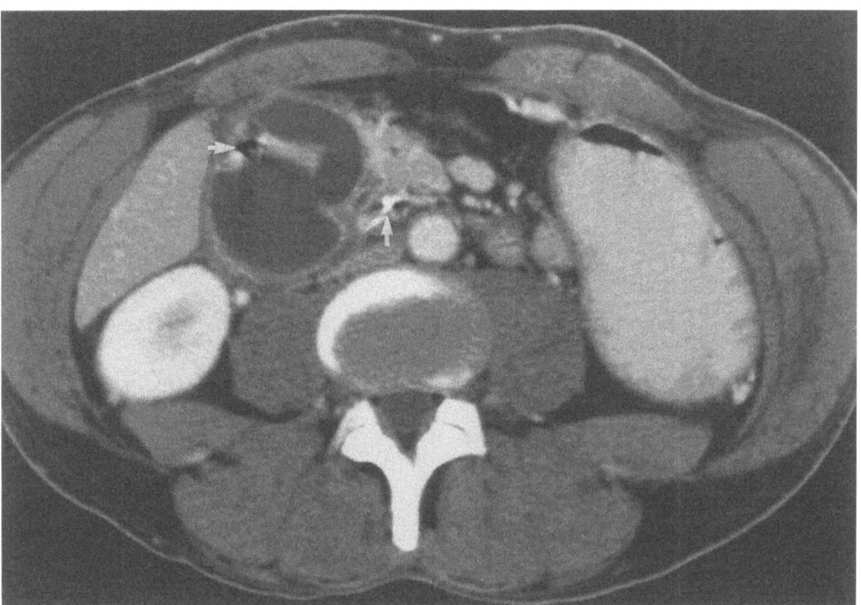

Fig. 18.2 b. Chronic pancreatitis with duodenal stenosis. Contrast-enhanced CT scan reveals a pseudocyst in the head of the pancreas compressing the descending duodenum. Air (*horizontal arrow*) and a small amount of contrast are visible in the descending duodenum. Several calculi (*vertical arrow*) are visible in the head of the pancreas. The patient underwent a Roux-en-Y cystojejunostomy and gastrojejunostomy and has remained pain-free during the past 8 years

ed in patients with chronic pancreatitis [70]. Chronic pancreatitis including tropical calcifying pancreatitis had not previously been included among precancerous conditions [28, 70]. Other studies have been confirmative [15, 36]. Interestingly, the risk of pancreatic carcinoma was also increased in patients with cystic fibrosis [86].

Unfortunately, it is very difficult to diagnose a pancreatic carcinoma in chronic pancreatitis. Carcinoma of the pancreas should be suspected in a patient with chronic pancreatitis if there is increasing abdominal discomfort, progressive weight loss, jaundice, and radiological evidence including nodularity of the duodenal sweep. On one occasion, pancreatic calcification was seen to recede, presumably as a result of erosion of calcific deposits by the expanding carcinoma [122]. However, this has not been confirmed [13]. Confirmation of carcinoma may be quite difficult in chronic calcific pancreatitis.

18.2.5.1
Treatment

Treatment of pancreatic carcinoma in chronic pancreatitis is the same as in idiopathic pancreatic carcinoma.

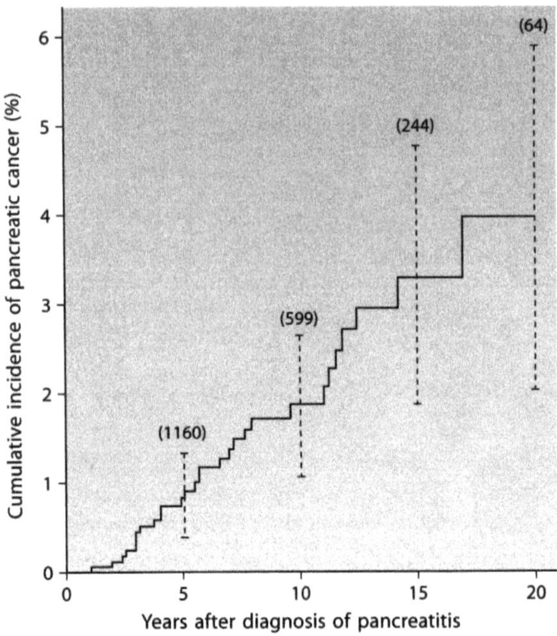

Fig. 18.3. Cumulative incidence of pancreatic cancer in 1552 subjects with chronic pancreatitis with a minimum of 2 years of follow-up. The *vertical lines* represent 95% confidence intervals. In *parentheses* are the numbers of subjects at risk. One additional case of cancer developed after 25 years of follow-up. (From [70] with permission)

18.3
Extrapancreatic Complications

18.3.1
Stenosis of Adjacent Viscera

18.3.1.1
Duodenal Stenosis

Duodenal stenosis complicating chronic pancreatitis may originate from prior severe inflammation of the pancreas that involves the wall of the contiguous duodenum, from extensive fibrosis of the head of the pancreas, or from a pancreatic pseudocyst that compresses the duodenal wall (Fig. 18.2 a, b). The frequency of this complication has been variously reported as 20% [75], 9% [93], and 5.1% [71]. It may be associated with upper abdominal pain, nausea, and vomiting sufficient to require pancreaticoduodenectomy [75]. Diagnosis is usually based on a barium meal examination showing marked narrowing of the descending duodenum. At times, reactive mucosal changes in the duodenum may simulate pancreatic carcinoma [20].

18.3.1.1.1
Treatment

If duodenal stenosis is due to an acute inflammation of the head of the pancreas, treatment of this acute attack may lead to spontaneous resolution. If duodenal stenosis is a fixed obstruction, treatment depends on the accompanying complication. Some patients have vomiting only and can be treated with a gastrojejunostomy. Others have associated common bile duct stenosis and require decompression of the common bile duct in addition to therapy for duodenal stenosis. Finally, another group has intractable pain when there is marked swelling of the head of the pancreas; this requires a Whipple's operation.

18.3.1.2
Colonic Stenosis

Partial or complete stenosis of the colon, mostly below the splenic flexure, may occur in chronic pancreatitis as a result of pancreatic exudate in a preceding episode of an acute attack passing from the anterior surface of the pancreas through the leaves of the transverse mesocolon into the colon. Although more frequent in acute pancreatitis, this complication may also occur in the chronic form of the disease and sometimes mimic carcinoma of the colon [41, 48, 63, 95, 96, 107].

18.3.1.2.1
Treatment

If colonic stenosis is due to an acute attack of chronic pancreatitis, medical treatment of this condition is the same as in acute pancreatitis (see Sects. 11.1.2, 11.1.3) and may result in spontaneous resolution. However, if the stenosis persists and leads to obstructive symptoms or signs (colicky pain, fever, prestenotic dilatation of the colon), surgical resection of the colonic stenosis is necessary.

18.3.2
Stenosis of the Common Bile Duct

The distal portion of the common bile duct may be affected by inflammation of the pancreas because it traverses the head of the pancreas, or just behind it, before entering the duodenum. In chronic pancreatitis, this portion of the common bile duct may be obstructed by an acute inflammatory exacerbation, by fibrosis of the head of the pancreas (Fig. 18.4 a, b), or by an adjacent pancreatic pseudocyst. Occurrence rates for this complication as given in earlier reports varied from 10% to 62% [22, 23, 109, 132, 133]. A study of 2481 patients with chronic pancreatitis described partial biliary obstruction in 5.2% [114], a persistently elevated serum alkaline phosphatase activity in 82.5% of the patients, and elevated serum bilirubin levels in 66.3%.

Cholangitis in early stages and secondary biliary cirrhosis in long-standing cases of biliary obstruction present serious problems [1, 49, 109].

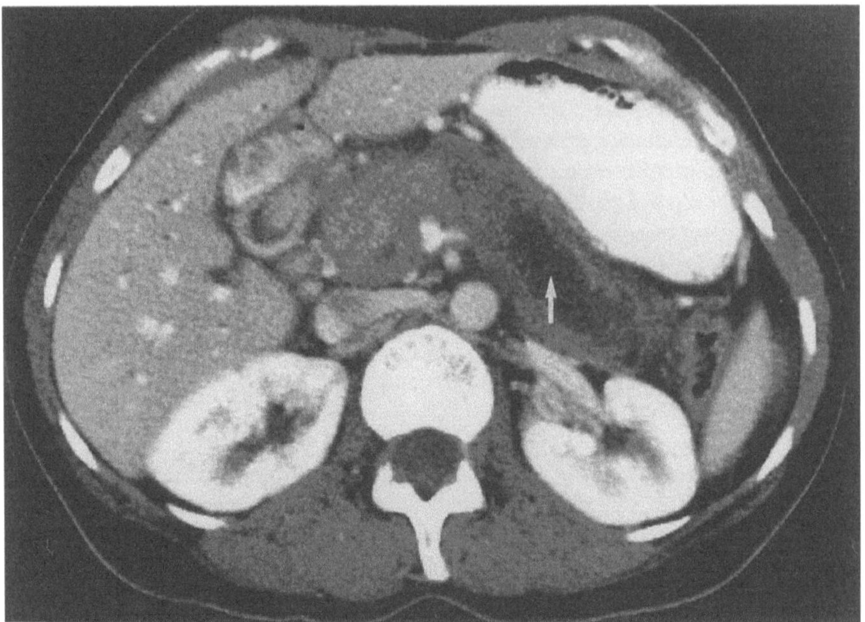

Fig. 18.4a. Chronic pancreatitis with stenosis of both the pancreatic duct and distal common bile duct. Dynamic contrast-enhanced CT scan shows massive dilatation of the pancreatic duct in the body and tail of the pancreas (*arrow*). This 44-year-old woman has been experiencing intractable abdominal pain for more than 1 year. A series of CT scans had revealed progressive dilatation of the pancreatic duct

18.3.2.1
Treatment

An endoscopically placed biliary stent may relieve transient obstruction and allow the inflammatory process to heal [54]. However, in long-standing bile duct stenosis, biliary stents provide only temporary relief. Metal stents should not be used. If the patient develops symptoms, i.e., intractable pain, progressive jaundice, or sepsis, surgical treatment is indicated and involves usually a choledochojejunostomy or rarely a cholecystojejunostomy.

18.3.3
Peptic Ulcer

The coexistence of peptic ulcer disease and chronic pancreatitis has been documented in 6.3% to 37.5% of patients [32, 43, 71, 82, 85, 123]. Olsen [89], however, found a frequency rate of only 6%, not different from that in patients who died of other diseases. Employing a different approach, Marks et al. [77] documented gastrointestinal

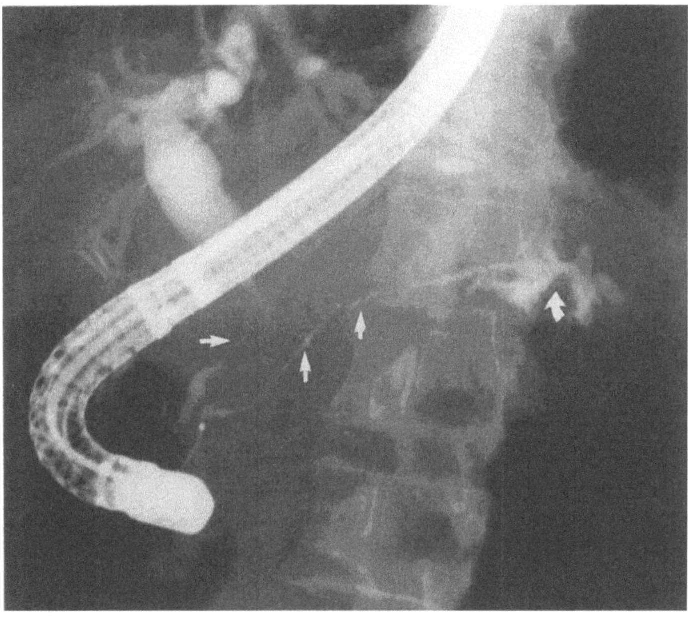

Fig. 18.4 b. Chronic pancreatitis with stenosis of both the pancreatic duct and distal common bile duct. ERCP reveals considerable narrowing of the main pancreatic duct (*vertical arrows*) with contrast partially opacifying dilated ducts in the tail of the pancreas (*curved arrow*). The distal common bile duct has a lengthy stricture (*horizontal arrow*) causing massive dilatation of the more proximal duct. Because of intractable symptoms, she underwent a Whipple operation, which revealed very severe chronic pancreatitis but no tumor. Her postoperative course was uneventful, and she has remained pain-free. The final diagnosis was idiopathic chronic pancreatitis

bleeding in about 20% of 429 patients with chronic pancreatitis, 3.5% of whom had an ulcer. Whatever the precise occurrence rate, the clinician would be well advised to suspect peptic ulcer disease in patients with chronic pancreatitis, who have recurrent episodes of upper abdominal pain, and to perform upper gastrointestinal endoscopy.

Why peptic ulcers develop in patients with chronic pancreatitis is unclear. One explanation is that the deterioration of pancreatic exocrine function results in a reduction of bicarbonate concentration in the pancreatic juice, thereby lowering the pH in the duodenum [82, 106].

18.3.3.1
Treatment

Treatment of peptic ulcer complicating chronic pancreatitis is the same as in peptic ulcer disease, including H_2-blockers or proton pump inhibitors.

18.3.4
Gastrointestinal Bleeding

Gastrointestinal bleeding in chronic pancreatitis may have pancreatic causes or result from associated diseases. Possible causes include alcohol- and aspirin-related gastritis, esophageal tear from vomiting, gastric and duodenal ulcers, variceal bleeding due to segmental portal hypertension, or tryptic digestion of large vessels in the wall of pancreatic pseudocysts [3, 14, 38, 46, 60, 92]. In addition, diffuse mucosal bleeding of the duodenum may occur when there is contiguous inflammation from the head of the pancreas.

Hemorrhage from pseudoaneurysm complicating chronic pancreatitis is a rare but very severe and often life-threatening complication (Fig. 18.5 a–c) [74].

Two types of clinical presentation are possible when bleeding occurs from a pseudoaneurysm located within the wall of a pancreatic pseudocyst. When the cyst has no connection with the pancreatic duct, distension of the pseudocyst by blood can cause severe abdominal pain and a tender abdominal mass [74]. When the cyst has a sufficient connection to the pancreatic duct, a brisk flow of blood into the duodenum may lead to the predominant symptom of hematemesis or melena [2, 58, 104]. Occasionally, arterial pulsation may be visible through the abdominal wall and auscultation may reveal a murmur (i.e., a bruit) caused by turbulence as blood gushes out of the pseudoaneurysm into the pseudocyst. Usually, dynamic contrast-enhanced CT is sufficient to identify a pseudoaneurysm. In selected cases, angiography may be necessary and may be used for the embolization of the vessel. The use of a side-viewing endoscope to document bleeding from the papilla is recommended.

18.3.4.1
Treatment

In case of acute massive bleeding from a pseudoaneurysm, immediate intervention is necessary. This may entail an emergency operation or a selective angiography with embolization of the bleeding vessel. According to the specific findings, either the vessel should be intraoperatively repaired by ligation, or the affected part of the pancreas should be resected. The successful embolization of the vessel may be performed as a definite therapy or to achieve a preoperative standstill of the bleeding. Hitherto, it has been a matter of debate which therapeutical procedure should be favored. We recommend selective angiography with embolization as the first step, surgical intervention as the last resort.

Fig. 18.5 a–c. This 67-year-old retired male nurse, an alcoholic, suffered from chronic pancreatitis. Shortly before a planned discharge from hospital when the patient felt well, he developed acute abdominal pain. The CT after bolus showed signs of an acute attack of chronic pancreatitis with ill-defined parenchyma, peripancreatic reaction, multiple pseudocysts (**a, c** ➡) and duct dilatation (**b** →), and a large encapsulated cyst with bright marginal gastroduodenal pseudoaneurysm (**b, c** ▲). (From [74] with permission)

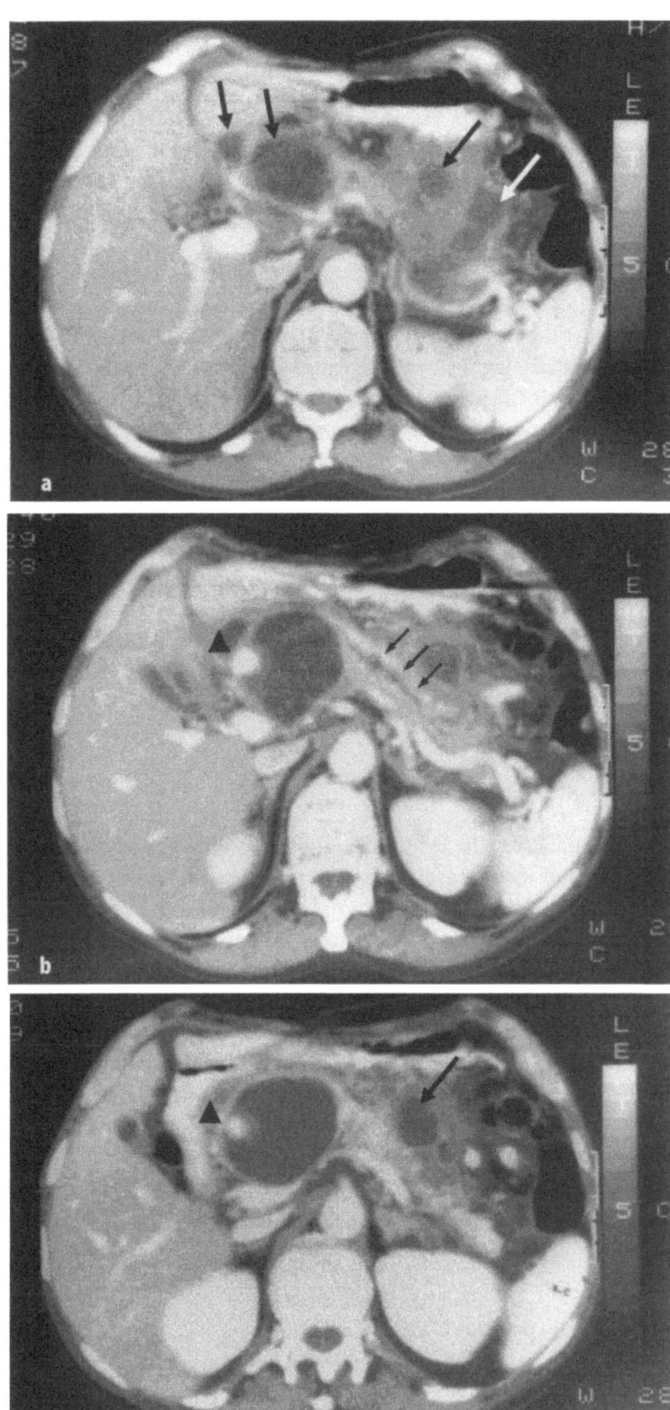

18.3.5
Pleural Effusion

Fluid accumulation in the pleural space traceable to chronic pancreatitis is, as a rule, caused by leakage from a poorly walled-off pseudocyst, or disruption of the pancreatic duct, or a main tributary (see Fig. 17.21). When the pancreatic juice leaks posteriorly into the retroperitoneum, it may enter the mediastinum or pleural space through the diaphragmatic foramina.

A chest film reveals unilateral or bilateral pleural effusion, and analysis of aspirated pleural fluid nearly always shows amylase levels higher than serum. A pancreaticopleural fistula may be demonstrated by ERCP followed by CT [56].

Differential diagnosis must include a pulmonary malignant neoplasm that secretes amylase [8]. If the pleural effusion contains a high concentration of lipase as well as of amylase, a pancreatic source is most likely.

18.3.5.1
Treatment

In contrast to acute pancreatitis, pleural effusion rarely vanishes in chronic pancreatitis and treatment is usually necessary. The best approach is to do an ERCP to identify the disruption of the duct, and then place a pancreatic stent across it.

18.3.6
Ascites

In acute pancreatitis, ascites develops following the acute attack and resolves during the course of the disease. In chronic pancreatitis, ascites may be insidious at the onset without any other signs and symptoms of chronic pancreatitis. It is probably a rare complication, but its true incidence is not known [25, 31, 53]. As with pleural effusions, leakage from a pseudocyst and disruption of, or leakage from, the pancreatic duct with subsequent leakage of pancreatic fluid in an anterior direction, first entering the lesser sac and then reaching the peritoneal cavity, are the likely operative mechanisms.

Differential diagnosis of ascites includes infectious processes such as tuberculosis, diffuse intraabdominal malignancy, and cirrhosis with portal hypertension. The diagnosis of pancreatic ascites is made on the basis of an elevated amylase (and lipase) concentration in ascitic fluid, usually many times higher than in serum, and an elevated albumin concentration (>3 g%). Fluid is usually clear or straw-colored, but may also be chylous or bloody [31]. ERCP is indicated to localize a suspected leakage.

18.3.6.1
Treatment

As with intractable pleural effusion, the best treatment is stenting if the disruption of the pancreatic duct is identified by ERCP. If the stent fails and the duct is dilated, a lateral pancreaticojejunostomy is effective. If the blow-out is near the tail, sometimes a distal pancreatectomy is required.

18.3.7
Splenic Changes

Because of the geographic proximity of the pancreas and the spleen, splenic changes complicate pancreatic inflammatory disease more often than was thought [60].

The most frequently encountered splenic change with chronic pancreatitis is probably splenic vein thrombosis. Extrinsic compression of the vein secondary to edema, cellular infiltration, and subsequent fibrosis are much more characteristic of acute than of chronic pancreatitis [83].

Incomplete or complete splenic vein thrombosis has been reported in frequencies between 22% and 54% of patients [51, 66, 98, 101, 102].

Occlusion of the superior mesenteric vein or portal vein may also occur in chronic pancreatitis, frequently in association with splenic vein occlusion [127].

Splenic complications due to expanding pancreatic pseudocysts may occur in patients with acute rather than chronic pancreatitis [124]. Rupture of the spleen in the absence of pseudocysts, however, has been reported in patients with chronic pancreatitis [24, 27, 40, 131]. Fibrous fixation of the splenic hilum may be a predisposing factor [40, 128].

18.3.7.1
Treatment

In asymptomatic splenic vein thrombosis and asymptomatic varices, a watch-and-wait-for-bleeding policy is reasonable. If complications occur such as erosion of a pancreatic pseudocyst into the spleen or a rupture of the spleen, splenectomy is required.

18.3.8
Osseous Lesions

In acute pancreatitis, osseous lesions are very rare and mainly consist of fat necrosis or septic metastases. In chronic pancreatitis, skeletal involvement is also very rare and can manifest itself as osteomalacia [16, 52, 59, 94, 115], idiopathic necrosis of the femoral head [118], bacterial osteomyelitis [125], or lesions in knees and feet [105].

18.3.8.1
Treatment

Osseous lesions are rare and should be individually treated. There are no data comprising large numbers of patients enabling general recommendations.

18.3.9
Metabolic Consequences

In chronic pancreatitis associated with steatorrhea, deficiencies of single or multiple fat-soluble vitamins (vitamins A, D, E, and K) are frequent, even in patients treated for pancreatic insufficiency [33]. However, these deficiencies are not generally of major clinical importance. Lower vitamin E levels have been reported in patients with decompensated exocrine pancreatic insufficiency [55], but the significance and clinical importance of this finding remain to be elucidated.

Vitamin B_{12} malabsorption can be documented by a Schilling test in 30%–50% of patients with severe chronic pancreatitis, but this, too, is only rarely of clinical importance. The prevailing postulate with respect to the mechanism of vitamin B_{12} malabsorption is that there are proteins in saliva and gastric juice (termed R-binders) that normally bind vitamin B_{12}. Once acid and pepsin digest this vitamin from dietary protein, pancreatic proteases then degrade the R-binders, permitting vitamin B_{12} to bind with intrinsic factor. The vitamin B_{12}-intrinsic factor complex then travels to the terminal ileum, attaches to specific ileal receptors and is absorbed. Deficiency in the secretion of pancreatic proteases in chronic pancreatitis presumably prevents the degradation of R-binders and hence prevents subsequent binding of intrinsic factor with vitamin B_{12}.

18.3.9.1
Treatment

The administration of potent pancreatic extracts normalizes vitamin B_{12} absorption [120].

18.3.10
Associated Diseases

An interesting but unanswered question is whether an alcoholic patient is more likely to develop alcohol-induced acute or chronic pancreatitis, alcoholic cirrhosis of the liver, or both. A report by Ammann [4] indicated that liver cirrhosis occurred in 5% of patients with chronic pancreatitis. However, Greiner et al. [42] found alcoholic liver cirrhosis in 30% of patients with pancreatic duct changes suggestive of chronic pancreatitis, and Dutta et al. [34] reported a frequency of liver cirrhosis in 19% of patients with chronic pancreatitis investigated retrospectively; a prospective study from the same group reported severe fatty liver, alcohol hepatitis, or cirrhosis in 43% of the patients [34]. Investigating patients with alcoholic liver disease at autopsy, Renner et al. [97] found that 20% of 1022 patients had chronic pancreatitis.

Gallstones were found in one survey [4] in 6.1% of patients with chronic pancreatitis. Primary sclerosing cholangitis has been found to be associated with exocrine pancreatic insufficiency [35, 45, 62, 91], and exocrine pancreatic insuffiency has been reported in patients with inflammatory bowel disease [39, 88, 108, 110].

Chronic pancreatitis is associated with a high prevalence of giardiasis [69] which has been found in 27% of patients with chronic pancreatitis and in 28% of patients with cystic fibrosis, indicating that exocrine pancreatic insufficiency may predispose to colonization with *Giardia lamblia,* implying in turn that pancreatic exocrine secretion may play a role in host defense against giardiasis [135]. Furthermore, chronic pancreatitis occurred among almost 1% of patients who experienced a *Yersinia enterocolitica* infection [103].

In 17.2% of patients with chronic pancreatitis, marked eosinophilia was observed. There was no difference between alcoholics and nonalcoholics, endocrine pancreatic function was maintained comparatively well, despite marked exocrine pancreatic insufficiency. Eosinophilia frequently developed in association with severe complications such as pleural effusion, pericarditis, and ascites [119].

Cardiovascular and pulmonary investigations showed that patients with chronic pancreatitis suffer more frequently from vascular diseases and early lung parenchymal damage then controls [44, 79].

18.3.10.1
Treatment

Treatment is dependent on the associated disease.

18.3.11
Extrapancreatic Carcinomas

Extrapancreatic carcinomas in chronic pancreatitis are not rare. They have been reported with varying incidence, reaching from 3.9% to 12.5% [10, 64, 82, 100, 117]. In some of these and other studies [10, 64, 78, 82], a considerable number of extrapancreatic carcinomas have involved the upper respiratory tract (oral cavity, larynx, bronchial tree). Since alcohol abuse is the dominating etiology of chronic pancreatitis, and many alcoholics are known to smoke, extrapancreatic carcinomas involving the upper respiratory tract may reflect the consequences of tobacco abuse.

18.3.11.1
Treatment

Treatment depends on the nature of the extrapancreatic carcinoma.

References

1. Afroudakis A, Kaplowitz N (1981) Liver histopathology in chronic common bile duct stenosis due to chronic alcoholic pancreatitis. Hepatology 1:65–72
2. Alexandre J-H, Guerrieri MT (1981) Role of total pancreatectomy in the treatment of necrotizing pancreatitis. World J Surg 5:369–377
3. Alwmark A, Gullstrand P, Ihse I, Joelsson B, Owman T (1981) Regional portal hypertension in chronic pancreatitis. Acta Chir Scand 147:155–157

4. Ammann R (1985) Diagnose und Therapie der alkoholischen chronischen Pankreatitis. Eine kritische Standortbestimmung. Schweiz Med Wochenschr 115 (Suppl 19):42–51
5. Ammann R, Münch R, Largiadèr F, Akovbiantz A, Marincek B (1992) Pancreatic and hepatic abscesses: a late complication in 10 patients with chronic pancreatitis. Gastroenterology 103: 560–565
6. Ammann RW (1980) Zur Klinik und Differentialdiagnose der chronischen Pankreatitis. Berücksichtigung des Langzeitverlaufs von 258 Patienten. Schweiz Med Wochenschr 110:1322–1327
7. Ammann RW, Akovbiantz A, Largiadèr F, Schueler G (1984) Course and outcome of chronic pancreatitis. Longitudinal study of a mixed medical-surgical series of 245 patients. Gastroenterology 86:820–828
8. Ammann RW, Berk JE, Fridhandler L, Ueda M, Wegmann W (1973) Hyperamylasemia with carcinoma of the lung. Ann Intern Med 78:521–525
9. Ammann RW, Hammer B, Fumagalli I (1973) Chronic pancreatitis in Zurich, 1963–1972. Clinical findings and follow-up studies of 102 cases. Digestion 9:404–415
10. Ammann RW, Knoblauch M, Möhr P, Deyhle P, Largiadèr F, Akovbiantz A, Schüler G, Schneider J (1980) High incidence of extrapancreatic carcinoma in chronic pancreatitis. Scand J Gastroenterol 15:395–399
11. Ammann RW, Muench R, Otto R, Buehler H, Freiburghaus AU, Siegenthaler W (1988) Evolution and regression of pancreatic calcification in chronic pancreatitis. A prospective long-term study of 107 patients. Gastroenterology 95:1018–1028
12. Aranha GV, Prinz RA, Esguerra AC, Greenlee HB (1983) The nature and course of cystic pancreatic lesions diagnosed by ultrasound. Arch Surg 118:486–488
13. Baltaxe HA, Leslie EV (1967) Vanishing pancreatic calcifications. A case report. Am J Roentgenol 99:642–644
14. Bank S (1986) Chronic pancreatitis: clinical features and medical management. Am J Gastroenterol 81:153–167
15. Bansal P, Sonnenberg A (1995) Pancreatitis is a risk factor for pancreatic cancer. Gastroenterology 109:247–251
16. Bars L, Soulé J-C, Morin T, Hioco D, Bader J-P (1978) Pancréatite chronique. Cause unique d'une ostéomalacie sévère. Gastroenterol Clin Biol 2:499–506
17. Barthet M, Sahel J, Bodiou-Bertel C, Bernard J-P (1995) Endoscopic transpapillary drainage of pancreatic pseudocysts. Gastrointest Endosc 42:208–213
18. Bartholomew LG, Comfort MW (1956) Chronic pancreatitis without pain. Gastroenterology 31: 727–745
19. Binmoeller KF, Seifert H, Walter A, Soehendra N (1995) Transpapillary and transmural drainage of pancreatic pseudocysts. Gastrointest Endosc 42:219–224
20. Blackstone MO, Mizuno H (1977) Reactive duodenal changes in chronic pancreatitis simulating the contiguous spread of pancreatic carcinoma. Am J Dig Dis 22:658–661
21. Bradley III EL, Clements JL Jr, Gonzalez AC (1979) The natural history of pancreatic pseudocysts: a unified concept of management. Am J Surg 137:135–141
22. Bradley III EL, Salam AA (1978) Hyperbilirubinemia in inflammatory pancreatic disease: natural history and management. Ann Surg 188:626–629
23. Bradley EL (1986) Parapancreatic biliary and intestinal obstruction in chronic obstructive pancreatitis. Is prophylactic bypass necessary? Am J Surg 151:256–258
24. Byrd BF Jr, Couch OA Jr (1955) Pancreatitis with rupture of spleen and hemorrhagic pleural effusion. JAMA 157:1112–1113
25. Cameron JL (1978) Chronic pancreatic ascites and pancreatic pleural effusions. Gastroenterology 74:134–140
26. Catalano MF, Geenen JE, Schmalz MJ, Johnson GK, Dean RS, Hogan WJ (1995) Treatment of pancreatic pseudocysts with ductal communication by transpapillary pancreatic duct endoprosthesis. Gastrointest Endosc 42:214–218
27. Catanzaro FP, Abiri M, Allegra S (1968) Spontaneous rupture of spleen and pleural effusion complicating pancreatitis. Rhode Island Med J 51:328–329
28. Chari ST, Mohan V, Pitchumoni CS, Viswanathan M, Madanagopalan N, Lowenfels AB (1994) Risk of pancreatic carcinoma in tropical calcifying pancreatitis: an epidemiologic study. Pancreas 9:62–66

29. Crass RA, Way LW (1981) Acute and chronic pancreatic pseudocysts are different. Am J Surg 142:660–663
30. Creutzfeldt W, Fehr H, Schmidt H (1970) Verlaufsbeobachtungen und diagnostische Verfahren bei der chronisch-rezidivierenden und chronischen Pankreatitis. Schweiz Med Wochenschr 100:1180–1189
31. DiMagno EP, Layer P, Clain JE (1993) Chronic pancreatitis. In: Go VLW, DiMagno EP, Gardner JD, Lebenthal E, Reber HA, Scheele GA (eds) The Pancreas: Biology, Pathobiology, and Disease, 2nd edn. Raven Press, New York, pp 665–706
32. Dreiling DA, Naqvi MA (1969) Peptic ulcer diathesis in patients with chronic pancreatitis. Am J Gastroenterol 51:503–510
33. Dutta SK, Bustin MP, Russell RM, Costa BS (1982) Deficiency of fat-soluble vitamins in treated patients with pancreatic insufficiency. Ann Intern Med 97:549–552
34. Dutta SK, Mobrahan S, Iber FL (1978) Associated liver disease in alcoholic pancreatitis. Am J Dig Dis 23:618–622
35. Epstein O, Chapman RWG, Lake-Bakaar G, Foo AY, Rosalki SB, Sherlock S (1982) The pancreas in primary biliary cirrhosis and primary sclerosing cholangitis. Gastroenterology 83:1177–1182
36. Fernandez E, La Vecchia C, Porta M, Negri E, d'Avanzo B, Boyle P (1995) Pancreatitis and the risk of pancreatic cancer. Pancreas 11:185–189
37. Ferrucci JT Jr, Wittenberg J, Black EB, Kirkpatrick RH, Hall DA (1979) Computed body tomography in chronic pancreatitis. Radiology 130:175–182
38. Fékété F, Laigneau P, Belghiti J (1980) Les hémorragies digestives au cours des pancréatites chroniques. Gastroenterol Clin Biol 4:551–555
39. Gallagher P, Chadwick P, Jones DM, Turner L (1981) Acute pancreatitis associated with campylobacter infection. Br J Surg 68:383
40. Gardner RJ, Preston FW (1961) Rupture of the spleen associated with pancreatitis. JAMA 177:784–785
41. Greiner L (1982) Kolonstenose infolge chronischer Pankreatitis. Seltene Differentialdiagnose einer Colitis regionalis Crohn. Med Welt 33:1632–1633
42. Greiner L, Schubert E, Franken FH (1983) Koinzidenz von chronischer Pankreatitis und Leberzirrhose bei Alkoholabusus. Eine röntgen- und histomorphologische Studie. Z Gastroenterol 21:526–532
43. Gullo L, Costa PL, Labò G (1977) Chronic pancreatitis in Italy. Aetiological, clinical and histological observations based on 253 cases. Rendic Gastroenterol 9:97–104
44. Gullo L, Stella A, Labriola E, Costa PL, Descovich G, Labò G (1982) Cardiovascular lesions in chronic pancreatitis. A prospective study. Dig Dis Sci 27:716–722
45. Gurian LE, Keeffe EB (1982) Pancreatic insufficiency associated with ulcerative colitis and pericholangitis. Gastroenterology 82:581–585
46. Hall RI, Lavelle MI, Venables CW (1982) Chronic pancreatitis as a cause of gastrointestinal bleeding. Gut 23:250–255
47. Hammel P, Levy P, Voitot H, Levy M, Vilgrain V, Zins M, Flejou J-F, Molas G, Ruszniewski P, Bernades P (1995) Preoperative cyst fluid analysis is useful for the differential diagnosis of cystic lesions of the pancreas. Gastroenterology 108:1230–1235
48. Hancock RJ, Christensen RM, Osler TR, Cassim MM (1973) Stenosis of the colon due to pancreatitis and mimicking carcinoma. Can J Surg 16:393–398
49. Harris AI, Korsten MA (1976) Acute suppurative cholangitis secondary to calcific pancreatitis. Gastroenterology 71:847–850
50. Hayakawa T, Kondo T, Shibata T, Sugimuto Y, Kitagawa M (1989) Chronic alcoholism and evolution of pain and prognosis in chronic pancreatitis. Dig Dis Sci 34:33–38
51. Hofer BO, Ryan JA Jr, Freeny PC (1987) Surgical significance of vascular changes in chronic pancreatitis. Surg Gynecol Obstet 164:499–505
52. Hoffbrand BI (1965) Chronic pancreatitis (? alcoholic) with osteomalacia. Proc Roy Soc Med 58:697–698
53. Hotz J, Goebell H, Herfarth C, Probst M (1977) Massive pancreatic ascites without carcinoma. Report of three cases. Digestion 15:200–216
54. Itani KMF, Taylor TV (1995) The challenge of therapy for pancreatitis-related common bile duct stricture. Am J Surg 170:543–546

55. Kalvaria I, Labadarios D, Shephard GS, Visser L, Marks IN (1986) Biochemical vitamin E deficiency in chronic pancreatitis. Int J Pancreatol 1:119–128
56. Kimura Y, Yamamoto T, Zenda S, Kawamura E, Suzuki E (1987) Pancreatic pleural fistula: demonstration by computed tomography after endoscopic retrograde pancreatography. Am J Gastroenterol 82:790–793
57. Kondo T, Hayakawa T, Noda A, Ito K, Yamazaki Y, Iinuma Y, Okumura N, Sakakibara A, Mizuno R, Naruse S (1981) Follow-up study of chronic pancreatitis. Gastroenterol Jpn 16:46–53
58. Köhler H, Becker HD (1984) Die Pancreaticorrhagie. Ein Beitrag zur Differentialdiagnose der oberen gastrointestinalen Blutung. Chirurg 55:526–527
59. Lamotte-Barrillon S, Bernier JJ, Tricoire J, Labrousse C (1964) Grande ostéomalacie et pancréatite calcifiante. Presse Med 72:3441–3445
60. Lankisch PG (1990) The spleen in inflammatory pancreatic disease. Gastroenterology 98:509–516
61. Lankisch PG, Burchard-Reckert S, Petersen M, Lehnick D, Schirren CA, Stöckmann F, Köhler H (1996) Etiology and age have only a limited influence on the course of acute pancreatitis. Pancreas 13:344–349
62. Lankisch PG, Creutzfeldt W (1987) Exokrine Pankreasinsuffizienz bei primär sklerosierender Cholangitis. Z Gastroenterol 25:175–181
63. Lankisch PG, Lopez E, Winckler K, Schuster R (1976) Kolonstenosen nach Pankreatitis. Schweiz Med Wochenschr 106:1243–1247
64. Lankisch PG, Löhr-Happe A, Otto J, Creutzfeldt W (1993) Natural course in chronic pancreatitis. Pain, exocrine and endocrine pancreatic insufficiency and prognosis of the disease. Digestion 54:148–155
65. Lankisch PG, Otto J, Löhr A, Schirren C-A, Schuster R (1989) Pancreatic calcifications in patients with normal pancreatic function. Int J Pancreatol 5:281–293
66. Lemaitre G, L'Herminé C, Maillard J-P, Toison F (1971) "L'hypertension portale segmentaire" des pancréatites. Aspects angiographiques. Lille Med 16:928–932
67. Lewandrowski K, Lee J, Southern J, Centeno B, Warshaw A (1995) Cyst fluid analysis in the differential diagnosis of pancreatic cysts: a new approach to the preoperative assessment of pancreatic cystic lesions. Am J Roentgenol 164:815–819
68. Lewandrowski KB, Southern JF, Pins MR, Compton CC, Warshaw AL (1993) Cyst fluid analysis in the differential diagnosis of pancreatic cysts. A comparison of pseudocysts, serous cystadenomas, mucinous cystic neoplasms, and mucinous cystadenocarcinoma. Ann Surg 217:41–47
69. Lopez JJ, Wright JA, Hammer RA, Ertan A (1992) Chronic pancreatitis is associated with a high prevalence of giardiasis. Can J Gastroenterol 6:73–76
70. Lowenfels AB, Maisonneuve P, Cavallini G, Ammann RW, Lankisch PG, Andersen JR, DiMagno EP, Andrén-Sandberg Å, Domellöf L, International Pancreatitis Study Group (1993) Pancreatitis and the risk of pancreatic cancer. N Engl J Med 328:1433–1437
71. Löhr A (1990) Der natürliche Verlauf der chronischen Pankreatitis. Die Entwicklung der Leitsymptome Schmerzen, exokrine und endokrine Pankreasinsuffizienz und die Prognose der Erkrankung. Med Diss Göttingen
72. Löhr-Happe A, Peiper M, Lankisch PG (1994) Natural course of operated pseudocysts in chronic pancreatitis. Gut 35:1479–1482
73. Machado MCC, Monteiro da Cunha JE, Bacchella T, de Barros Mott C, Duarte I, Bettarello A (1984) Acute pancreatic necrosis in chronic alcoholic pancreatitis. Dig Dis Sci 29:709–713
74. Mahlke R, Elbrechtz F, Petersen M, Schafmayer A, Lankisch PG (1995) Acute abdominal pain in chronic pancreatitis: hemorrhage from a pseudoaneurysm? Z Gastroenterol 33:404–407
75. Makrauer FL, Antonioli DA, Banks PA (1982) Duodenal stenosis in chronic pancreatitis. Clinicopathological correlations. Dig Dis Sci 27:525–532
76. Marks IN, Bank S, Barbezat GO (1976) Alkoholpankreatitis – Ätiologie, klinische Formen, Komplikationen. Leber Magen Darm 6:257–270
77. Marks IN, Bank S, Louw JH, Farman J (1967) Peptic ulceration and gastrointestinal bleeding in pancreatitis. Gut 8:253–259
78. Marks IN, Girdwood AH, Bank S, Louw JH (1980) The prognosis of alcohol-induced calcific pancreatitis. S Afr Med J 57:640–643
79. Masoero G, Spinaci S, Arossa W, Andriulli A, Gaia E, de Pretis G, Dobrilla G, de la Pierre M (1984) Pulmonary involvement in chronic pancreatitis. Dig Dis Sci 29:896–901

80. Mathai V, Banerjee Jesudason SR, Muthusami JC, Kuruvilla R, Idikula J, Sada P (1994) Chronic pancreatitis caused by intraductal hydatic cysts of the pancreas. Br J Surg 81:1029

81. McConnell DB, Gregory JR, Sasaki TM, Vetto RM (1982) Pancreatic pseudocyst. Am J Surg 143: 599–601

82. Miyake H, Harada H, Kunichika K, Ochi K, Kimura I (1987) Clinical course and prognosis of chronic pancreatitis. Pancreas 2:378–385

83. Moossa AR, Gadd MA (1985) Isolated splenic vein thrombosis. World J Surg 9:384–390

84. Möhr P, Ammann R, Largiadèr F, Knoblauch M, Schmid M, Akovbiantz A (1975) Pankreaskarzinom bei chronischer Pankreatitis. Schweiz Med Wochenschr 105:590–592

85. Mörl M, Piechulek H (1987) Leberschäden bei chronisch-kalzifizierter, alkoholinduzierter Pankreatitis. Z Gastroenterol 25:325–330

86. Neglia JP, FitzSimmons SC, Maisonneuve P, Schöni MH, Schöni-Affolter F, Corey M, Lowenfels AB, Cystic Fibrosis and Cancer Study Group (1995) The risk of cancer among patients with cystic fibrosis. N Engl J Med 332:494–499

87. Neher M, Mangold G, Schönborn H (1977) Akute hämorrhagisch-nekrotisierende Verlaufsformen der chronisch rezidivierenden Pankreatitis. Münch Med Wochenschr 119:191–192

88. Niemelä S, Lehtola J, Karttunen T, Lähde S (1989) Pancreatitis in patients with chronic inflammatory bowel disease. Hepatogastroenterology 36:175–177

89. Olsen TS (1978) The incidence and clinical relevance of chronic inflammation in the pancreas in autopsy material. Acta Pathol Microbiol Scand A 86:361–365

90. Owens JL Jr, Howard JM (1958) Pancreatic calcification: a late sequel in the natural history of chronic alcoholism and alcoholic pancreatitis. Ann Surg 147:326–338

91. Palmer KR, Cotton PB, Chapman M (1984) Pancreatogram in cholestasis. Gut 25:424–427

92. Pedrazzoli S, Petrin P, De Marchi L, Miotto D, Bonadimani B, Costantino V (1986) An unusual complication of chronic pancreatitis: a recanalized portal tree communicating with a pancreatic pseudocyst. Am J Gastroenterol 81:698–701

93. Petrozza JA, Dutta SK, Latham PS, Iber FL, Gadacz TR (1984) Prevalence and natural history of distal common bile duct stenosis in alcoholic pancreatitis. Dig Dis Sci 29:890–895

94. Prost A, Hanniche M, Bordier P, Miravet L, de Sèze S, Rambaud J-C (1975) Ostéomalacie et pancréatite chronique associée. Cinq observations. Nouv Presse Med 4:1561–1566

95. Ravey M, Mouktar M (1973) Sténose de l'angle colique gauche secondaire à une pancréatite chronique. J Chir (Paris) 105:553–560

96. Remington JH, Mayo CW, Dockerty MB (1947) Stenosis of the colon secondary to chronic pancreatitis. Proc Staff Meet Mayo Clin 22:260–264

97. Renner IG, Savage III WT, Stace NH, Pantoja JL, Schultheis WM, Peters RL (1984) Pancreatitis associated with alcoholic liver disease. A review of 1022 autopsy cases. Dig Dis Sci 29:593–599

98. Rignault D, Mine J, Moine D (1968) Splenoportographic changes in chronic pancreatitis. Surgery 63:571–575

99. Ring EJ, Eaton SB Jr, Ferrucci JT Jr, Short WF (1973) Differential diagnosis of pancreatic calcification. Am J Roentgenol 117:446–452

100. Rocca G, Gaia E, Iuliano R, Caselle MT, Rocca N, Calcamuggi G, Emanuelli G (1987) Increased incidence of cancer in chronic pancreatitis. J Clin Gastroenterol 9:175–179

101. Rösch J, Herfort K (1962) Contribution of splenoportography to the diagnosis of diseases of the pancreas. I. Tumorous diseases. Acta Med Scand 171:251–261

102. Rösch J, Herfort K (1962) Contribution of splenoportography to the diagnosis of diseases of the pancreas. II. Inflammatory diseases. Acta Med Scand 171:263–272

103. Saebø A, Lassen J (1992) Acute and chronic pancreatic disease associated with Yersinia enterocolitica infection: a Norwegian 10-year follow-up study of 458 hospitalized patients. J Intern Med 231:537–541

104. Sandblom P (1970) Gastrointestinal hemorrhage through the pancreatic duct. Ann Surg 171: 61–66

105. Sarles H, Capitaine Y (1973) Complications ostéo-articulaires au cours de deux cas de pancréatite chronique calcifiante. Traitement par wirsungo-jéjunostomie. Arch Franc Maladies Appareil Dig 62:61–65

106. Schulze S, Thorsgaard Pedersen N, Jørgensen MJ, Møllmann K-M, Rune SJ (1983) Association between duodenal bulb ulceration and reduced exocrine pancreatic function. Gut 24:781–783

107. Schwartz S, Nadelhaft J (1957) Simulation of colonic obstruction at the splenic flexure by pancreatitis: Roentgen features. Am J Roentgenol 78:607–616
108. Schwartz SI, Dale WA (1958) Primary sclerosing cholangitis. Review and report of six cases. Arch Surg 77:439–450
109. Scott J, Summerfield JA, Elias E, Dick R, Sherlock S (1977) Chronic pancreatitis: a cause of cholestasis. Gut 18:196–201
110. Seyrig J-A, Jian R, Modigliani R, Golfain D, Florent C, Messing B, Bitoun A (1985) Idiopathic pancreatitis associated with inflammatory bowel disease. Dig Dis Sci 30:1121–1126
111. Smits ME, Rauws EAJ, Tytgat GNJ, Huibregtse K (1995) The efficacy of endoscopic treatment of pancreatic pseudocysts. Gastrointest Endosc 42:202–207
112. Sorgman JA, Langevin E, Banks PA (1992) Urinoma masquerading as pancreatic pseudocyst. Int J Pancreatol 11:195–198
113. Sperti C, Pasquali C, Costantino V, Perasole A, Liessi G, Pedrazzoli S (1995) Solitary true cyst of the pancreas in adults. Report of three cases and review of the literature. Int J Pancreatol 18:161–167
114. Stahl TJ, O'Connor Allen M, Ansel HJ, Vennes JA (1988) Partial biliary obstruction caused by chronic pancreatitis. An appraisal of indications for surgical biliary drainage. Ann Surg 207:26–32
115. Steinbach HL, Kolb FO, Crane JT (1959) Unusual roentgen manifestations of osteomalacia. Am J Roentgenol 82:875–886
116. Tenner S, Roston A, Lichtenstein D, Sica G, Carr-Locke D, Banks PA (1995) Von Hippel-Lindau disease complicated by acute pancreatitis and Evan's syndrome. Int J Pancreatol 18:271–275
117. Thorsgaard Pedersen N, Andersen BN, Pedersen G, Worning H (1982) Chronic pancreatitis in Copenhagen. A retrospective study of 64 consecutive patients. Scand J Gastroenterol 17:925–931
118. Tim LO, Segal I (1978) Exocrine pancreatic function in patients with idiopathic necrosis of the femoral head. S Afr Med J 54:441–442
119. Tokoo M, Oguchi H, Kawa S, Homma T, Nagata A (1992) Eosinophilia associated with chronic pancreatitis: an analysis of 122 patients with definite chronic pancreatitis. Am J Gastroenterol 87:455–460
120. Toskes PP, Deren JJ, Fruiterman J, Conrad ME (1973) Specificity of the correction of vitamin B_{12} malabsorption by pancreatic extract and its clinical significance. Gastroenterology 65:199–204
121. Toskes PP, Greenberger NJ (1983) Acute and chronic pancreatitis. Disease-a-Month 29:1–81
122. Tucker DH, Moore IB (1963) Vanishing pancreatic calcification in chronic pancreatitis. A sign of pancreatic carcinoma. N Engl J Med 268:31–33
123. Vantini I, Piubello W, Scuro LA, Benini P, Talamini G, Benini L, Micciolo R, Cavallini G (1982) Duodenal ulcer in chronic relapsing pancreatitis. Digestion 24:23–28
124. Vogel H, Sjiariel M, Maas R, Klapdor R (1983) Pankreaspseudozysteneinbruch in Abdominalorgane. Inn Med 10:243–246
125. Wallner B, Friedrich JM, Pietrzyk C (1988) Knöcherne Läsionen bei chronischer Pankreatitis. Fortschr Röntgenstr 149:289–293
126. Warshaw AL, Compton CC, Lewandrowski K, Cardenosa G, Mueller PR (1990) Cystic tumors of the pancreas. New clinical, radiologic, and pathologic observations in 67 patients. Ann Surg 212:432–445
127. Warshaw AL, Jin G, Ottinger LW (1987) Recognition and clinical implications of mesenteric and portal vein obstruction in chronic pancreatitis. Arch Surg 122:410–415
128. Warshaw AL, McC.Chesney T, Evans GW, McCarthy HF (1972) Intrasplenic dissection by pancreatic pseudocysts. N Engl J Med 287:72–75
129. Warshaw AL, Rutledge PL (1987) Cystic tumors mistaken for pancreatic pseudocysts. Ann Surg 205:393–398
130. Weissmann D, Lewandrowski K, Godine J, Centeno B, Warshaw A (1994) Pancreatic cystic islet-cell tumors. Clinical and pathologic features in two cases with cyst fluid analysis. Int J Pancreatol 15:75–79
131. Whalley RC (1967) Pseudopancreatic cyst. Report of a case of spontaneous intra-gastric rupture associated with ruptured spleen. Br J Clin Pract 21:567–568
132. Wilson C, Auld CD, Schlinkert R, Hasan AH, Imrie CW, Macsween RNM, Carter DC (1989) Hepatobiliary complications in chronic pancreatitis. Gut 30:520–527

133. Wisløff F, Jakobsen J, Osnes M (1982) Stenosis of the common bile duct in chronic pancreatitis. Br J Surg 69:52–54
134. Worning H (1984) Chronic pancreatitis: pathogenesis, natural history and conservative treatment. Clin Gastroenterol 13:871–894
135. Wright JA, Lopez J, Daum RS, Ertan A (1988) Chronic pancreatitis is associated with a high prevalence of giardiasis. Gastroenterology 94:A503 (abstr)

19 Chronic Pancreatitis: Treatment

19.1
Pain

19.1.1
Definition and Mechanisms

Although pain is the most common symptom of chronic pancreatitis, there are no specific features which easily distinguish pain caused by pancreatitis from that caused by other abdominal conditions. The cause of abdominal pain in chronic pancreatitis is not clear, and pancreatic and extrapancreatic reasons are discussed (Table 19.1).

19.1.1.1
Pancreatic Causes

19.1.1.1.1
Acute Inflammation

Acute inflammation is clearly apparent when there is abdominal pain and tenderness, elevation of serum amylase and lipase and evidence of pancreatic and/or peripancreatic inflammation by ultrasound or computed tomography (CT) [10]. The patho-

Table 19.1. Causes of abdominal pain in chronic pancreatitis

Pancreatic causes
- Acute inflammation
- Neural inflammation
- Increased intrapancreatic pressure
  Ducts
  Parenchyma
  Pseudocyst

Extrapancreatic causes
- Stenosis of the distal common bile duct
- Stenosis of the descending duodenum
- Peptic ulcer
- Stenosis of the colon

genesis of an acute exacerbation of chronic pancreatitis is presumably the same as in acute pancreatitis.

19.1.1.1.2
Increased Intrapancreatic Pressure

Endoscopic retrograde cholangiopancreatography (ERCP) may show a variety of ductal abnormalities (Fig. 19.1; see also Figs. 17.15 a, b, 17.16 a, b, 17.21 a, b, 18.4 a, b) which have been carefully classified by the Cambridge meeting [8].

However, it is not certain that such duct changes are responsible for the pain, and it is still unclear why pain is continuous only in the minority of patients and occurs at different time intervals. When, for example, dilatation of the pancreatic duct occurs on the basis of a ductal stenosis, focal obstruction, irregular dilatation, or the presence of occluding stones, increased intraductal pressure appears to be the cause of pain. When, however, the duct is generally dilated without these irregularities, or is not dilated at all, increased ductal pressure as the underlying cause of pain is less probable. The same applies for pancreatic pseudocysts. When they communicate with the stenotic duct, increased intracystic pressure may be present and may cause pain, but in a noncommunicating pseudocyst, increased pressure is less plausible [10]. None of these anatomic derangements in chronic pancreatitis indicates whether a patient has, or will experience, pain [21, 69, 100, 142]. Nonetheless, when a patient with pain is found to harbor duct changes or cysts, we tend to hold these abnormalities responsible and recommend surgical procedures to relieve the pain [10].

At present, it is not even proven that ductal abnormalities lead to an increased intraductal pressure. Measurements in a few patients without pancreatic diseases have recorded pressures between 7 mm Hg (direct puncture at surgery) [59] and 10–16 mm Hg (ERCP) [24, 163, 193]. In patients with ductal abnormalities, endoscopically measured intraductal pressure was between 18–48 mm Hg [24, 59, 140]. However, in

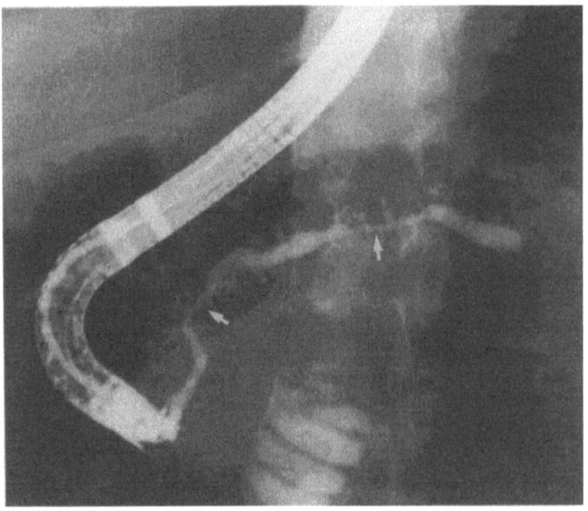

Fig. 19.1. Chronic pancreatitis with ductal stenosis. ERCP reveals two areas of marked narrowing of the main pancreatic duct (*arrows*) followed by areas of dilatation. Numerous secondary branches are dilated. This 24-year-old man with idiopathic chronic pancreatitis has experienced episodes of moderately severe abdominal pain every 4–6 months lasting only 2–3 days

another study, there was no difference in ductal pressure between patients with alcohol-induced chronic pancreatitis and normal controls [161]. Furthermore, intraductal pressure measured by endoscopic manometry was even higher in normal subjects than in patients with chronic pancreatitis [177]. These pressure studies were made endoscopically and may not really reflect intraductal pressure, especially if there are stones or stricture.

The impact of intraductal stones on intraductal pressure and pain is unclear since the removal of stones has led to pain relief in some but has failed to do so in others (see below).

19.1.1.1.3
Parenchymal Abnormalities

More recently, parenchymal abnormalities probably related to fibrosis of the gland and capsule have attracted considerable interest as one cause of pain. Ebbehøj et al. [60], using a thin needle for recording intraparenchymal pressure, reported a significant correlation between percutaneously and intraoperatively recorded pressures. The group found significantly higher elevated pressures in patients with chronic pancreatitis and pain and/or pseudocysts compared with those without pain or such a complication. Pressure recordings were independent of the degree of exocrine pancreatic insufficiency and the presence or absence of calcifications [57]. After decompression by pancreaticogastrostomy, pressure fell in the majority of patients [58].

Further studies are required to clarify how increased tissue pressure causes pain and why some patients respond to decompressive therapy and others not.

19.1.1.1.4
Pancreatic Pseudocysts

Pain in patients with pancreatic pseudocysts may be due to increased pressure in the cysts communicating with the ductal system (see Sect. 19.1.1.1.2). The size of a pancreatic pseudocyst plays a role since large pseudocysts are most frequently linked to severe pain (see Figs. 18.1, 18.2) [142].

19.1.1.1.5
Neural Inflammation

Analysis of nerves in pancreatic tissue removed from patients with chronic pancreatitis has shown that the nerves are preferentially retained, while the parenchyma degenerates and is replaced by fibrosis. The retained nerves, however, remained in an altered condition, i.e., the perineural sheath is altered in a way that it no longer provides a barrier between the surrounding connective tissue and the internal neural components (perineural disruption). Increased mean diameters argue against pain being caused by constriction due to fibrosis [20]. Further investigations showed an intensification of the immunostaining for calcitonin gene-related peptide and substance P in numerous nerve fibers. Since both of these peptides are generally regarded as pain transmitter candidates, Büchler and coworkers [26] suggested that changes in pancreatic nerves might be responsible for the long-lasting pain syndrome in chronic pancreatitis. Another factor which may explain pain due to neural inflammation could be the increase of eosinophils in the perineurial space. There was a significant correlation between the percentage of eosinophilic infiltrate and pain severity and the timing of alcohol consumption [103].

Further studies are required for more detailed information on how neural inflammation may contribute to pancreatic pain.

19.1.1.2
Extrapancreatic Causes

Extrapancreatic complications such as stenosis of the distal common bile duct, the descending duodenum and the colon (see Sects. 18.3.1. 18.3.2), or peptic ulcer (see Sect. 18.3.3) are not infrequent and may certainly cause pain. However, the incidence of pain due to these complications and their influence on the symptoms of chronic pancreatitis is still to be established.

19.1.2
Conservative Treatment

Treatment of active inflammation of the gland is the same as for acute pancreatitis (see Sects. 11.1.2, 11.1.3).

When the acute attack subsides, medical treatment aims to prevent recurring episodes and to treat residual pain. There is a variety of narcotics orally, intramuscularly, or as patches, which are usually effective in controlling pain. A pain service can provide valuable insight into the choice of narcotic and the frequency of administration as well as monitoring to avoid narcotic addiction. Alcohol abstinence must be recommended since it may reduce pain attacks in about 50% of chronic pancreatitis patients [183]. Certain dietary precautions (listed in Table 19.2) may also be helpful. Short term inhibition of pancreatic secretion by octreotide had no influence on pain [143].

Table 19.2. Dietary recommendations in exocrine pancreatic insufficiency due to chronic pancreatitis

- Abstinence from alcohol (strict and lifelong)
- Limited fat content in the food (40–60 g/day; < 30% of total calories)
- Frequent small meals
- As little fat as possible in food preparation (e.g., aluminium foil, earthenware cooking pot, grill)
- Avoidance of hard-to-digest foods such as legumes, cold drinks, or ice cream
- In cases of noncompensable steatorrhea and weight loss, replacement of dietary fat by medium-chain triglycerides

When pain persists and requires analgesics on a frequent basis, morphological examination of the gland including ERCP and CT is mandatory to exclude ductal or other abnormalities which may be responsible for pain and which may be corrected endoscopically or surgically.

19.1.2.1
Oral Pancreatic Enzyme Therapy

There has been considerable interest in the use of oral pancreatic enzymes to curb pancreatic pain and possibly to prevent acute exacerbation of chronic pancreatitis. This is based on the assumption of a feedback regulation of pancreatic secretion.

Briefly, it is assumed that low intraduodenal protease activities stimulate, whereas high activities inhibit pancreatic enzyme secretion. In chronic pancreatitis with pain relapses and low intraduodenal protease activities, oral pancreatic enzyme therapy is assumed to increase these activities, to inhibit pancreatic secretion, and, by lowering intraductal pressure, to put the pancreas at rest, thus bringing pain relief.

Since the first description of a patient in whom the feedback regulation could be demonstrated [96], several investigations using different study designs have reached different results. According to recent studies, a feedback mechanism seems to exist in humans [6, 125, 132, 164]. Whether it exists under true physiological and not just under experimental conditions, and whether it is cholecystokinin-(CCK-)mediated, is still a matter of discussion [153]. Under experimental conditions, the protease inhibitor camostate interferes with feedback regulation of basal pancreatic secretion in humans, which seems predominantly mediated by the cholinergic system [5, 6].

Until recently, there were only 4 studies involving a total of 69 patients, which evaluated the effectiveness of oral pancreatic enzymes in relieving pain in alcoholic chronic pancreatitis, idiopathic chronic pancreatitis, and chronic pancreatitis of other etiologies [83, 97, 171, 190]. Three of the studies were double-blinded [83, 97, 190], one was not [171]; three of the studies showed some benefit [97, 171, 190], one did not [83]. In the latter study, the failure was attributed to the use of a pancreatic preparation (pancrease) in the form of microspheres, which, presumably, might release active enzymes beyond the duodenum. Because feedback control of pancreatic secretion is a phenomenon that may be restricted to the duodenum, it is preferable to use preparations that predictably release the enzymes within the duodenum [11]. However, in one of the 3 studies in which benefit was noted [171], pancrease was also used, but since this study was not double-blinded, the results are not conclusive.

In 2 other double-blinded studies that demonstrated therapeutic benefit [97, 190], there are some concerns. In one, although benefit was noted with a resulting decrease of analgesic tablets, this decrease was not significant [97]. In the other, only 3 of 10 patients with alcoholic pancreatitis responded [190]. All 3 had minimal or no steatorrhea, whereas the remaining 7 had steatorrhea. The implication was that pancreatic pain in association with milder forms of alcoholic pancreatitis might respond to oral pancreatic enzymes, but that far advanced alcoholic pancreatitis would not [11]. In the same study, 8 of 10 patients with idiopathic pancreatitis clearly responded to oral pancreatic enzymes. In these patients, the diagnosis of chronic pancreatitis was based on an abnormal secretin test, whereas all of them showed a normal pancreatic duct system upon ERCP.

Recently, in addition to the above described 4 studies, 3 large prospective and placebo-controlled studies were published, which all showed no significant effect on pain [121, 141, 152]. Thus, further studies are needed to establish the benefits of oral pancreatic enzymes in improving pancreatic pain.

Recommendation. At present, there is no convincing evidence that pancreatic enzymes are generally effective in treating pain in patients with chronic pancreatitis. In some, enzyme treatment could reduce abdominal bloating which may contribute to the pain of the patients. We recommend pancreatic enzymes for a period of 2–3 months and ask the patient to record his pain on a daily visual analogue scale.

19.1.2.2
Endoscopic Treatment

To avoid more invasive surgical therapy, endoscopic techniques have been developed for treating chronic pancreatitis. Most commonly, a stent is inserted into either the major or the minor papilla to overcome intraductal obstruction caused by ductal stricture, pancreatic stone, or hypertensive sphincter of Oddi, or to retrieve stones and to drain pancreatic pseudocysts which communicate with the main pancreatic duct [67, 93, 104, 105, 189].

An important concern has been raised about stenting since pancreatic stents can induce ductal changes consistent with chronic pancreatitis. 36% of all patients and 72% of patients who had an initially normal pancreatogram showed ductal changes subsequent to pancreatic duct stent placement. Although these changes seem to cause no impairment of pancreatic function [178] and are reversible after removal [39, 178], there is concern about the safety of such a procedure.

Endoscopic biliary drainage in chronic pancreatitis was found to be an effective treatment for cholangitis or jaundice in patients with chronic pancreatitis and biliary stenosis, but the results of definitive endoscopic drainage for these patients are less satisfactory because resolution of the stricture after removal of the stent is rarely obtained [40].

Recently, pancreatic stone lithotrypsy has been introduced in the endoscopic treatment of pain, thought to derive from stones in the pancreatic duct.

With an electromagnetic lithotryptor after endoscopic pancreatic sphincterotomy in a large series, the success rate of disintegration was 99%, a decrease of duct dilatation was observed in 82%, and a complete clearance of the main pancreatic duct in 54%. Whereas continuous pain disappeared in all patients in this series [37], another report showed no improvement in the intensity and frequency of pain in half of the patients in a smaller series [186].

Randomized prospective trials for all endoscopic treatment procedures of chronic pancreatitis are needed.

Lithotrypsy and ductal clearance may also be successfully performed by inducing miniscopes into the pancreatic duct [158]. Further studies are required.

Recommendation. The described techniques may be utilized in centers with a particular interest and expertise in the treatment of patients with chronic pancreatitis for the purposes of evaluating safety and and efficacy. Although stenting has been done in many centers, and although efficacy has been suggested, efficacy has not been proven in scientific studies. Randomized prospective trials will be required to assess the safety and efficacy. These studies should provide information pertaining to quality of life, pain, and cost.

19.1.2.3
Nerve Block

Nerve block is considered to be the simplest, most effective and least hazardous method for pain relief in patients with pancreatic carcinoma and may also be used in selected cases of chronic pancreatitis [15]. The success rate of this procedure in chronic pancreatitis varies considerably between 50% to almost 100% of all cases [36, 129, 139, 165]. However, the beneficial effect lasts only for a few months.

Recommendation. Nerve block in patients with chronic pancreatitis is a last resort in desperate cases. Two new techniques of nerve block include endoscopical ultrasound-(EUS-)guided injection of the celiac plexus and thoracoscopic clipping of the splanchnic nerves. Studies are underway to evaluate both of these modalities.

19.1.3
Surgical Treatment

Surgery is not a primary treatment for chronic pancreatitis and cannot cure the disease. Surgery is used only when conservative treatment has proven to be inadequate. Surgical treatment may reduce symptoms or deal with specific complications (Table 19.3), but there is little evidence that it will halt the progression of the disease or improve function (see Sect. 19.4).

Table 19.3. Indication for surgical intervention in chronic pancreatitis

- Intractable pain
- Complications
  Pancreatic pseudocyst
  Pancreatic abscess
  Biliary obstruction
  Duodenal obstruction
  Colonic obstruction
  Splenic vein occlusion with variceal bleeding
  Hemosuccus pancreaticus/intracystic bleeding (rupture of pancreatic pseudoaneurysm)
  Internal pancreatic fistula(s)
  – Ascites
  – Pleural effusion
- Suspicion of pancreatic carcinoma

However, when indicated, surgery should be contemplated before the patient becomes addicted to narcotic drugs. Furthermore, surgery should be considered before nutritional or metabolic disturbances arise due to postprandial pain, gastric outlet obstruction, biliary stasis, or internal pancreatic fistulas. Finally, surgery should be considered whenever suspicion of pancreatic carcinoma persists despite adequate diagnostic investigation. There is no ideal standard surgical procedure for the treatment of chronic pancreatitis. Therefore, the choice of surgical procedure should be tailored to the condition of the patient. The aim of surgery in chronic pancreatitis is to relieve symptoms while preserving as much exocrine and endocrine pancreatic function as possible.

Based on the assumption that obstruction of pancreatic secretion with increased intraductal pressure is an important cause of pain, different duct-decompressing procedures have been tried. The most frequent and recommended surgical procedure is lateral pancreaticojejunostomy for patients with dilated duct (>8 mm on ERCP) and/or for patients with symptomatic pancreatic pseudocysts (Fig. 19.2a, b; see also Fig. 17.14a–d). In short, an anastomosis is performed between the dilated pancreatic duct and a jejunal loop (Roux principle). The complication rate of this procedure is between 10% and 20%, the mortality rate between 1% and 3% (Fig. 19.3) [28].

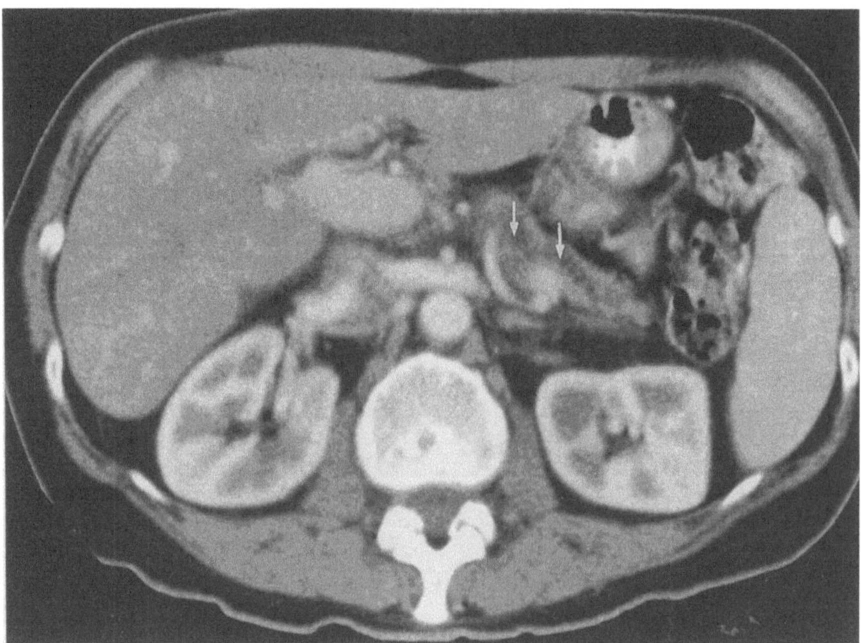

Fig. 19.2a. Ductal dilatation in chronic pancreatitis. Dynamic contrast-enhanced CT scan showing a dilated duct in the body and tail of the pancreas (*arrows*) in a 46-year-old woman with alcoholic chronic pancreatitis who was experiencing intractable abdominal pain

Resective procedures for pain in chronic pancreatitis are reserved by most surgeons for patients with nondilated pancreatic duct and localized extensive glandular fibrosis. If this complication is located in the tail of the pancreas, a left-sided resection is indicated with preserving as much exocrine and endocrine tissue as possible.

If there is an inflammatory process or a complication in the head of the pancreas, a classic Whipple's operation may be performed (Fig. 19.4 a, b; see also Fig. 18.4 a, b). The pancreatic gland right to the portal vein, including the duodenum, the gallbladder, and the extrahepatic bile ducts, and 30%–50% of the distal part of the stomach are removed. The reconstruction is done in the upper jejunum (pancreaticojejunostomy), choledochojejunostomy, and an anastomosis with the postpyloric duodenum or the distal stomach. The postoperative complication rate is 30%–50%, especially due to the anastomosis of the pancreatic body. The mortality rate is less than 5% [28]. To reduce postoperative syndromes (see Sect. 19.4), modifications have been developed: pylorus-preserving pancreaticoduodenectomy (Fig. 19.5 a, b) and duodenum-preserving resection of the pancreatic head (Fig. 19.6 a–d [14]; see also Fig. 18.4 a, b). In short, during pylorus-preserving partial duodenopancreatectomy, the head of the pancreas left to the portal vein, the duodenum, the extrahepatic bile ducts, and the gallbladder are removed. Reconstruction is performed by a jejunal loop to anastomose the pancre-

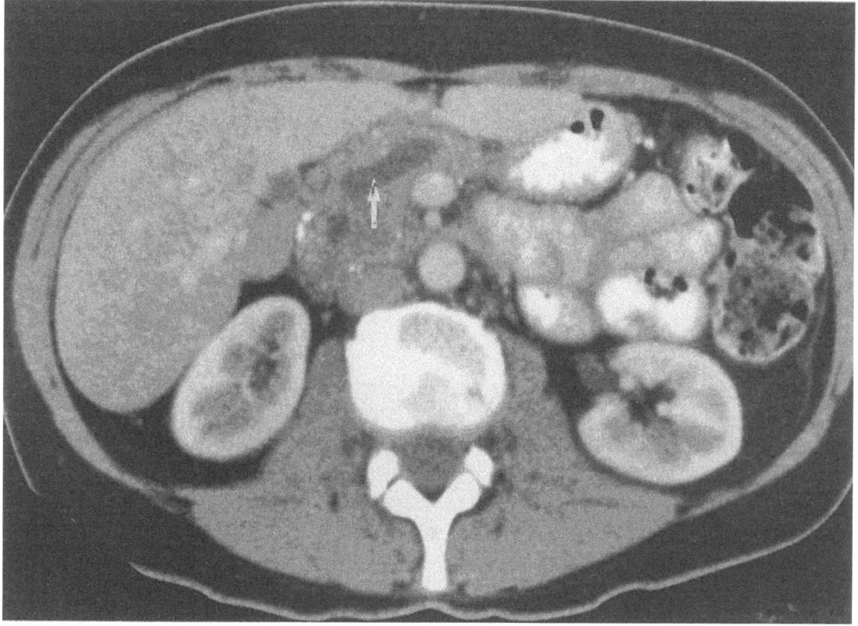

Fig. 19.2 b. Ductal dilatation in chronic pancreatitis. At a lower level, the head of the pancreas is somewhat enlarged. A dilated duct is once again visualized (*arrow*). Small calcifications are also visible. Following failure of medical strategy and inability to insert a pancreatic stent because of a large stone occluding the duct, she underwent a lateral pancreaticojejunostomy and remains pain-free 6 months later

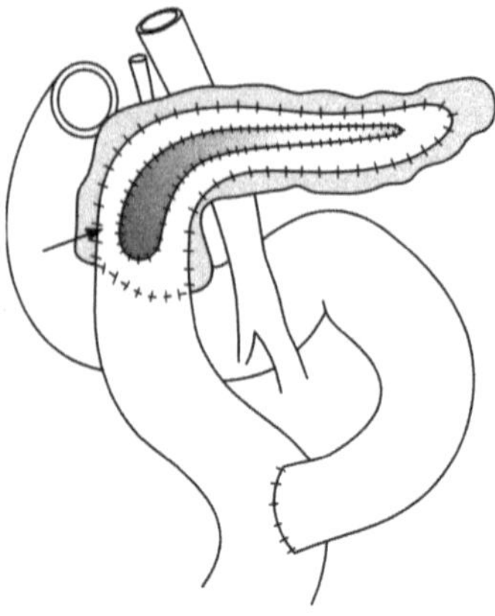

Fig. 19.3. Lateral pancreaticojejunostomy (Puestow/Partington-Rochelle operation). Anastomosis of the dilated pancreatic duct with an excluded jejunal loop (*arrow*). (From [28] with permission)

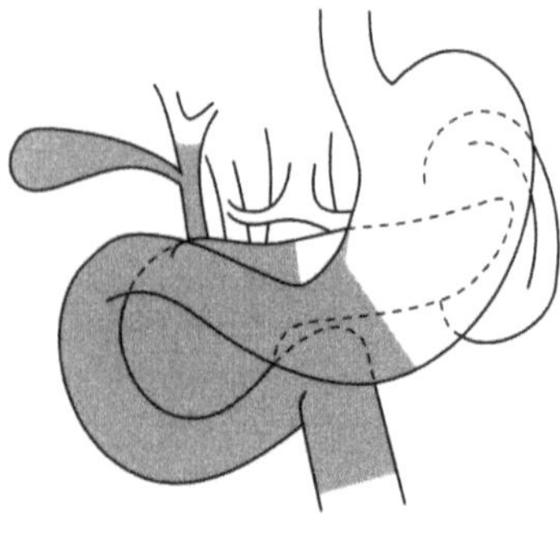

a

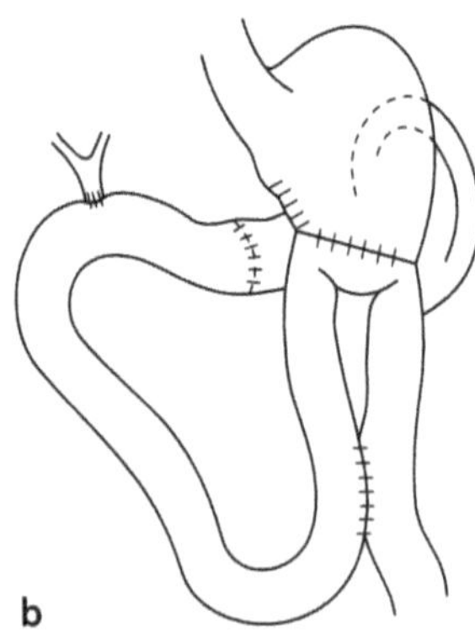

b

Fig. 19.4a, b. Classical Whipple operation. **a** *Shaded organs* are partially or totally resected. **b** Reconstruction scheme. (From [28] with permission)

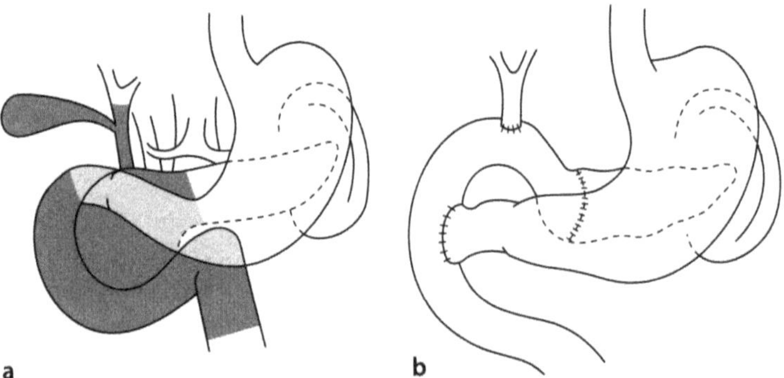

a   b

Fig. 19.5 a, b. Pylorus-preserving partial duodenopancreatectomy. **a** *Shaded organs* are partially or totally removed. **b** Reconstruction scheme. (From [28] with permission)

as, the common bile duct and the postpyloric duodenum (Fig. 19.5 a, b). The complication rate is between 30% and 50% and the mortality rate less than 5% [28].

In the course of the duodenum-preserving resection of the head of the pancreas, the head of the gland is resected from the body and the tail of the organ. At the duodenum, a small part of the pancreatic parenchyma, about 0.5 cm, is left to ensure blood circulation of the duodenum. Thus, the duodenum, the common bile, and the pancreatic duct as well as the retropancreatic vessels are decompressed. Reconstruction is done using an excluded jejunal loop (Roux principle) (Fig. 19.6 a–d) [14]. When there is a stenosis of the common bile duct or a dilatation or stenosis of the pancreatic duct in the tail of organ, the operation is modified by an internal anastomosis of the bile duct and/or a pancreaticojejunostomy of the remaining pancreatic duct (Fig. 19.6 a–d). The complication rate is 20% and the mortality rate less than 1% in experienced hands [28].

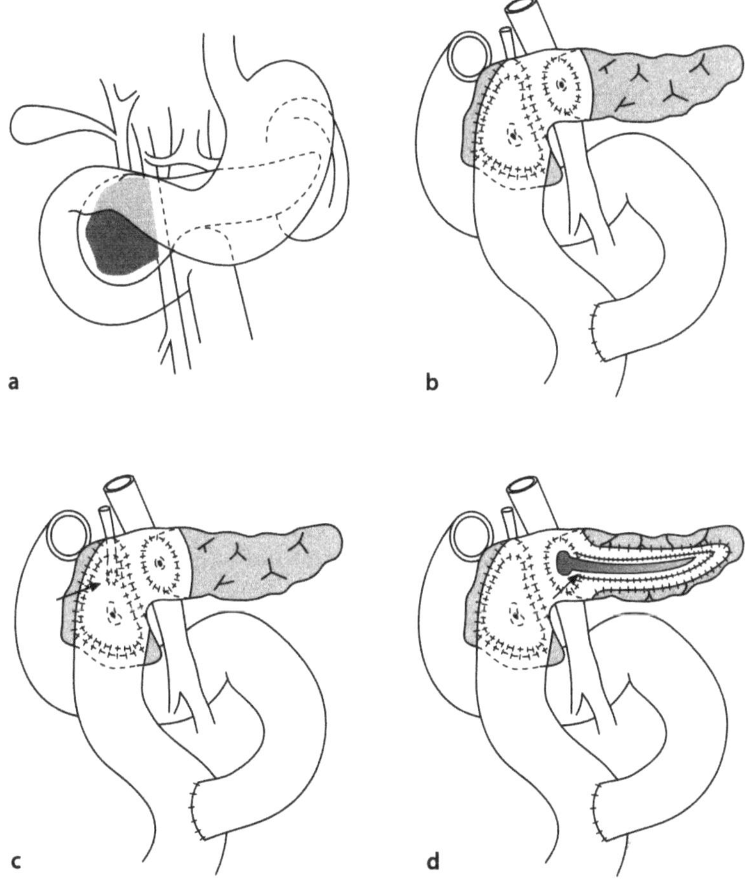

Fig. 19.6 a–d. Duodenum-preserving resection of the head of the pancreas. a *Shaded area* represents resection of part of the head of the organ. **b** Reconstruction scheme using an excluded jejunal loop. **c** Modification with additional anastomosis of the internal bile duct (*arrow*). **d** Modification with additional longitudinal anastomosis of the pancreatic duct (*arrow*). (From [14] with permission)

An alternative procedure is the local resection of the head of the pancreas combined with longitudinal pancreaticojejunostomy, an operation developed by Frey and Akimura [62].

Finally, in cases of endstage pancreatitis and intractable pain, total pancreatectomy may be a last desperate attempt to help the patient.

Whereas the role of surgical procedures in the treatment of pain in chronic pancreatitis may be debatable regarding the short-term effect (see Sect. 19.4.2 and also Table 19.8), its role in the treatment of complications is indisputable, e.g., to treat severe complications such as biliary stasis, severe bleeding from splenic vein occlusion and varices, or rupture of pancreatic pseudoaneurysm either directly into the pancreatic duct or a pancreatic pseudocyst, or ascites, or pleural effusion due to internal pancreatic fistulas.

Finally, there will be some cases in which even after extensive diagnostic procedures showing the contrary, pancreatic carcinoma is still suspected and a laparotomy is indicated either to confirm or to exclude this suspicion.

Recommendation. We recommend surgical treatment in therapy-resistant pain and in symptomatic common bile duct stenosis, duodenal stenosis, and pancreatic pseudocysts (causing pain or stenosis of the common bile duct or the duodenum). Furthermore, surgery is indicated when a pseudocyst is infected or ruptured, or bleeding has occurred into the cyst. In case of bleeding from varices into the esophagus and the stomach caused by splenic vein thrombosis, splenectomy should be performed.

19.2
Exocrine Pancreatic Insufficiency

19.2.1
Definition and Mechanisms

Exocrine pancreatic insufficiency may result from a general or isolated reduction in pancreatic enzymes or from a failure of enzyme activation in the small intestine (Table 19.4). The leading cause is chronic pancreatitis.

The substantial pancreatic reserve capacity, however, allows for significant impairment of the pancreatic secretion of digestive enzymes of up to 90% without manifestation of overt malabsorption [182]. Only when pancreatic lipase and trypsin fall below 10% of normal are steatorrhea and azotorrhea manifest (see Fig. 17.9) [44]. Although recent studies have confirmed this finding for the majority of patients with chronic pancreatitis, there are two further groups of patients: (a) those with pancreatic secretion higher than 10% but with steatorrhea; and (b) those with almost nonexistent lipase secretion, but normal daily fat excretion [118, 204]. Whereas (a) may be due to the large variability in exocrine pancreas reserve capacity, (b) may be due to the action of nonpancreatic lipases. Nonpancreatic lipases may come from lingual serous glands and from the gastric mucosa, where lipase activity is higher in the upper greater curvature than in the upper smaller curvature, and lowest in the antral area of both curvatures [3]. Accordingly, patients with exocrine pancreatic insufficiency may absorb more than 50% of dietary fat in the absence of measurable pancreatic lipase

Table 19.4. Causes of exocrine pancreatic insufficiency

General enzyme reduction
- Chronic pancreatitis
- Acute pancreatitis (mostly short-term insufficiency)
- Carcinoma obstructing the pancreatic duct
- Major pancreatic resection
- Pancreatic trauma (mostly short-term insufficiency)
- Mucoviscidosis
- Primary sclerosing cholangitis
- Kwashiorkor
- Shwachman syndrome
- Congenital insufficiency (cystic pancreas)

Isolated enzyme deficiency
- Lipase
- Trypsin
- Amylase

Failure of enzyme activation in the small intestine
- Enterokinase insufficiency

activity. Abrams et al. [1] found that pancreatic insufficiency was associated with significantly higher nonpancreatic lipolytic activity in the duodenum under conditions of fasting. However, no significant difference between the groups tested was found in postprandial, nonpancreatic lipolytic activity. Nonpancreatic lipolytic activity accounted for more than 90% of total lipolytic activity of the ligament of Treitz in patients with exocrine pancreatic insufficiency, as opposed to 7% in the control subjects. The latter may also explain why some patients do not need enzyme substitution after total pancreatectomy [33].

On the other hand, in pancreatic carcinoma, pancreatic insufficiency rapidly occurs and usually coincides with ductal obstruction in the head of the pancreas. Nonetheless, the proximal 40% of the pancreas can maintain maximal enzyme secretion [45].

In comparison, secretion of lipase may decrease more rapidly than that of proteolytic enzymes and hence steatorrhea is often a more serious problem than azotorrhea [46]. However, even when steatorrhea occurs in severe chronic pancreatitis, 20–50 g of a daily intake of 100 g of fat can still be absorbed without pancreatic enzyme replacement [173].

19.2.2
Salient Clinical Features

Mild to moderate steatorrhea may not be clinically apparent and may not cause diarrhea or weight loss.

Even if steatorrhea is severe, there may be only 1–3 bowel movements per day, and there are rarely more than 6 per day. In our series, diarrhea was absent in 41% of the patients at the time of diagnosis, whereas 18% had mild diarrhea (≤ 3 bowel movements/day), 31% had moderate diarrhea (4–6 bowel movements/day), and only 10% suffered from severe diarrhea (> 6 bowel movements/day) [137].

Besides the frequency of the bowel movements, the patients may report that their stools are usually bulky and difficult to flush down the toilet. There may be passage of oil droplets causing soilage of underwear. At that stage, weight loss may be severe and the patient may become quite cachectic.

One of the contributing factors to pancreatogenic steatorrhea may be the presence of bacterial overgrowth [9, 127]. The frequency of this complication is not well established. Furthermore, giardiasis occurs in a considerable number of patients with chronic pancreatitis (27%). An investigation for giardiasis should be undertaken in every patient with pancreatic insufficiency where diarrhea is difficult to control by dietary pancreatic enzymes [210].

Clinically important deficiencies of fat-soluble vitamins A, D, E, and K rarely occur in chronic pancreatitis even when steatorrhea is severe. There may be two protective mechanisms: (1) unabsorbed dietary fat does not bind fat-soluble vitamins and (2) food intake and hence vitamin intake is not limited in chronic pancreatitis unless there is severe abdominal pain [10]. Nonetheless, if measured, deficiency of these fat-soluble vitamins at a subclinical stage may be documented [54].

19.2.3
Pancreatic Enzyme Replacement

19.2.3.1
Aim

The aims of pancreatic enzyme replacement therapy are to compensate for exocrine pancreatic insufficiency and to abolish or ameliorate symptoms due to exocrine function loss.

19.2.3.2
Indications

Therapy of exocrine pancreatic insufficiency includes treatment for malabsorption of fat, protein and starch. The major problem, however, is how to deal effectively with steatorrhea.

Mild steatorrhea may not manifest any symptoms. In the absence of abdominal pain, weight loss is frequently minimal if the patient's food intake continues to be adequate. There is no information available to demonstrate precisely at what stage of steatorrhea pancreatic enzyme replacement should be initiated. As a rule, enzyme replacement is necessary only when daily fat excretion exceeds 15 g and/or the patient is losing weight and/or has diarrhea or dyspeptic symptoms.

Treatment of exocrine pancreatic insufficiency consists of diet [110] and pancreatic enzyme replacement therapy, the first supporting the latter.

19.2.3.3
Choice of Enzyme Preparations

A great number of pancreatic enzyme preparations is available in the form of powder (only restricted availability), tablets, or capsules. Capsules contain many microspheres or microtablets and ensure as so-called multi-unit dose preparations, much better mixing with the chyme compared to single-unit dose preparations like tablets.

To correct malabsorption, the amount and concentration of enzymes delivered into the duodenum must be 5%–10% of the quantities usually present after maximal stimulation of the pancreas [44, 173]. Under optimal conditions, i.e., if no inactivation of supplemental enzymes occurs in the stomach or duodenum, approximately 30 000 IU of lipase must be taken with each meal (this is about 5–10 g of pancreatin/day) [42]. There is a high activity loss along the gastrointestinal tract such that only 22% of trypsin and 8% of lipase activity delivered by pancreatin were found postprandially at the ligament of Treitz [47].

Given the instability of lipase during the postprandial transit, lipase is the most important determinant of the effectiveness of pancreatic preparations. Most prescribed enzyme preparations in the United States and in Europe are summarized in Tables 19.5 and 19.6. Since enzyme preparations available vary considerably in their lipase content [50, 74, 89, 95, 175, 176] and the price of pancreatic preparations is high, consideration should be given to the *unit price* of the lipase content in a given preparation.

19.2.3.4
Choice of Administration Schedule

The optimal dosage schedule for the administration of pancreatic extracts has been studied. Early studies found that hourly dosages were superior to ingestion of enzymes with meals [101], but a subsequent study established no difference between hourly and prandial dosage schedules [102]. Later, DiMagno et al. [47] evaluated 2 dosage schedules by means of intestinal intubation and perfusion methods. Pancreatin was given in the form of 8 tablets with a standard meal, or as 2 tablets hourly. Medication with meals was as effective as hourly administration and thus recommended for the convenience of patients.

The lipase dosage necessary is about 100 000 Ph.Eur. (= European Pharmacopoeia) units/day, equivalent to 20 000 to 40 000 Ph.Eur. units/meal. Depending on the pancreatic enzyme preparation, this entails 2–4 capsules for a main meal and 1–2 capsules for a snack. It should be noted here that these are only rough guidelines, and enzyme replacement therapy must be adjusted to the individual patient; daily dosages exceeding 250 000 Ph.Eur. units are not uncommon. The success of treatment clearly depends on the careful instruction of and the compliance by the patient.

19.2.4
Interactions, Contraindications and Side Effects

Pancreatic enzymes should not be given together with a fiber-enriched diet since fiber has been shown to inhibit pancreatic enzymes in vitro and in vivo [51, 84–86, 98, 99, 188].

Most pancreatic concentrates are of porcine origin. A person with a history of hypersensitivity to pork protein may react unfavorably. Immediate hypersensitivity reac-

Table 19.5. Most prescribed enzyme preparations in the United States (enzyme content in U.S.P.[a] units) (MT = microtablets)

		Lipase	Amylase	Proteases
Pancrease	MT 4 (McNeil)	4000	12000	12000
	MT 10	10000	30000	30000
	MT 16	16000	48000	48000
	MT 20	20000	56000	44000
Pancrease	(McNeil)	4500	20000	25000
Creon	Minimicrospheres (Solvay)			
Creon	5	5000	16600	18750
	10	10000	33200	37500
	20	20000	66400	75000
Ultrase	MT 20 (Scandipharm)	20000	65000	65000
Viokase	(Robins)	8000	30000	30000

[a] U.S.P = United States Pharmacopoeia.

Enzyme declaration. Quality and content of a product or formulation must conform to the description laid out in the relevant pharmacopoeia. Different pharmacopoeia and methods of analysis exist (see below) for pancreatic enzyme preparations.

Enzymes are sensitive proteins and their activity is degraded with time and under biological conditions. Measured enzyme activities are generally higher than the declared activities, to ensure the required minimum activity at the end of the shelf-life.

In the *European Pharmacopoeia* (1984) 1 mg of pancreatin contains not less than 1 European Pharmacopoeia (Ph.Eur.) unit of total proteolytic activity, 15 Ph.Eur. units of lipolytic activity, and 12 Ph.Eur. units of amylolytic activity.

Ph.Eur. units of protease, lipase and amylase activity are equivalent to F.I.P. (Fédération Internationale Pharmaceutique) units and B.P. (British Pharmacopoeia) units.

Enzyme declaration according to different pharmacopoeia: Creon 25000

	Lipase	Amylase	Protease
Ph.Eur. units	25000	18000	1000
F.I.P. units	25000	18000	1000

The B.P. method for pancreatin measures only free protease activity because the step of activation with enterokinase, necessary for release of zymogen bound protease, is not included in this method. However, for pancreatic extract B.P. total protease activity is measured.

The Ph.Eur. method measures the free and zymogen bound protease forms, i.e., the total protease activity.

The U.S.P. differs substantially and the equivalent values in the conversion table should be regarded as approximate values only [167].

Conversion table for units of enzyme activity [167]

Amylase	1 Ph.Eur. unit	= 1 F.I.P. unit	= 1 B.P. unit	= 4.15	U.S.P. units
Lipase	1 Ph.Eur. unit	= 1 F.I.P. unit	= 1 B.P. unit	= 1	U.S.P. unit
Protease	1 Ph.Eur. unit	= 1 F.I.P. unit	= 1 B.P. unit[a]	= 62.5	U.S.P. units

[a] Only free protease for pancreatin, total protease for pancreatic extract

Table 19.6. Most prescribed enzyme preparations in Europe (enzyme content in Ph.Eur.[a] units)

		Lipase	Amylase	Proteases
Creon	10 000 (Solvay)	10 000	8 000	600
	25 000	25 000	18 000	1 000
Eurobiol	25 000 (Jouveinal)	25 000	22 500	12 500
Panzytrat	10 000 (BASF)	10 000	9 000	500
	25 000	25 000	12 000	800
Enzym-Lefax	N (Schering)	2 200	1 800	100
			+ Simethicone 41.2 mg	
Pankreon	10 000 (Solvay)	10 000	8 000	550
Pankreon forte	28 000	28 000	22 000	1 500

[a] Ph.Eur. = European Pharmacopoeia
Enzyme declaration: see Table 19.5

tions to powdered pancreatic extracts have occurred among patients with exocrine pancreatic insufficiency and among persons administering the enzymes, especially relatives and nurses [12, 16, 48, 90, 134, 181, 203]. Furthermore, in patients with cystic fibrosis, high doses of pancreatic extracts have been found to lead to hyperuricosuria [160, 192]. A later study, however, questioned the role of pancreatic extracts in the development of hyperuricosuria observed in these patients. A clear-cut relationship between the urinary urate concentration and the severity of the disease has been demonstrated [159].

Recently, several reports have been published on the development of colonic strictures among children with cystic fibrosis who consumed considerable amounts of high-strength pancreatic enzymes [22, 107, 135, 146, 191, 198]. The cause at present is not clear, but thickening of colon wall, especially the cecum or ascending colon, has been found [128, 138]. Excessive amounts of pancreatic enzymes should be applied with caution in children. Such an association has not been observed in adult patients with chronic pancreatitis.

Finally, oral pancreatic extracts form insoluble complexes with folic acid and may, therefore, impair folate absorption [55]. More recently, a significant impairment of iron absorption was detected in patients with cystic fibrosis and in controls after administration of pancreatic enzymes [212].

19.2.5
Control of Response

In general, sufficient information on the efficacy of enzyme treatment can be obtained by questioning the patient as to improvement of weight and reduction in diarrhea, abdominal pain and bloating. For the scientific trial, fecal weight and fat estimations are necessary.

Azotorrhea is more frequently eliminated by pancreatic extracts than steatorrhea [43, 47, 75, 173]. There appear to be at least two reasons for this. First, protease secretion may be better preserved than lipase secretion in chronic pancreatitis [46], as recent investigations in healthy persons suggest [122, 200]. Second, when potent pancreatic extracts are administered, more trypsin (22%) than lipase (8%) reaches the ligament of Treitz in an active form [47], possibly because trypsin is inactivated not by acid, but only by pepsin.

19.2.6
Failure to Respond

In the vast majority of patients, modern enzyme preparations lead to clinical improvement and reduction of steatorrhea. Failure to respond to exogenous pancreatic enzymes may have different reasons:

- *Patient's compliance.* The patient may occasionally forget to take medication or may inadvertently take it before or after the meal (postcibal asynchrony) and not in the middle of the meal.
- *Incorrect diagnosis.* One of the first questions should be whether the diagnosis is in error, i.e., whether steatorrhea is of nonpancreatic origin. There are other diseases which may also lead to steatorrhea, for example celiac sprue, giardiasis, or bacterial overgrowth. Their coexistence with chronic pancreatitis seems to be high, but still remains to be established more precisely [9, 136, 172, 210]. Furthermore, enzyme substitution will be difficult when gastrointestinal transit disturbances occur, for example in coexisting diabetes mellitus or following vagotomy.
- *Incorrect prescription of the medication.* Physicians throughout the world are being urged to reduce costs and, therefore, may be inclined to prescribe inadequate amounts of pancreatic enzymes. Moreover, the pharmacist should always check the expiration date to determine whether the enzyme preparation has lost its potency.
- *Incorrect choice of pancreatic enzyme preparation.* Recent investigations have shown that pancreatic enzyme preparations may be inactivated by gastric acid (see Sect. 19.2.7) and that nonsimultaneous gastric emptying of pancreatic enzyme preparations with food may play a role in the failure of enzyme substitution (see Sect. 19.2.8).

19.2.7
Gastric Acid Inactivation of Pancreatic Enzyme Preparations

Inactivation of pancreatic supplements by gastric acid has been known for many years [88]. Recent studies in patients with chronic pancreatitis have shown that gastric hypersecretion is more frequent than previously reported [81, 187]. Pancreatic lipase is irreversibly inactivated by gastric acid at a pH of 4.0 and below. Such a pH, also present in the duodenum, stimulates release of duodenal secretin. However, pancreatic insufficiency hinders normal bicarbonate secretion from the pancreas, and the duodenum thus may remain much more acidic than normal [47, 55, 56, 173, 174, 213], therefore inactivating the oral pancreatic extracts in the duodenum. Finally, a persisting acid milieu in the duodenum causes the secretion of large amounts of biliary and pancreatic fluids which dilute the intraduodenal contents.

Measures to prevent inactivation of enzymes by gastric acid include ingestion of antacids, H_2-receptor antagonists, or protein pump inhibitors, as well as the use of protective covering of the enzymes (enteric-coated). Efforts to neutralize or inhibit gastric acid and to protect pancreatic enzymes against inactivation have been made with differing success. For a variety of antacids, only the additional administration of aluminium hydroxide resulted in a greater reduction of steatorrhea than enzyme treatment alone [76]). While sodium bicarbonate was not beneficial in one series [173]), another study showed limited benefit [76], probably because it had been taken with the meals. Administration of magnesium and aluminium hydroxides, or of calcium carbonate, leads to increased fecal fat excretion [49]. This may be explained by the formation of calcium soaps or precipitation of glycine-conjugated bile salts [77].

An antacid capable of protecting enzymes from inactivation by acid must maintain the gastric pH above 4.0 for at least 60 min postprandially, and the duodenal pH above 4.0 for at least 90 min [41, 74]. However, this may lead to an increase in intragastric volumes and thereby to a dilution of enzyme concentrations below the critical level of 5%–10% of normal [173].

Studies on the effect of cimetidine show contradictory results. Cimetidine supplementation has been reported to reduce steatorrhea (Fig. 19.7) [23, 32, 52, 115, 173], or to have no effect [76, 194], when added to conventional enzyme preparations. Cimetidine has also been shown to eliminate steatorrhea when given together with a microencapsulated compound [71]. An analysis of these studies revealed that the benefit of

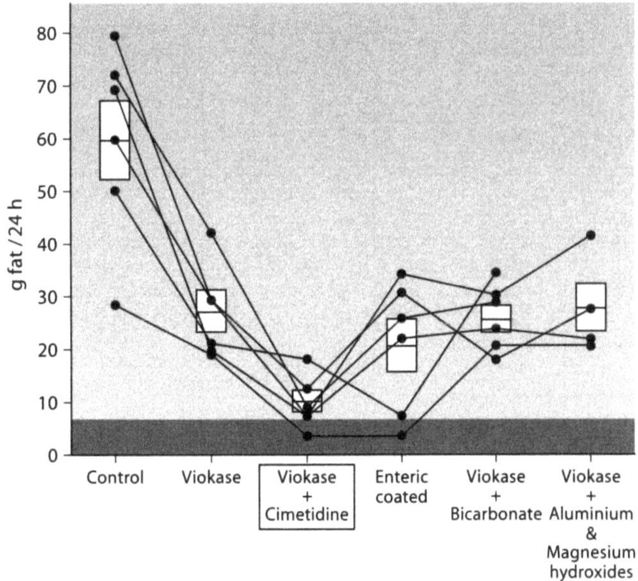

Fig. 19.7. Effect of different modes of treatment on steatorrhea due to pancreatic insufficiency in six patients. Regimens were administered in randomized order. Normal levels for fecal fat excretion (<7 g/24 h) are represented by *dark-shaded areas. Rectangles* represent the mean ± SEM. (From [173] with permission)

cimetidine strongly depended on the amount of lipase given orally [42]. In several trials involving cystic fibrosis patients, cimetidine was not always effective [23, 32, 52, 71]. Since these patients often had increased gastric secretion [32], one possible reason for the failure of cimetidine might have been an inadequate reduction of gastric activity [42].

The need for H_2-blocking agents prior to meals and enzyme preparations places great demands on the patient to ingest a large number of tablets. The acid-protected enzyme preparations were therefore a welcome development. In these preparations, enzyme activity is released from acid-protected granules at a pH level of 5.5 and above, thus protecting against gastric acid and permitting an even mixture of enzymes with the food. In a controlled study on adults with chronic pancreatitis and normal gastric secretion, Creon® (Solvay Pharmaceuticals, Germany) was found to be superior to conventional enzyme preparations, and just as effective as a combination of cimetidine and a conventional enzyme preparation (Fig. 19.8) [115]. Subsequent studies confirmed that this new type of enzyme preparation simplifies and improves treatment of exocrine pancreatic insufficiency [61, 115, 195, 196].

More recently, in vitro experiments have shown that lipolytic activity of bacterial lipase survives better than that of porcine lipase in human gastric and duodenal content [170]. The development of further enzyme preparations using bacterial lipase would, therefore, be of interest.

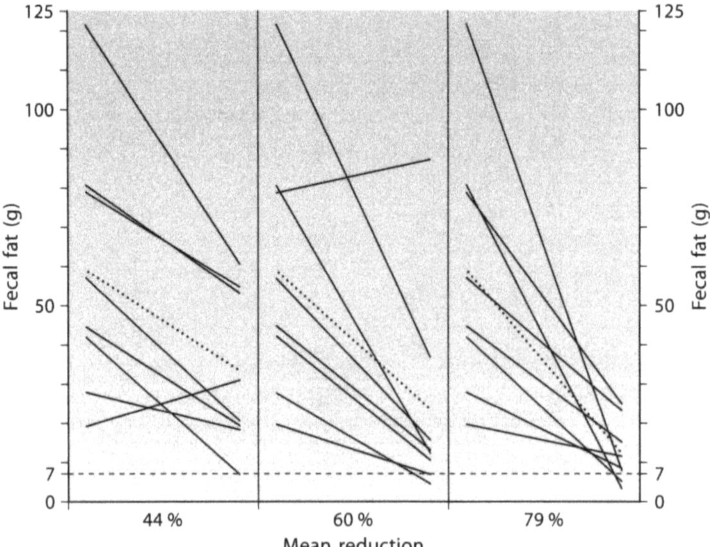

Fig. 19.8. Effect of three different modes of pancreatic enzyme replacement therapy [Pankreon 700 (*left column*); Pankreon 700 plus cimetidine, 300 mg 30 min before the three main meals (*middle column*); Creon (*right column*)] on daily fecal fat. The *broken horizontal line* represents a fecal fat excretion of 7 g/day (upper limit of normal). The *dotted lines* represent the mean values of all patients before and during treatment. (From [115] with permission)

19.2.8
Nonsimultaneous Gastric Emptying of Pancreatic Enzyme Preparations With the Food

Meyer et al. [149] showed that postprandial gastric emptying of pancreatic enzymes is decisive for the effectiveness of enzyme therapy. Independent of the size of the meal, spheres of 1 mm emptied faster than spheres of 2.4 mm and 3.2 mm (Fig. 19.9 a, b). All studies have indicated that spheres should be 1.4 mm to empty at about the same rate as the chyme.

Various pancreatic enzyme preparations contain microspheres of different diameters, which may explain why some microsphere preparations are more effective than others.

Using a cholesteryl octanoate breath test for monitoring enzyme replacement therapy in exocrine pancreatic insufficiency, Mundlos et al. [154] demonstrated that acid-protected pellets of 2 mm size were retained in the stomach and did not empty simultaneously with the chyme. Subsequently, the same group studied the effect of pancreatin microspheres (Creon®) of 1.0–1.2 mm and 1.8–2.0 mm [108]. The breath test showed a distinctly earlier rise of $^{14}CO_2$ excretion in 3 of 10 patients, whereas the differences in the remaining patients were not as clear (Fig. 19.10). The authors assumed the presence of factors other than gastric transit affecting acid-protected preparations. More recently, Layer et al. [123] showed that in the early postprandial period (≤ 30 min) duodenal lipase delivery and triglyceride digestion were greater with the smaller microspheres (1.0–1.2 mm) than with the larger (1.8–2.0 mm). Both were equally effective in the later period (> 30 min). They concluded that adaptating the size of pancreatin micropellets to that required for normal prandial gastric emptying of solid particles remarkably improved the digestive efficacy in pancreatic insufficiency.

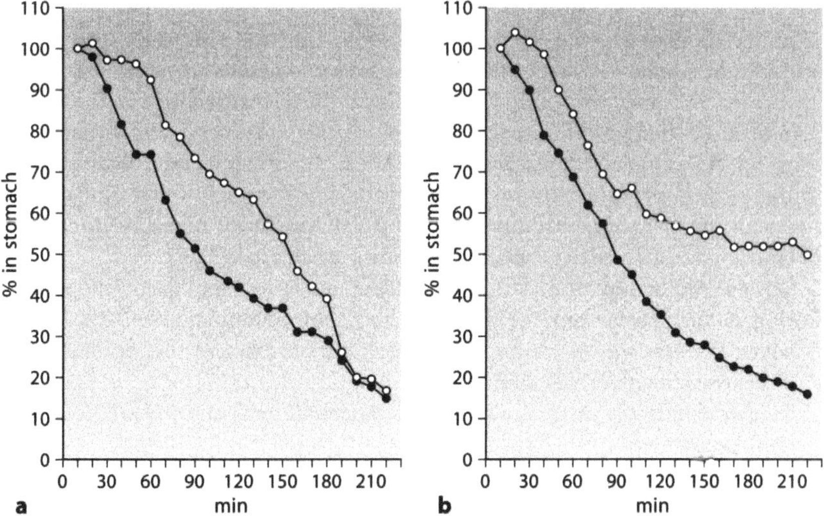

Fig. 19.9 a, b. Average emptying time of 1-mm (*lines with open circles*) and 2.4-mm spheres (*lines with closed circles*) taken as capsules with **a** small and **b** large test meals. Averages from six healthy volunteers. (From [149] with permission)

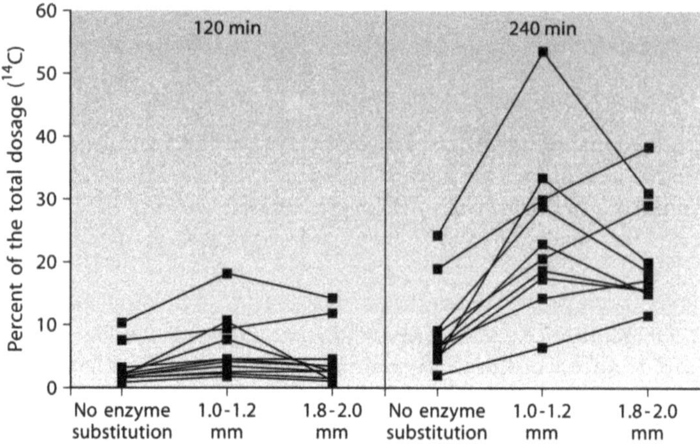

Fig. 19.10. Cumulative $^{14}CO_2$ excretion after 120 and 240 min without enzyme substitution and with enzyme substitution using 1.0- to 1.2- and 1.8- to 2.0-mm enzyme particles. (From [108] with permission)

Further studies are necessary to demonstrate the clinical importance of these findings. Earlier studies using fecal fat estimation as the parameter of treatment efficacy have not shown differences between enteric-coated enzyme preparations of different sizes when lipase-equivalent dosages were used [17, 116, 117].

19.2.9
Factors Preventing Total Elimination of Steatorrhea

Elimination of steatorrhea by exogenous replacement of pancreatic enzymes would seem to be a relatively easy task when sufficient amounts of potent pancreatic enzymes are consumed with each meal. However, clinical experience with pancreatic enzymes shows that *partial* compensation of exocrine pancreatic insufficiency may be easy, but *full* compensation seems impossible in a number of cases. Neither the application of acid-protected enzyme preparations small enough to be transported with the food, nor an increased dosage [106], or direct instillation of pancreatin into the duodenum, have succeeded in totally eliminating steatorrhea [214].

Several studies have dealt with this problem and found that one or more of the following factors may be responsible for hindering total elimination of steatorrhea:
- Other diseases may be causing steatorrhea, such as celiac sprue, giardiasis and bacterial overgrowth [9, 127, 136, 172, 210]
- Nonsimultaneous gastric emptying of pancreatic enzyme preparations with the food (see above)
- Low micellar concentration of bile salts due to the precipitation of bile salts in the abnormally acidic duodenal contents [53, 174]
- Susceptibility of lipase to gastric acidity (see above) and chymotrypsin hydrolysis. Layer and coworkers [122] have shown that during postprandial and aboral transit in healthy subjects only 1% of lipase arrives in the ileum, whereas 74% of amylase

and 22% of trypsin survive the transit. Later, Thiruvengadam and DiMagno [200] demonstrated that chymotrypsin is a more potent inactivator of human lipase than trypsin. Chymotrypsin inactivates lipase in the absence of trypsin, but trypsin inactivation of lipase requires chymotrypsin. Thus, ineffective lipase activity in pancreatic enzymes may be due not only to inactivation by gastric acid but also to chymotrypsin hydrolysis in the enzyme preparation
– Poor mixing of lipase with nutrients [150]

19.2.10
Conclusions, Recommendations, and Future Aspects

For patients with proven exocrine pancreatic insufficiency and normal gastric acid secretion, pancreatic enzymes should be substituted in multi-unit, acid-protected dosages. For patients with gastric hyposecretion and for those who underwent partial or total gastrectomy, enzyme substitution should be administered as granules to enable mixing and simultaneous transport of enzymes with the chyme.

For practical purposes we recommend pancreatin microspheres containing lipase concentrations of 25 000–40 000 units. Parameters for success control are improvement of weight and decrease of diarrhea, abdominal pain, bloating, fecal weight and fecal fat excretion. If these parameters are not fulfilled and treatment is unsuccessful, the pancreatin dosage should be increased to 2–3 times of the initial dosage. If treatment still remains unsuccessful, the patient's compliance should be checked by asking appropriate questions or by estimating fecal chymotrypsin. If the patient is compliant, the diagnosis should be reevaluated (is it really exocrine pancreatic insufficiency?), and evidence of giardiasis, bacterial overgrowth, and blind loop in operated patients should be saught. If such a search is negative, other intestinal absorption disorders should be excluded. If this again is negative, a last resort is to decrease fat intake to 40–60 g/day or to add H_2-blockers or protein pump inhibitors to the treatment (Fig. 19.11; modification of similar recommendations [124]).

Further studies are necessary to determine whether pancreatic enzyme replacement therapy with lingual lipase improves fat absorption to a greater extent than the pancreatic preparations currently in use [2].

Finally, one needs to know more about on how to coordinate the duodenal delivery of enzymes with gastric emptying of the substrate and the gastrointestinal transit of fat [148].

19.3
Endocrine Pancreatic Insufficiency

19.3.1
Definition and Mechanisms

Endocrine pancreatic insufficiency, that is, diabetes mellitus, is explained by the simultaneous damage of endocrine and exocrine pancreatic tissue. The diabetic syn-

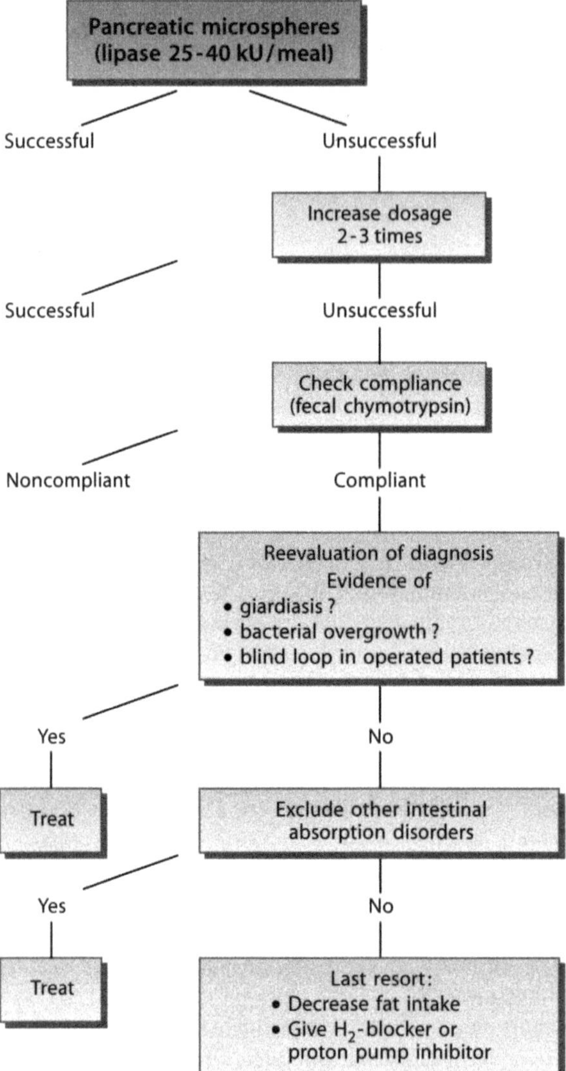

Fig. 19.11. Suggested treatment of exocrine pancreatic insufficiency

drome secondary to pancreatic disease is an example of acquired β- and α-cell insufficiency, and shows some clinical and metabolic features which differentiate it from type I diabetes.

Both insulin and glucagon deficiencies have important consequences. In healthy people, hypoglycemia leads to prompt pancreatic glucagon secretion, which converts liver glycogen to glucose. When there is a lack of glucagon as is in severe chronic pancreatitis, even a small quantity of insulin may induce severe hypoglycemia. In endocrine pancreatic insufficiency due to chronic pancreatitis, diabetic ketoacidosis is rare [38, 130]. This may be due to diminished but never totally absent secretion of insulin in chronic pancreatitis. Only a small amount of insulin is required to prevent the release of fatty acids from adipose tissue and their subsequent metabolism in the liver to ketone bodies.

The symptoms of diabetes secondary to chronic pancreatitis are similar to those of type I diabetes mellitus, with the above mentioned exceptions of the special tendency to hypoglycemia and the rarity of diabetic coma.

Retinopathy and nephropathy, as complications of diabetes secondary to chronic pancreatitis, have similar incidences as among patients with type I diabetes mellitus [31, 82, 131].

19.3.2
Treatment of Endocrine Pancreatic Insufficiency

Diabetes mellitus secondary to pancreatic insufficiency is managed with diet and insulin. The pancreatogenic diabetes of chronic pancreatitis responds only briefly, if at all, to oral antidiabetics of the sulphonylurea type. After total pancreatectomy, these preparations are ineffective.

Insulin-dependent diabetes mellitus in chronic pancreatitis is usually insulin-sensitive and, therefore, hyperglycemia is easily controlled. The proneness of hypoglycemic reactions is a serious problem, especially in alcoholics who do not comply with their therapeutic scheme or even may have additionally alcoholic hypoglycemia [133]. Management of diabetes mellitus in patients with chronic pancreatitis must not aim at normoglycemic control. Mean blood glucose levels should be between 120 and 150 mg/dl. The daily insulin requirement is usually between 20 U and 30 U, and, although low, should be divided into 2 or 3 injections. The patient must comply with his dietary scheme of several meals, each taken together with pancreatic enzymes in order to avoid absorption irregularities.

Owing to the marked tendency to develop hypoglycemia, major pancreatic resection should be avoided in alcoholics who are unlikely to comply with these instructions [34].

There have been attempts to treat pancreatogenic diabetes by autotransplantation of islet cells [34, 155]. However, postoperative septic complications [201], disseminated intravascular coagulation [29, 147, 201], and portal hypertension [29, 147] have been observed. These intra- or postoperative problems can frequently be overcome [147], but several studies indicate that islet cell autotransplantation is not helpful in the treatment of pancreatogenic diabetes since normal or near-normal preoperative islet cell function is necessary for successful grafting [29, 79, 91, 202]. In patients with severe chronic pancreatitis, islet cell reserve has usually decreased beyond the level at which the isolation of a sufficient amount of β-cells is possible [34]. Pancreatic transplantation may be the ultimate answer.

19.4
Postoperative Syndromes

19.4.1
Definition

Besides surgery-specific postoperative syndromes following surgical treatment for chronic pancreatitis, there are other disease-related syndromes which make the evaluation of surgical treatment difficult:
- More than two-thirds of alcoholics continue drinking after the diagnosis of chronic pancreatitis and possibly also following surgical treatment. Therefore, the benefit of surgery on the disease may be countered by the symptoms of alcohol abuse.
- The natural course of chronic pancreatitis and especially that of pain, exocrine and endocrine pancreatic insufficiency varies and is not predictable [119]. It is, therefore, impossible to decide whether the natural course of the disease in operated patients has really been influenced by surgery itself.
- Following some operations, it is not possible to repeat preoperative pancreatic function tests for evaluation of the course of the disease. This is especially the case after Whipple's operation, which requires gastric resection. Because of the gastric resection, a secretin-pancreozymin test – the gold standard test for exocrine pancreatic function testing (see Sect. 17.2.2.2.3) [109] – is no longer possible. Indirect, less sensitive procedures as the pancreolauryl test and fecal chymotrypsin estimation may lead to false-abnormal results possibly due to postcibal asynchrony following gastric resection [112]. The role of elastase-1 estimation in feces under this condition has not yet been evaluated. For postoperative evaluation of exocrine pancreatic function mostly fecal fat analysis is used which shows only major changes in exocrine pancreatic function and may show steatorrhea due to postcibal asynchrony after gastric resection in patients with normal pancreatic function.

19.4.2
Disease-related Postoperative Pain Symptoms

For the patient, pain is the most important symptom. During the course of the disease in every second to fourth patient, surgery for pain and/or organ complications such as pancreatic pseudocysts is necessary [7, 119]. The influence of surgery on pain is difficult to evaluate, and comparison among different studies is also difficult due to the following reasons:
- Definition of pain is often vague and pain symptoms are not measured, for example, according to a visual analogue scale.
- Not all patients with the same indication for surgery receive the same surgical treatment. Due to the difficult postoperative treatment of endocrine pancreatic insufficiency, resection operation – even when indicated – is often refused for alcoholics [64, 208].
- While patients continuing alcohol abuse have had distinctly worse operative results [30, 92, 126], it is difficult to decide whether postoperative deterioration is due to the natural course of the disease, to continuous alcohol abuse, or to surgery.

Table 19.7. Percentage of patients who were free of pain 6 months, 2, and 5 years after different surgical procedures because of chronic pancreatitis [199]

Follow-up	Whipple's operation (%)	Pancreatico-jejunostomy (%)	Left-sided resection (%)
Alcohol-induced pancreatitis			
6 months	82	87	60
2 years	74	53	39
5 years	71	54	26
Idiopathic pancreatitis			
6 months	50	80	77
2 years	50	60	46
5 years	33	60	20

- The study of Taylor et al. [199] (Table 19.7) shows clearly that during the course of a longer follow-up pain recurs. This casts doubt on the favorable impression gained after a short postoperative follow-up.

The choice of surgical procedure certainly depends on the special condition of each patient with chronic pancreatitis. Previous reports on postoperative results show that relief of pain after surgery does not always take place following a variety of operative techniques (Table 19.8).

It is of concern that in the long run the course of pain has been the same in operated and nonoperated patients [119, 137].

19.4.3
Exocrine Pancreatic Insufficiency

The effect of surgical treatment on exocrine pancreatic function in chronic pancreatitis is not well known due to the following reasons:
- The primary aim of surgical treatment is freedom of pain; therefore, pancreatic function is only rarely considered
- Exocrine pancreatic function tests, such as the secretin-pancreozymin test and the Lundh test, require the intubation of the duodenum which is impossible after right-sided resective and difficult after drainage operations

In conservatively treated patients with chronic pancreatitis, spontaneous amelioration of exocrine pancreatic function is possible [119] and has also been found postoperatively in a few patients [114, 185]. Concerning the Göttingen patients, postoperative exocrine pancreatic function has improved in 6% and even normalized in 6%. In 50%, there was no change in exocrine pancreatic insufficiency, whereas 38% showed deterioration [114, 137].

When surgical results were analysed according to the type of surgery, drainage and resection (Table 19.9), it was found that deterioration of exocrine pancreatic function was significantly more frequent after resective operations [137]. Other investigators,

Table 19.8. Reports on pain relief after different surgical procedures in chronic pancreatitis: Further evaluation of the postoperative beneficial effect on pain was not considered. Closure of literature research March 1996

References	Surgical procedure	Mean observation time (years)		n	Pain relief (%)
Way et al. [207]	Drainage/resection	5 (approx.)		37	64
Lankisch et al. [114]	Drainage/resection	2	1/12	40	60
Mangold et al. [144]	Partial duodenopancreatectomy	1	8/12	44	73
	Total duodenopancreatectomy	2	10/12	18	91
	Partial left-sided resection	3	5/12	37	60
	Subtotal left-sided resection	2	10/12	17	83
Proctor et al. [169]	Pancreaticojejunostomy		11/12	22	50
Rosenberger et al. [179]	Resection	6		67	69
	Nonresective procedures	6		40	50
Lankisch et al. [113]	Pancreaticojejunostomy	3	1/12	17	76
	Resection	3	1/12	22	64
Prinz and Greenlee [168]	Pancreaticojejunostomy	6	1/12		
		≤7	11/12	91	35
Sato et al. [185]	Pancreaticojejunostomy	6	6/12	38	68
	Left-sided resection	6	6/12	14	79
	Whipple's operation	6	6/12	9	67
Gall et al. [68]	Whipple's operation, duct occlusion	>1		67	93
Morrow et al. [151]	Ductal drainage	4–13		46	46
	40%–80% left-sided resection	4–13		21	33
	80%–95% left-sided resection	4–13		8	100
	Drainage	6		46	80
	Subtotal pancreatectomy	7		21	24
Sato et al. [184]	Left-sided resection	>	6/12	21	91
	Whipple's operation	>	6/12	11	55
	Pancreaticojejunostomy	>	6/12	43	91
Bradley III [25]	Lateral pancreaticojejunostomy	5	9/12	46	28
	Caudal pancreaticojejunostomy	5	9/12	18	17
Frick et al. [65, 66]	Left-sided resection	6	6/12	74	50
	Partial duodenopancreatectomy	6	6/12	62	45
	Total duodenopancreatectomy	6	6/12	22	55
	Drainage	4	7/12	156	48
Rossi et al. [180]	Whipple's operation		6/12	61	72
		2		44	61
		5		33	61
		10		18	61
		15		6	83
Mannell et al. [145]	Drainage/resection	8	6/12	100	77
Stone et al. [197]	Whipple's operation	6	2/12	15	27
	Total duodenopancreatectomy	9	1/12	15	27
Beger et al. [13]	Duodenum-preserving resection of the head of the pancreas	3	8/12	128	77
Peiper and Köhler [166]	Resection	10		51	79
	Drainage	10		24	65
Lankisch et al. [119]	Drainage/resection	6		70	57
Büchler et al. [27]	Duodenum-preserving resection of the head of the pancreas		6/12	15	40
	Pylorus-preserving Whipple's operation		6/12	16	75
Adams et al. [4]	Lateral pancreaticojejunostomy	6	4/12	62	42

Table 19.9. Pre- and postoperative exocrine and endocrine pancreatic function in 34 and 109 patients, respectively, with chronic pancreatitis treated by drainage ($n=94$) or resection operation ($n=49$). Median of the observation time 1.7 years [137]

Exocrine pancreatic insufficiency	Drainage operation ($n=22$)	Resection operation ($n=12$)
Improvement	3 (14%)	1 (8%)
No change	14 (63%)	3 (25%)
Deterioration	5 (23%)	8 (67%)
$p=0.0394$, significant		

Endocrine pancreatic insufficiency	Drainage operation ($n=72$)	Resection operation ($n=37$)
Improvement	0 (0%)	0 (0%)
No change	28 (39%)	15 (40%)
Deterioration	44 (61%)	22 (60%)
Not significant		

too, found postoperative deterioration of exocrine pancreatic insufficiency more frequently following resective than drainage operations [70, 169]. The extent of deterioration depends on the extent of resection [64] (Table 19.10).

A beneficial influence of the drainage operation on exocrine and endocrine pancreatic function is obviously to be expected when patients are operated in an early stage. One group [156, 157] defined the severity of chronic pancreatitis by means of ERCP, oral glucose tolerance test, measurement of pancreatic polypeptide following stimulation, fecal fat analysis over 3 days and bentiromide test according to a scoring system. Patients who had mild to moderate severe chronic pancreatitis, showed postoperatively a significantly less frequent deterioration of pancreatic function than those treated conservatively (13% vs. 78%). In patients with severe chronic pancreatitis, there were postoperatively no changes in pancreatic function. The authors concluded that the progressive functional loss in chronic pancreatitis may be at least temporarily halted by pancreaticojejunostomy. The postoperative preservation of pancreatic function, however, could not be explained by cessation of alcohol abuse, since both operated and nonoperated patients continued drinking. Possibly, the postoperative lowering of pancreatic duct pressure plays a favorable role.

Table 19.10. Pre- and postoperative frequency of clinically relevant steatorrhea in 198 patients with chronic pancreatitis treated by different surgical procedures [64]

Surgical procedure	n	Clinically relevant steatorrhea	
		Preoperative	Postoperative
40%–80% left-sided resection	53	2 (3.7%)	10 (19.0%)
80%–95% left-sided resection	77	7 (9.0%)	29 (37.6%)
Whipple's operation	19	1 (5.2%)	10 (53.0%)

19.4.3.1
Treatment

An indication for pancreatic enzyme substitution in exocrine pancreatic insufficiency is steatorrhea exceeding 15 g/day and/or progressive weight loss. In patients with normal gastric secretion and gastric emptying, acid-protecting small-sized particles containing enzyme preparations leaving the stomach synchronously with the meals should be prescribed. When gastric resection is performed for purposes of right-sided resection (Whipple's operation), enzyme preparations that are not acid-protected may be satisfactory if gastric secretion is minimal [110, 111].

19.4.4
Endocrine Pancreatic Insufficiency

Little is known about the influence of pancreatic surgery on endocrine pancreatic function.

Improvement of endocrine pancreatic function seldomly follows drainage and resective operations [113, 114, 185], but is more frequent after duodenum-preserving resection of the head of the pancreas [18]. As a rule, the percentage of insulin-dependent diabetes increases after drainage [78] and resective operations [70, 144, 185, 199], but it is difficult to decide whether this is due to surgery or the natural course of the disease (Table 19.9). However, after resective operations, the frequency as well as the insulin requirement of diabetes mellitus increase with the extent of pancreatic resection. Therefore, Frey et al. [64], who initially had favored an extensive resection of the organ, now recommends a limited resection in order to avoid a postoperative insulin-dependent diabetes mellitus, especially in alcoholics. Several of their operated alcoholics had to be postoperatively institutionalized because of hypoglycemia-induced brain damage. In another study, almost every third postoperative death was due to diabetes and its complications [184].

19.4.4.1
Treatment

Postoperatively, insulin sensitivity increases after resective operations, probably as a result of a simultaneous decrease in glucagon secretion. This renders the postoperative treatment of diabetes mellitus difficult. Severe, even life-threatening hypoglycemia may occur if food intake and/or pancreatic enzyme substitution are erratic. Large amounts of insulin should be avoided.

Following total pancreatectomy, pancreatic enzyme substitution poses no problem. Treatment of postoperative insulin-dependent diabetes mellitus is difficult, because glucagon-producing α-cells are completely removed. Contrary to other species, humans have no extrapancreatic glucagon. Prevention of hypoglycemia due to glucagon deficiency in patients undergoing total pancreatectomy requires not only very careful use of insulin but also the observance of a strict diet. Alcoholics usually are not able to do so [34]. Therefore, the aim of surgical procedure in alcoholics is to preserve as much endocrine tissue as possible.

19.4.5
Surgery-related Sequelae

Peptic ulcer, disturbance of gastric emptying, intestinal bacterial overgrowth, and relapsing cholangitis are important postoperative problems.

19.4.5.1
Sequelae of Gastric Resection

As a consequence of Whipple's operation or pancreatic resection, peptic ulcer may occur.

The reason for this relative frequent complication is unclear. From the surgeon's point of view, the limited gastric resection (usually only hemigastrectomy), and from the internist's point of view, smoking and alcohol abuse have been held responsible for the development of peptic ulcer.

Another reason for the development of gastric or duodenal ulcer may be a decreased bicarbonate secretion in the course of chronic pancreatitis and the consequent transformation in the duodenum of the alkaline into the acidic milieu.

It has been suggested that gastric resection should be combined with a selective gastric vagotomy [162]. Several studies have shown, however, that vagotomy is of limited influence on postoperative ulceration [35, 72, 73, 205].

Comparative investigations in patients after Whipple's operation and after 40%–80% or 80%–95% left-sided resection show that peptic ulcers occurred in 5,2%, 5,6%, and 16% patients, respectively [64]. Follow-up after duodenum-preserving resection of the head of the pancreas and Whipple's operation has shown that peptic ulcers occur more frequently after the latter operation [72].

The remaining postoperative syndromes after gastric resection such as dumping, reflux disease, gastritis, etc. are of minor consequence following pancreatic resection.

After Whipple's operation, and also after duodenum-preserving resection of the head of the pancreas, disturbed gastric emptying has been observed in 40% of the cases [206, 209, 211]. This disturbed gastric emptying persists for a short interval and can be treated either with gastric feeding tubes [94, 206], or by the administration of erythromycin, or another prokinetic agent. Long-term problems do not occur [72].

19.4.5.2
Sequelae of Biliodigestive Anastomosis

After Whipple's operation and total pancreatectomy, a connection between bile ducts and a small intestinal loop is necessary. Theoretically, reflux of intestinal fluid could lead to cholangitis. Based on clinical experience, cholangitis develops only when a stricture of anastomosis leads to stasis in the bile duct. The more narrow the lumen of the common bile duct at the time of resection of the head of the pancreas, the more frequent are strictures of anastomosis. Septic cholangitis as a sequela of these complications may lead to a severe course or fatal outcome [120].

19.4.5.3
Sequelae of Duct Drainage

After resection of the head of the pancreas, and also after pancreaticojejunostomy, a blind loop with bacterial overgrowth may develop. Bacterial overgrowth results in the deconjugation of bile acids. Because conjugated bile acids are required for micellar formation in the duodenum and jejunum, deconjugation leads to inadequate formation of micelles and thereby to steatorrhea.

Bacterial overgrowth can be diagnosed by the H_2-glucose breath test and be treated by appropriate antibiotics [120].

19.5
Evaluation of Follow-up Results

19.5.1
Quality of Life

Whereas criteria have already been developed to evaluate functional and morphological changes, defining quality of life for a patient with chronic pancreatitis is more difficult. It certainly depends on freedom from symptoms, especially pain, and the patient's performance capacity at work, home, play, and sport, as well as the patient's general well-being, including the psychological state. The answers of the questions of whether or not the patient is free of symptoms and able to perform a normal life and feels generally well sum up of whether or not the patient is satisfied with his life.

The quality-of-life assessment should be brief, easy to score and to interpret.

Current approaches rely on a validated questionnaire, which is not easy in case of alcoholics and very ill patients, and on a standardized interview which is feasible when kept short.

Mandatory questions for such an interview are listed in Table 19.11. A future approach to assessment of quality-of-life should consist of a scale based on signs and symptoms and a disease-specific grading scale. At present, a quality of life questionnaire of the European Organization for Research and Treatment of Cancer seems to be valid also in patients suffering from chronic pancreatitis [19].

Another important question is who should perform the assessment and thus define the patient's quality of life. The best choice is obviously the patient's physician, who may, however, be biased because of having recommended the therapy. Another physician and nurse could perform the interview. A nonmedical person would not be

Table 19.11. Questions for standardized interview to evaluate treatment results

Did you
- Have pain?
- Lose weight?
- Lose your appetite?
- Have diarrhea?
- Interrupt work, home activities, play or sport?
- Resume or reduce your activities?

Table 19.12. Questions to evaluate capacity of performance

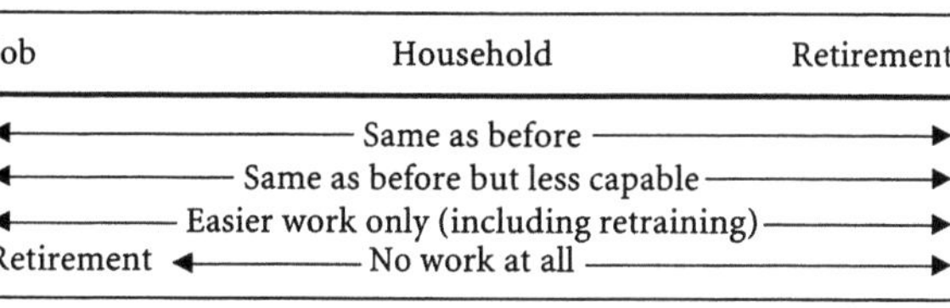

acceptable to all doctors and patients, and not all patients may accept answering a computerized questionnaire.

To determine the patient's capacity to perform, it should be established whether the patient is still employed, or retired, or still active in the household.

It is also important to evaluate whether the disease has had any implications for the performance capacity, i.e., whether or not the patient has the same work capacity as before the onset of the disease (Table 19.12). It may be that the patient required retraining for another employment if the disease had reduced his performance capacity, and that should be stated.

Finally, it should be recorded whether a patient, who had worked until the onset of the disease, has since retired.

If a patient was already retired before the onset of the disease, it should be determined as to whether the patient is still capable of doing any work.

An assessment of the state of well-being can be made only by the patients themselves. Categorizations could be *very good, good, fair,* and *poor,* but should include whether there is a frequent fluctuation from one state to another.

19.5.2
Evaluation of Conservative and Surgical Treatment Results

Conservative treatment results may be evaluated according to the staging of the disease. However, there are some difficulties concerning the assessment of operative results, which should be mentioned briefly.

Necessary data for postoperative assessment include the preoperative staging of the disease to find out to what extent the operation was beneficial to the patient. Early and late mortality have to be stated and whether they are due to pancreatitis or nonpancreatic diseases.

A patient's failure to appear for follow-up evaluations is not necessarily a sign of successful surgery!

The exact role of alcohol abstinence on the progression of the disease still remains to be established, but since some studies [7, 80, 87] showed that alcohol abstinence had at least some benefit, continued postoperative drinking or abstinence should be reported.

Further elements for postoperative evaluation are early and late surgery-dependent complications, or morbidity and postoperative staging of exocrine and endocrine pancreatic function.

Assessment of postoperative exocrine and endocrine pancreatic function, however, may be difficult. Direct exocrine pancreatic function tests (tube tests) are sometimes not feasible due to changed anatomical conditions after resective operations, or difficult to assess after drainage operations. Indirect (tubeless) pancreatic function tests and fecal fat estimation are usually possible, but small improvements may be overlooked.

Endocrine pancreatic function test results are difficult to evaluate, at least after resective operations, because in case of deterioration, this may be due to the operation or to the natural progress of the disease.

All imaging procedures have the limitation that it may be difficult to decide whether the postoperative pathological and morphological results are a complication of the disease or of the operation. Also, due to possibly changed anatomical conditions following resective operations, it may be difficult to demonstrate relapse or progression of the disease or disease-dependent complications.

Finally, it has to be decided at which time intervals the results of operative treatment of pancreatitis should be reported. Frey and Braasch [63] recommended that such follow-up results should be reported at 2-, 5- and 10-year intervals, and the minimal acceptable time for follow-up should be 2 years. The same time intervals should be followed for conservative treatment results.

19.5.3
Outlook

A global evaluation index of treatment results in chronic pancreatitis should include pain, work performance, well-being, symptoms other than pain, and systemized follow-up intervals. However, the order of importance for each factor on a grading scale remains to be established.

Recently, a quality-of-life questionnaire that evaluated postoperative results in patients with chronic pancreatitis has shown to be a reliable valid measure of quality of life in these patients [19]. Further studies are required.

References

1. Abrams CK, Hamosh M, Dutta SK, Hubbard VS, Hamosh P (1987) Role of nonpancreatic lipolytic activity in exocrine pancreatic insufficiency. Gastroenterology 92:125–129
2. Abrams CK, Hamosh M, Hubbard VS, Dutta SK, Hamosh P (1984) Lingual lipase in cystic fibrosis. Quantitation of enzyme activity in the upper small intestine of patients with exocrine pancreatic insufficiency. J Clin Invest 73:374–382

3. Abrams CK, Hamosh M, Lee TC, Ansher AF, Collen MJ, Lewis JH, Benjamin SB, Hamosh P (1988) Gastric lipase: localization in the human stomach. Gastroenterology 95:1460–1464

4. Adams DB, Ford MC, Anderson MC (1994) Outcome after lateral pancreaticojejunostomy for chronic pancreatitis. Ann Surg 219:481–489

5. Adler G, Müllenhoff A, Koop I, Bozkurt T, Göke B, Beglinger C, Arnold R (1988) Stimulation of pancreatic secretion in man by a protease inhibitor (camostate). Eur J Clin Invest 18:98–104

6. Adler G, Reinshagen M, Koop I, Göke B, Schafmayer A, Rovati LC, Arnold R (1989) Differential effects of atropine and a cholecystokinin receptor antagonist on pancreatic secretion. Gastroenterology 96:1158–1164

7. Ammann RW, Akovbiantz A, Largiadèr F, Schueler G (1984) Course and outcome of chronic pancreatitis. Longitudinal study of a mixed medical-surgical series of 245 patients. Gastroenterology 86:820–828

8. Axon ATR, Classen M, Cotton PB, Cremer M, Freeny PC, Lees WR (1984) Pancreatography in chronic pancreatitis: international definitions. Gut 25:1107–1112

9. Balgha V, Pap A (1991) Bacterial overgrowth of small intestine demonstrated by H2 test in patients with chronic pancreatitis. Digestion 49:6 (abstr)

10. Banks PA (1990) Pain in chronic pancreatitis: pathomechanism and clinical presentation. In: Beger HG, Büchler M, Ditschuneit H, Malfertheiner P (eds) Chronic Pancreatitis. Springer, Berlin-Heidelberg, pp 213–217

11. Banks PA (1991) Management of pancreatic pain. Pancreas 6, Suppl. 1:S52–S59

12. Baur X, Wießmann KJ, Wüthrich B (1984) Enzyme sind die allergenwirksamen Komponenten von inhaliertem Pankreatin. Dtsch Med Wochenschr 109:257–260

13. Beger HG, Büchler M, Bittner RR, Oettinger W, Roscher R (1989) Duodenum-preserving resection of the head of the pancreas in severe chronic pancreatitis. Early and late results. Ann Surg 209:273–278

14. Beger HG, Krautzberger W, Bittner R, Büchler M, Limmer J (1985) Duodenum-preserving resection of the head of the pancreas in patients with severe chronic pancreatitis. Surgery 97:467–473

15. Bengtsson M, Löfström JB (1990) Nerve block in pancreatic pain. Acta Chir Scand 156:285–291

16. Bergner A, Bergner RK (1975) Pulmonary hypersensitivity associated with pancreatin powder exposure. Pediatrics 55:814–817

17. Beverley DW, Kelleher J, MacDonald A, Littlewood JM, Robinson T, Walters MP (1987) Comparison of four pancreatic extracts in cystic fibrosis. Arch Dis Child 62:564–568

18. Bittner R, Büchler M, Butters M, Leibl B, Nägele S, Roscher R, Beger HG (1992) Der Einfluß der duodenumerhaltenden Pankreaskopfresektion (DPKR) auf die endokrine Pankreasfunktion bei Patienten mit chronischer Pankreatitis. Z Gastroenterol 30:12–16

19. Bloechle C, Izbicki JR, Knoefel WT, Kuechler T, Broelsch CE (1995) Quality of life in chronic pancreatitis – Results after duodenum-preserving resection of the head of the pancreas. Pancreas 11:77–85

20. Bockman DE, Buchler M, Malfertheiner P, Beger HG (1988) Analysis of nerves in chronic pancreatitis. Gastroenterology 94:1459–1469

21. Bornman PC, Marks IN, Girdwood AH, Clain JE, Narunsky L, Clain DJ, Wright JP (1980) Is pancreatic duct obstruction or stricture a major cause of pain in calcific pancreatitis? Br J Surg 67:425–428

22. Borowitz DS, Grand RJ, Durie PR, Consensus Committee (1995) Use of pancreatic enzyme supplements for patients with cystic fibrosis in the context of fibrosing colonopathy. J Pediatr 127:681–684

23. Boyle BJ, Long WB, Balistreri WF, Widzer SJ, Huang N (1980) Effect of cimetidine and pancreatic enzymes on serum and fecal bile acids and fat absorption in cystic fibrosis. Gastroenterology 78:950–953

24. Bradley III EL (1982) Pancreatic duct pressure in chronic pancreatitis. Am J Surg 144:313–316

25. Bradley III EL (1987) Long-term results of pancreatojejunostomy in patients with chronic pancreatitis. Am J Surg 153:207–213

26. Büchler M, Weihe E, Friess H, Malfertheiner P, Bockman E, Müller S, Nohr D, Beger HG (1992) Changes in peptidergic innervation in chronic pancreatitis. Pancreas 7:183–192

27. Büchler MW, Friess H, Müller MW, Wheatley AM, Beger HG (1995) Randomized trial of duodenum-preserving pancreatic head resection versus pylorus-preserving Whipple in chronic pancreatitis. Am J Surg 169:65–70

28. Büchler MW, Uhl W, Malfertheiner P (1996) Pankreaserkrankungen. Akute Pankreatitis, chronische Pankreatitis, Tumore des Pankreas. Karger, Basel

29. Cameron JL, Mehigan DG, Broe PJ, Zuidema GD (1981) Distal pancreatectomy and islet autotransplantation for chronic pancreatitis. Ann Surg 193:312–317

30. Capitaine Y, Roche B, Wiesner L, Hahnloser P (1988) Pancréatite chronique: histoire naturelle et évolution en relation avec l'alcoolisme. Schweiz Med Wochenschr 118:817–820

31. Couet C, Genton P, Pointel JP, Louis J, Gross P, Saudax E, Debry G, Drouin P (1985) The prevalence of retinopathy is similar in diabetes mellitus secondary to chronic pancreatitis with or without pancreatectomy and in idiopathic diabetes mellitus. Diabetes Care 8:323–328

32. Cox KL, Isenberg JN, Osher AB, Dooley RR (1979) The effect of cimetidine on maldigestion in cystic fibrosis. J Pediatr 94:488–492

33. Creutzfeldt W, Kern E, Kümmerle F, Schumacher J (1961) Die radikale Entfernung der Bauchspeicheldrüse beim Menschen – Indikationen, Ergebnisse, Folgeerscheinungen. In: Heilmeyer L, Schoen R, de Rudder B (eds) Ergebnisse der Inneren Medizin, Vol. 16. Springer, Berlin–Göttingen–Heidelberg, pp 79–124

34. Creutzfeldt W, Lankisch PG (1980) Totale Duodenopankreatektomie bei chronischer Pankreatitis. Z Gastroenterol 18:641–643

35. Crist DW, Sitzmann JV, Cameron JL (1987) Improved hospital morbidity, mortality, and survival after the Whipple procedure. Ann Surg 206:358–365

36. Delhaye M, Hennart D, Bredas P, Engelman E, Cremer M (1994) Steroid and alcohol coeliac plexus block in chronic pancreatitis. Eur J Gastroenterol Hepatol 6:553–558

37. Delhaye M, Vandermeeren A, Gabbrielli A, Cremer M (1990) Lithotripsie and endoscopy for pancreatic calculi: the first 104 patients. Gastroenterology 98:A216 (abstr)

38. Dellwyler W (1964) Le diabète des pancréatopathies. Sem Hop Paris 40:1676–1682

39. Derfus GA, Geenen JE, Hogan WJ (1989) Alterations in pancreatic duct morphology associated with endoscopic stent placement. Pancreas 4:613 (abstr)

40. Devière J, Devaere S, Baize M, Cremer M (1990) Endoscopic biliary drainage in chronic pancreatitis. Gastrointest Endosc 36:96–100

41. DiMagno EP (1979) Medical treatment of pancreatic insufficiency. Mayo Clin Proc 54:435–442

42. DiMagno EP (1982) Controversies in the treatment of exocrine pancreatic insufficiency. Dig Dis Sci 27:481–484

43. DiMagno EP, Bell JS, Perez MM, Regan PT, Go VLW, Moertel CG (1981) Malabsorption can be abolished in pancreatic insufficiency. Gastroenterology 80:1136 (abstr)

44. DiMagno EP, Go VLW, Summerskill WHJ (1973) Relations between pancreatic enzyme outputs and malabsorption in severe pancreatic insufficiency. N Engl J Med 288:813–815

45. DiMagno EP, Malagelada J-R, Go VLW (1979) The relationships between pancreatic ductal obstruction and pancreatic secretion in man. Mayo Clin Proc 54:157–162

46. DiMagno EP, Malagelada JR, Go VLW (1975) Relationship between alcoholism and pancreatic insufficiency. Ann N Y Acad Sci 252:200–207

47. DiMagno EP, Malagelada JR, Go VLW, Moertel CG (1977) Fate of orally ingested enzymes in pancreatic insufficiency. Comparison of two dosage schedules. N Engl J Med 296:1318–1322

48. Dolan TF Jr, Meyers A (1974) Bronchial asthma and allergic rhinitis associated with inhalation of pancreatic extracts. Am Rev Respir Dis 110:812–813

49. Drube HC, Büttner H (1964) Über die Wirkung oraler Kalziumgaben auf die Stuhlfettausscheidung bei Gesunden und Kranken mit Steatorrhoe. Med Klin 59:1234–1236

50. Drummond S, Saunders JHB, Leach R, Wormsley KG (1977) Enzymic activities of commercial preparations of pancreatic enzymes. Scot Med J 22:221–224

51. Dunaif G, Schneeman BO (1981) The effect of dietary fiber on human pancreatic enzyme activity in vitro. Am J Clin Nutr 34:1034–1035

52. Durie PR, Bell L, Linton W, Corey ML, Forstner GG (1980) Effect of cimetidine and sodium bicarbonate on pancreatic replacement therapy in cystic fibrosis. Gut 21:778–786

53. Dutta SK, Anand K, Gadacz TR (1986) Bile salt malabsorption in pancreatic insufficiency secondary to alcoholic pancreatitis. Gastroenterology 91:1243–1249

54. Dutta SK, Bustin MP, Russell RM, Costa BS (1982) Deficiency of fat-soluble vitamins in treated patients with pancreatic insufficiency. Ann Intern Med 97:549–552

55. Dutta SK, Russell RM, Iber FL (1979) Impaired acid neutralization in the duodenum in pancreatic insufficiency. Dig Dis Sci 24:775–780
56. Dutta SK, Russell RM, Iber FL (1979) Influence of exocrine pancreatic insufficiency on the intraluminal pH of the proximal small intestine. Dig Dis Sci 24:529–534
57. Ebbehøj N, Borly L, Bülow J, Grønvall Rasmussen S, Madsen P, Matzen P, Owre A (1990) Pancreatic tissue fluid pressure in chronic pancreatitis. Relation to pain, morphology, and function. Scand J Gastroenterol 25:1046–1051
58. Ebbehøj N, Borly L, Madsen P, Matzen P (1990) Pancreatic tissue fluid pressure during drainage operations for chronic pancreatitis. Scand J Gastroenterol 25:1041–1045
59. Ebbehøj N, Borly L, Madsen P, Svendsen LB (1986) Pancreatic tissue pressure and pain in chronic pancreatitis. Pancreas 1:556–558
60. Ebbehøj N, Svendsen LB, Madsen P (1984) Pancreatic tissue pressure: techniques and pathophysiological aspects. Scand J Gastroenterol 19:1066–1068
61. Freise J, Horstkotte H (1986) Exokrine Pankreasinsuffizienz. Vergleich einer Substitutionstherapie mit nichtsäureresistenten und einer säureresistenten Enzympräparation. Fortschr Med 104:625–628
62. Frey CF, Amikura K (1994) Local resection of the head of the pancreas combined with longitudinal pancreaticojejunostomy in the management of patients with chronic pancreatitis. Ann Surg 220:492–507
63. Frey CF, Braasch J (1984) Surgical management of chronic pancreatitis: the need to improve our observations and assessment of results. Am J Surg 147:189–190
64. Frey CF, Child III CG, Fry W (1976) Pancreatectomy for chronic pancreatitis. Ann Surg 184:403–414
65. Frick S, Ebert M, Rückert K (1987) Chirurgie der chronischen Pankreatitis. II. Spätergebnisse nach nicht resezierenden Operationen. Dtsch Med Wochenschr 112:832–837
66. Frick S, Jung K, Rückert K (1987) Chirurgie der chronischen Pankreatitis. I. Spätergebnisse nach Resektionsbehandlung. Dtsch Med Wochenschr 112:629–635
67. Fuji T, Amano H, Ohmura R, Akiyama T, Aibe T, Takemoto T (1989) Endoscopic pancreatic sphincterotomy – technique and evaluation. Endoscopy 21:27–30
68. Gall FP, Gebhardt C, Zirngibl H (1982) Chronic pancreatitis – results in 116 consecutive, partial duodenopancreatectomies combined with pancreatic duct occlusion. Hepatogastroenterology 29:115–119
69. Girdwood AH, Marks IN, Bornman PC, Kottler RE, Cohen M (1981) Does progressive pancreatic insufficiency limit pain in calcific pancreatitis with duct stricture or continued alcohol insult? J Clin Gastroenterol 3:241–245
70. Gooszen HG, Schmidt JM, Van Heurn LWE, Jansen JBMJ, Lamers CBHW, Terpstra JL (1988) Surgical treatment for pain relief in chronic pancreatitis. Scand J Gastroenterol 23, Suppl. 154:98–102
71. Gow R, Bradbear R, Francis P, Shepherd R (1981) Comparative study of varying regimens to improve steatorrhoea and creatorrhoea in cystic fibrosis: effectiveness of an enteric-coated preparation with and without antacids and cimetidine. Lancet 2:1071–1074
72. Grace PA, Pitt HA, Longmire WP (1990) Pylorus preserving pancreatoduodenectomy: an overview. Br J Surg 77:968–974
73. Grace PA, Pitt HA, Tompkins RK, DenBesten L, Longmire WP Jr (1986) Decreased morbidity and mortality after pancreatoduodenectomy. Am J Surg 151:141–149
74. Graham DY (1977) Enzyme replacement therapy of exocrine pancreatic insufficiency in man. Relation between in vitro enzyme activities and in vivo potency in commercial pancreatic extracts. N Engl J Med 296:1314–1317
75. Graham DY (1979) An enteric-coated pancreatic enzyme preparation that works. Dig Dis Sci 24:906–909
76. Graham DY (1982) Pancreatic enzyme replacement. The effect of antacids or cimetidine. Dig Dis Sci 27:485–490
77. Graham DY, Sackman JW (1982) Mechanism of increase in steatorrhea with calcium and magnesium in exocrine pancreatic insufficiency: an animal model. Gastroenterology 83:638–644
78. Greenlee HB, Prinz RA, Aranha GV (1990) Long-term results of side-to-side pancreaticojejunostomy. World J Surg 14:70–76

79. Grodsinsky C, Malcom S, Goldman J, Dienst S, Oh HK, Westrick P (1981) Islet cell autotransplantation after pancreatectomy for chronic pancreatitis. Its limitations. Arch Surg 116:511–516

80. Gullo L, Barbara L, Labò G (1988) Effect of cessation of alcohol use on the course of pancreatic dysfunction in alcoholic pancreatitis. Gastroenterology 95:1063–1068

81. Gullo L, Corinaldesi R, Casadio R, Vezzadini P, Tomassetti P, Ventrucci M, Priori P, Labò G (1983) Gastric acid secretion in chronic pancreatitis. Hepatogastroenterology 30:60–62

82. Gullo L, Parenti M, Monti L, Pezzilli R, Barbara L (1990) Diabetic retinopathy in chronic pancreatitis. Gastroenterology 98:1577–1581

83. Halgreen H, Thorsgaard Pedersen N, Worning H (1986) Symptomatic effect of pancreatic enzyme therapy in patients with chronic pancreatitis. Scand J Gastroenterol 21:104–108

84. Hansen WE (1986) Effect of dietary fiber on proteolytic pancreatic enzymes in vitro. Int J Pancreatol 1:341–351

85. Hansen WE (1987) Effect of dietary fiber on pancreatic lipase activity in vitro. Pancreas 2:195–198

86. Hansen WE, Schulz G (1982) The effect of dietary fiber on pancreatic amylase activity in vitro. Hepatogastroenterology 29:157–160

87. Hayakawa T, Kondo T, Shibata T, Sugimuto Y, Kitagawa M (1989) Chronic alcoholism and evolution of pain and prognosis in chronic pancreatitis. Dig Dis Sci 34:33–38

88. Heizer WD, Cleaveland CR, Iber FL (1965) Gastric inactivation of pancreatic supplements. Bull Johns Hopkins Hosp 116:261–270

89. Hendeles L, Dorf A, Stecenko A, Weinberger M (1990) Treatment failure after substitution of generic pancrelipase capsules. Correlation with in vitro lipase activity. JAMA 263:2459–2461

90. Hill D (1975) Pancreatic extract lung sensitivity. Med J Aust 2:553–555

91. Hinshaw DB, Jolley WB, Hinshaw DB, Kaiser JE, Hinshaw K (1981) Islet autotransplantation after pancreatectomy for chronic pancreatitis with a new method of islet preparation. Am J Surg 142:118–122

92. Holmberg JT, Isaksson G, Ihse I (1985) Long term results of pancreticojejunostomy in chronic pancreatitis. Surg Gynecol Obstet 160:339–346

93. Huibregtse K, Schneider B, Vrij AA, Tytgat GNJ (1988) Endoscopic pancreatic drainage in chronic pancreatitis. Gastrointest Endosc 34:9–15

94. Hunter JG, White TW (1991) Gastrostomy and jejunostomy using a transgastric tube for early enteral nutrition after pylorus-preserving pancreaticoduodenectomy. Surg Gynecol Obstet 173:316–318

95. Ihse I, Lilja P (1979) Pancreatic enzymic activities of commercial pancreatic enzyme preparations incubated in human small intestinal juice. Digestion 19:48–51

96. Ihse I, Lilja P, Lundquist I (1977) Feedback regulation of pancreatic enzyme secretion by intestinal trypsin in man. Digestion 15:303–308

97. Isaksson G, Ihse I (1983) Pain reduction by an oral pancreatic enzyme preparation in chronic pancreatitis. Dig Dis Sci 28:97–102

98. Isaksson G, Lilja P, Lundquist I, Ihse I (1983) Influence of dietary fiber on exocrine pancreatic function in the rat. Digestion 27:57–62

99. Isaksson G, Lundquist I, Ihse I (1982) Effect of dietary fiber on pancreatic enzyme activity in vitro. The importance of viscosity, pH, ionic strength, adsorption, and time of incubation. Gastroenterology 82:918–924

100. Jensen AR, Matzen P, Malchow-Møller A, Christoffersen I, The Copenhagen Pancreatitis Study Group (1984) Pattern of pain, duct morphology, and pancreatic function in chronic pancreatitis. A comparative study. Scand J Gastroenterol 19:334–338

101. Jordan PH, Grossman MI (1959) Effect of dosage schedule on the efficacy of substitution therapy in pancreatic insufficiency. Gastroenterology 36:447–451

102. Kalser MH, Leite CA, Warren WD (1968) Fat assimilation after massive distal pancreatectomy. N Engl J Med 279:570–576

103. Keith RG, Keshavjee SH, Kerenyi NR (1985) Neuropathology of chronic pancreatitis in humans. Can J Surg 28:207–211

104. Kozarek RA (1990) Pancreatic stents can induce ductal changes consistent with chronic pancreatitis. Gastrointest Endosc 36:93–95

105. Kozarek RA, Patterson DJ, Ball TJ, Traverso LW (1989) Endoscopic placement of pancreatic stents and drains in the management of pancreatitis. Ann Surg 209:261–266

106. Kölbel C, Layer P, Hotz J, Goebell H (1986) Der Einfluß eines säuregeschützten, mikroverkapselten Pankreatinpräparats auf die pankreatogene Steatorrhö. Med Klin 81:85–86
107. Kremer H, Dobrinski W, Schreiber MA, Zöllner N (1984) Sonographie des Abdomens als Screeningmethode. Ultraschall 5:272–276
108. Kühnelt P, Mundlos S, Adler G (1991) Einfluß der Pelletgröße eines Pankreasenzympräparates auf die duodenale lipolytische Aktivität. Z Gastroenterol 29:417–421
109. Lankisch PG (1984) Secretin test or secretin-CCK test – gold standard in pancreatic function testing? In: Gyr KE, Singer MV, Sarles H (eds) Pancreatitis – Concepts and classification. Excerpta Medica, ICS 642, Amsterdam–New York, pp 247–259
110. Lankisch PG (1991) Differential treatment of exocrine pancreatic insufficiency in chronic pancreatitis. In: Lankisch PG (ed) Pancreatic Enzymes in Health and Disease. Springer, Berlin–Heidelberg, pp 191–208
111. Lankisch PG (1993) Enzyme treatment of exocrine pancreatic insufficiency in chronic pancreatitis. Digestion 54 (Suppl 2):21–29
112. Lankisch PG (1993) Function tests in the diagnosis of chronic pancreatitis. Critical evaluation. Int J Pancreatol 14:9–20
113. Lankisch PG, Fuchs K, Peiper H-J, Creutzfeldt W (1981) Pancreatic function after drainage or resection for chronic pancreatitis. In: Mitchell CJ, Kelleher J (eds) Pancreatic disease in clinical practice. Pitman Books, London, pp 362–369
114. Lankisch PG, Fuchs K, Schmidt H, Peiper H-J, Creutzfeldt W (1975) Ergebnisse der operativen Behandlung der chronischen Pankreatitis mit besonderer Berücksichtigung der exokrinen und endokrinen Funktion. Dtsch Med Wochenschr 100:1048–1060
115. Lankisch PG, Lembcke B, Göke B, Creutzfeldt W (1986) Therapy of pancreatogenic steatorrhoea: does acid protection of pancreatic enzymes offer any advantage? Z Gastroenterol 24:753–757
116. Lankisch PG, Lembcke B, Kirchhoff S, Creutzfeldt W (1987) Therapy of pancreatogenic steatorrhea: a comparison between two acid-protected enzyme preparations. Dig Dis Sci 32:1174 (abstr)
117. Lankisch PG, Lembcke B, Kirchhoff S, Hilgers R, Creutzfeldt W (1988) Therapie der pankreatogenen Steatorrhoe. Dtsch Med Wochenschr 113:15–17
118. Lankisch PG, Lembcke B, Wemken G, Creutzfeldt W (1986) Functional reserve capacity of the exocrine pancreas. Digestion 35:175–181
119. Lankisch PG, Löhr-Happe A, Otto J, Creutzfeldt W (1993) Natural course in chronic pancreatitis. Pain, exocrine and endocrine pancreatic insufficiency and prognosis of the disease. Digestion 54:148–155
120. Lankisch PG, Siewert R (1982) Postoperative Syndrome nach operativen Eingriffen am Pankreas. Internist 23:494–502
121. Larvin M, McMahon MJ, Thomas WEG, Puntis MCA (1991) Creon (enteric coated pancreatin microspheres) for the treatment of pain in chronic pancreatitis. A double blind randomised placebo controlled crossover study. Gastroenterology 100:A283 (abstr)
122. Layer P, Go VLW, DiMagno EP (1986) Fate of pancreatic enzymes during small intestinal aboral transit in humans. Am J Physiol 251:G475–G480
123. Layer P, Gröger G, Dicke D, v.d.Ohe M, Goebell H (1992) Enzyme pellet size and luminal nutrient digestion in pancreatic insufficiency. Digestion 52:100–101 (abstr)
124. Layer P, Holtmann G (1994) Pancreatic enzymes in chronic pancreatitis. Int J Pancreatol 15:1–11
125. Layer P, Jansen JBMJ, Cherian L, Lamers CBHW, Goebell H (1990) Feedback regulation of human pancreatic secretion. Effects of protease inhibition on duodenal delivery and small intestinal transit of pancreatic enzymes. Gastroenterology 98:1311–1319
126. Leger L, Lenriot JP, Lemaigre G (1974) Five to twenty year followup after surgery for chronic pancreatitis in 148 patients. Ann Surg 180:185–191
127. Lembcke B, Kraus B, Lankisch PG (1985) Small intestinal function in chronic relapsing pancreatitis. Hepatogastroenterology 32:149–151
128. Lembcke B, Pohl M, Krackhardt B, Posselt HG (1995) A unique pattern of ileocaecal gut wall morphology related to pancreatic enzyme replacement therapy: an ultrasonography study in 200 cystic fibrosis patients. Gastroenterology 108:A369 (abstr)
129. Leung JWC, Bowen-Wright M, Aveling W, Shorvon PJ, Cotton PB (1983) Coeliac plexus block for pain in pancreatic cancer and chronic pancreatitis. Br J Surg 70:730–732

130. Lev-Ran A (1978) Clinical observation on brittle diabetes. Arch Intern Med 138:372–376
131. Levitt NS, Adams G, Salmon J, Marks INS, Musson G, Swanepoel C, Levy M, Byrne MJ (1995) The prevalence and severity of microvascular complications in pancreatic diabetes and IDDM. Diabetes Care 18:971–974
132. Liener IE, Goodale RL, Deshmukh A, Satterberg TL, Ward G, DiPietro CM, Bankey PE, Borner JW (1988) Effect of a trypsin inhibitor from soybeans (Bowman-Birk) on the secretory activity of the human pancreas. Gastroenterology 94:419–427
133. Linde J, Nilsson LH, Bárány FR (1977) Diabetes and hypoglycemia in chronic pancreatitis. Scand J Gastroenterol 12:369–373
134. Lipkin GW, Vickers DW (1987) Allergy in cystic fibrosis nurses to pancreatic extract. Lancet 1:392
135. Lloyd-Still JD (1995) Editorial: Cystic fibrosis and colonic strictures. A new "iatrogenic" disease. J Clin Gastroenterol 21:2–5
136. Lopez JJ, Wright JA, Hammer RA, Ertan A (1992) Chronic pancreatitis is associated with a high prevalence of giardiasis. Can J Gastroenterol 6:73–76
137. Löhr A (1990) Der natürliche Verlauf der chronischen Pankreatitis. Die Entwicklung der Leitsymptome Schmerzen, exokrine und endokrine Pankreasinsuffizienz und die Prognose der Erkrankung. Med Diss Göttingen
138. Mac Sweeney EJ, Oades PJ, Buchdahl R, Rosenthal M, Bush A (1995) Relation of thickening of colon wall to pancreatic-enzyme treatment in cystic fibrosis. Lancet 345:752–756
139. Madsen P, Hansen E (1985) Coeliac plexus block versus pancreaticogastrostomy for pain in chronic pancreatitis. A controlled randomized trial. Scand J Gastroenterol 20:1217–1220
140. Madsen P, Winkler K (1982) The intraductal pancreatic pressure in chronic obstructive pancreatitis. Scand J Gastroenterol 17:553–554
141. Malesci A, Gaia E, Fioretta A, Bocchia P, Ciravegna G, Cantor P, Vantini I (1995) No effect of long-term treatment with pancreatic extract on recurrent abdominal pain in patients with chronic pancreatitis. Scand J Gastroenterol 30:392–398
142. Malfertheiner P, Büchler M, Stanescu A, Ditschuneit H (1987) Pancreatic morphology and function in relationship to pain in chronic pancreatitis. Int J Pancreatol 2:59–66
143. Malfertheiner P, Mayer D, Büchler M, Domínguez-Muñoz JE, Schiefer B, Ditschuneit H (1995) Treatment of pain in chronic pancreatitis by inhibition of pancreatic secretion with octreotide. Gut 36:450–454
144. Mangold G, Neher M, Oswald B, Wagner G (1977) Ergebnisse der Resektionsbehandlung der chronischen Pankreatitis. Dtsch Med Wochenschr 102:229–234
145. Mannell A, Adson MA, McIlrath DC, Ilstrup DM (1988) Surgical management of chronic pancreatitis: long-term results in 141 patients. Br J Surg 75:467–472
146. McHugh K, Thomson A, Tam P (1994) Case report: Colonic stricture and fibrosis associated with high-strength pancreatic enzymes in a child with cystic fibrosis. Br J Radiol 67:900–901
147. Mehigan DG, Bell WR, Zuidema GD, Eggleston JC, Cameron JL (1980) Disseminated intravascular coagulation and portal hypertension following pancreatic islet autotransplantation. Ann Surg 191:287–293
148. Meyer JH (1991) Delivery of pancreatin in microsphere preparations: transit, timing, physiological needs. In: Lankisch PG (ed) Pancreatic Enzymes in Health and Disease. Springer, Berlin–Heidelberg, pp 71–88
149. Meyer JH, Elashoff J, Porter-Fink V, Dressman J, Amidon GL (1988) Human postprandial gastric emptying of 1–3-millimeter spheres. Gastroenterology 94:1315–1325
150. Mizumoto A, Koike D, Sarr MG, DiMagno EP (1994) How important is mixing of lipase and nutrients in decreasing pancreatic steatorrhea? Gastroenterology 106:A308 (abstr)
151. Morrow CE, Cohen JI, Sutherland DER, Najarian JS (1984) Chronic pancreatitis: long-term surgical results of pancreatic duct drainage, pancreatic resection, and near-total pancreatectomy and islet autotransplantation. Surgery 96:608–616
152. Mössner J, Secknus R, Meyer J, Niederau C, Adler G (1992) Treatment of pain with pancreatic extracts in chronic pancreatitis: results of a prospective placebo-controlled multicenter trial. Digestion 53:54–66
153. Mössner J, Wresky HP, Back T (1990) Does feedback regulation exist in chronic pancreatitis? In: Beger HG, Büchler M, Ditschuneit H, Malfertheiner P (eds) Chronic Pancreatitis. Springer, Berlin–Heidelberg, pp 198–209

154. Mundlos S, Kühnelt P, Adler G (1990) Monitoring enzyme replacement treatment in exocrine pancreatic insufficiency using the cholesteryl octanoate breath test. Gut 31:1324–1328

155. Najarian JS, Sutherland DER, Baumgartner D, Burke B, Rynasiewicz JJ, Matas AJ, Goetz FC (1980) Total or near total pancreatectomy and islet autotransplantation for treatment of chronic pancreatitis. Ann Surg 192:526–542

156. Nealon WH, Thompson JC (1993) Progressive loss of pancreatic function in chronic pancreatitis is delayed by main pancreatic duct decompression. A longitudinal prospective analysis of the modified Puestow procedure. Ann Surg 217:458–468

157. Nealon WH, Townsend CM Jr, Thompson JC (1988) Operative drainage of the pancreatic duct delays functional impairment in patients with chronic pancreatitis. A prospective analysis. Ann Surg 208:321–329

158. Neuhaus H, Hoffmann W, Classen M (1992) Laser lithotripsy of pancreatic and biliary stones via 3.4 mm and 3.7 mm miniscopes: first clinical results. Endoscopy 24:208–214

159. Niessen KH, Wolf A (1982) Studies on the cause of hyperuricosuria in cystic fibrosis patients. J Pediatr Gastroenterol Nutr 1:349–354

160. Nousia-Arvanitakis S, Stapleton FB, Linshaw MA, Kennedy J (1977) Therapeutic approach to pancreatic extract-induced hyperuricosuria in cystic fibrosis. Pediatrics 90:302–305

161. Novis BH, Bornman PC, Girdwood AW, Marks IN (1985) Endoscopic manometry of the pancreatic duct and sphincter zone in patients with chronic pancreatitis. Dig Dis Sci 30:225–228

162. Ogden JM, O'Keefe SJD, Louw JA, Adams G, Marks IN (1993) Duodenal juice total protein and pancreatic enzyme synthesis, turnover, and secretion in patients after acute pancreatitis. Gut 34:1261–1266

163. Okazaki K, Yamamoto Y, Kagiyama S, Tamura S, Sakamoto Y, Morita M (1988) Pressure of papillary sphincter zone and pancreatic main duct in patients with alcoholic and idiopathic chronic pancreatitis. Int J Pancreatol 3:457–468

164. Owyang C, Louie DS, Tatum D (1986) Feedback regulation of pancreatic enzyme secretion. Suppression of cholecystokinin release by trypsin. J Clin Invest 77:2042–2047

165. Pap A, Nauss LA, DiMagno EP (1990) Is percutaneous celiac plexus block (PCPB) associated with pain relief in chronic pancreatitis? A comparison among analgesic, alcohol and steroid PCPB. Pancreas 5:725 (abstr)

166. Peiper H-J, Köhler H (1989) Chirurgische Therapie der chronischen Pankreatitis. Schweiz Med Wochenschr 119:712–716

167. Peschke GJ (1991) Active components and galenic aspects of enzyme preparations. In: Lankisch PG (ed) Pancreatic Enzymes in Health and Disease. Springer, Berlin–Heidelberg, pp 55–64

168. Prinz RA, Greenlee HB (1981) Pancreatic duct drainage in 100 patients with chronic pancreatitis. Ann Surg 194:313–320

169. Proctor HJ, Mendes OC, Thomas CG Jr, Herbst CA (1979) Surgery for chronic pancreatitis. Drainage versus resection. Ann Surg 189:664–671

170. Raimondo M, DiMagno EP (1994) Lipolytic activity of bacterial lipase survives better than that of porcine lipase in human gastric and duodenal content. Gastroenterology 107:231–235

171. Rämö OJ, Puolakkainen PA, Seppälä K, Schröder TM (1989) Self-administration of enzyme substitution in the treatment of exocrine pancreatic insufficiency. Scand J Gastroenterol 24:688–692

172. Regan PT, DiMagno EP (1980) Exocrine pancreatic insufficiency in celiac sprue: a cause of treatment failure. Gastroenterology 78:484–487

173. Regan PT, Malagelada J-R, DiMagno EP, Glanzman SL, Go VLW (1977) Comparative effects of antacids, cimetidine and enteric coating on the therapeutic response to oral enzymes in severe pancreatic insufficiency. N Engl J Med 297:854–858

174. Regan PT, Malagelada J-R, DiMagno EP, Go VLW (1979) Reduced intraluminal bile acid concentrations and fat maldigestion in pancreatic insufficiency: correction by treatment. Gastroenterology 77:285–289

175. Ribet A, Balas D, Bommelaer G, Pradayrol L, Varignon M (1979) Activité enzymatique "in vitro" de différents extraits pancréatiques. Gastroenterol Clin Biol 3:515–520

176. Roberts IM (1989) Enzyme therapy for malabsorption in exocrine pancreatic insufficiency. Pancreas 4:496–503

177. Rolny P, Ärlebäck A, Järnerot G, Andersson T (1986) Endoscopic manometry of the sphincter of Oddi and pancreatic duct in chronic pancreatitis. Scand J Gastroenterol 21:415–420

178. Rolny P, Ferstenberg R, Hogan WJ, Geenen JE (1990) Pancreatic exocrine function in patients with ductal alterations associated with endoscopic stent placement. Gastroenterology 98:A232 (abstr)

179. Rosenberger J, Stock W, Altmann P, Pichlmaier H (1980) Spätergebnisse nach organerhaltenden und resezierenden Eingriffen wegen chronischer Pankreatitis. Leber Magen Darm 10:22–27

180. Rossi RL, Rothschild J, Braasch JW, Munson JL, ReMine SG (1987) Pancreatoduodenectomy in the management of chronic pancreatitis. Arch Surg 122:416–420

181. Sakula A (1977) Bronchial asthma due to allergy to pancreatic extract. Lancet 2:193

182. Sarles H, Pastor J, Pauli AM, Barthelemy M (1963) Determination of pancreatic function. A statistical analysis conducted in normal subjects and in patients with proven chronic pancreatitis (duodenal intubation, glucose tolerance test, determination of fat content in the stools, sweat test). Gastroenterologia 99:279–300

183. Sarles H, Sahel J (1976) Die chronische Pankreatitis. In: Forell M (ed) Handbuch der Inneren Medizin, Vol. 3/6, Pankreas. 5th edn. Springer, Berlin–Heidelberg–New York, pp 737–844

184. Sato T, Miyashita E, Matsuno S, Yamauchi H (1986) The role of surgical treatment for chronic pancreatitis. Ann Surg 203:266–271

185. Sato T, Noto N, Matsuno S, Miyakawa K (1981) Follow-up results of surgical treatment for chronic pancreatitis. Present status in Japan. Am J Surg 142:317–323

186. Sauerbruch T, Holl J, Sackmann M, Paumgartner G (1989) Extracorporeal shock wave lithotripsy of pancreatic stones. Gut 30:1406–1411

187. Saunders JHB, Cargill JM, Wormsley KG (1978) Gastric secretion of acid in patients with pancreatic disease. Digestion 17:365–369

188. Schneider MU, Domschke S, Heptner G, Domschke W (1984) Einfluß von Pflanzenfasern auf die lipolytische und proteolytische exokrine Pankreasfunktion. Dtsch Med Wochenschr 109:250–253

189. Sherman S, Lehman GA, Hawes RH, Ponich T, Miller LS, Cohen LB, Kortan P, Haber GB (1991) Pancreatic ductal stones: frequency of successful endoscopic removal and improvement in symptoms. Gastrointest Endosc 37:511–517

190. Slaff J, Jacobson D, Tillman CR, Curington C, Toskes P (1984) Protease-specific suppression of pancreatic exocrine secretion. Gastroenterology 87:44–52

191. Smyth RL, van Velzen D, Smyth AR, Lloyd DA, Heaf DP (1994) Strictures of ascending colon in cystic fibrosis and high-strength pancreatic enzymes. Lancet 343:85–86

192. Stapleton FB, Kennedy J, Nousia-Arvanitakis S, Linshaw MA (1976) Hyperuricosuria due to high-dose pancreatic extract therapy in cystic fibrosis. N Engl J Med 295:246–248

193. Staritz M, Meyer zum Büschenfelde KH (1988) Elevated pressure in the dorsal part of pancreas divisum: the cause of chronic pancreatitis? Pancreas 3:108–110

194. Staub JL, Sarles H, Soule JC, Galmiche JP, Capron JP (1981) No effect of cimetidine on the therapeutic response to oral enzymes in severe pancreatic insufficiency. N Engl J Med 304:1364–1365

195. Stead RJ, Skypala I, Hodson ME (1988) Treatment of steatorrhea in cystic fibrosis: a comparison of enteric-coated microspheres of pancreatin versus non-enteric-coated pancreatin and adjuvant cimetidine. Aliment Pharmacol Ther 2:471–482

196. Stead RJ, Skypala I, Hodson ME, Batten JC (1987) Enteric coated microspheres of pancreatin in the treatment of cystic fibrosis: comparison with a standard enteric coated preparation. Thorax 42:533–537

197. Stone WM, Sarr MG, Nagorney DM, Mellrath DC (1988) Chronic pancreatitis. Results of Whipple's resection and total pancreatectomy. Arch Surg 123:815–819

198. Taylor CJ, Steiner GM (1995) Fibrosing colonopathy in a child on low-dose pancreatin. Lancet 346:1106–1107

199. Taylor RH, Bagley FH, Braasch JW, Warren KW (1981) Ductal drainage or resection for chronic pancreatitis. Am J Surg 141:28–33

200. Thiruvengadam R, DiMagno EP (1988) Inactivation of human lipase by proteases. Am J Physiol 255:G476–G481

201. Toledo-Pereyra LH (1983) Islet cell autotransplantation after subtotal pancreatectomy. Arch Surg 118:851–858

202. Traverso LW, Abou-Zamzam AM, Longmire WP Jr (1981) Human pancreatic cell autotransplantation following total pancreatectomy. Ann Surg 193:191–195

203. Twarog FJ, Weinstein SF, Khaw KT, Strieder DJ, Colten HR (1977) Hypersensitivity to pancreatic extracts in parents of patients with cystic fibrosis. J Allergy Clin Immunol 59:35–40
204. Ventrucci M, Gullo L, Costa PL, Bolondi L, Caletti GC, Corcioni E, Nesticò V (1980) Relation between pancreatic lipase and steatorrhoea in pancreatic disease. Ital J Gastroenterol 12:76–78
205. Walsh DB, Eckhauser FE, Cronenwett JL, Turcotte JG, Lindenauer SM (1982) Adenocarcinoma of the ampulla of Vater. Ann Surg 195:152–157
206. Warshaw AL, Torchiana DL (1985) Delayed gastric emptying after pylorus-preserving pancreaticoduodenectomy. Surg Gynecol Obstet 160:1–4
207. Way LW, Gadacz T, Goldman L (1974) Surgical treatment of chronic pancreatitis. Am J Surg 127:202–209
208. White TT (1981) Surgical treatment of chronic pancreatitis. Report of 227 cases. Jpn J Surg 11: 1–7
209. Williamson RCN, Bliouras N, Cooper MJ, Davies ER (1993) Gastric emptying and enterogastric reflux after conservative and conventional pancreatoduodenectomy. Surgery 114:82–86
210. Wright JA, Lopez J, Daum RS, Ertan A (1988) Chronic pancreatitis is associated with a high prevalence of giardiasis. Gastroenterology 94:A503 (abstr)
211. Yeo CJ, Barry MK, Sauter PK, Sostre S, Lillemoe KD, Pitt HA, Cameron JL (1993) Erythromycin accelerates gastric emptying after pancreaticoduodenectomy. A prospective, randomized, placebo-controlled trial. Ann Surg 218:229–238
212. Zempsky WT, Rosenstein BJ, Carroll JA, Oski FA (1989) Effect of pancreatic enzyme supplements on iron absorption. Am J Dis Child 143:969–972
213. Zentler-Munro PL, Fine DR, Northfield TC (1981) Mechanism whereby cimetidine enhances pancreatic enzyme therapy. Gastroenterology 80:1323
214. Zerega J, Lerner S, Meyer JH (1988) Duodenal instillation of pancreatin does not abolish steatorrhea in patients with pancreatic insufficiency. Dig Dis Sci 33:1245–1249

20 Chronic Pancreatitis: Prognosis

20.1
Introduction

The three leading problems of chronic pancreatitis are pain, exocrine and endocrine pancreatic insufficiency. They, along with numerous pancreatic complications and/or pancreatitis-associated diseases, affect the course and determine the prognosis of chronic pancreatitis. Their exact influence, however, has not yet been fully investigated. Only a few long-term studies have correlated the three leading problems with the course of the disease.

20.2
Pain

20.2.1
Painless Pancreatitis

Chronic pancreatitis takes a primarily painless course in a minority of patients, i.e., 5.8%–20% [5, 7, 17, 25, 26, 32, 41]. The leading symptoms for such patients are related to exocrine and endocrine pancreatic insufficiency.

For the majority of patients, however, pain is the decisive symptom, causing much discomfort in their daily lives.

20.2.2
Does Pain Decrease Differently in the Alcohol-induced
and Idiopathic Chronic Pancreatitis?

At present, this question cannot definitely be answered. Ammann et al. [4, 6] reported a high incidence of a painless clinical course of the disease in patients with nonalcoholic compared to patients with alcohol-induced chronic pancreatitis. Lankisch et al. [33] found no differences between alcoholics and nonalcoholics concerning the course of pain. Recently, Layer et al. [34] reported two distinct forms of idiopathic chronic pancreatitis. Patients with early-onset pancreatitis experienced a long course of severe pain, and developed morphological and functional pancreatic damage more slowly than patients with alcoholic pancreatitis. Patients with late-onset pancreatitis had a mild and often painless course. Both forms differed from alcoholic pancreatitis in that the gender distribution was equal and calcification occurred in a much slower rate. Further studies are required.

20.2.3
Does Pain Decrease With the Duration of the Disease?

Whether progressive parenchymal destruction (burning-out of the gland) leads, in the long run, to a decrease of pain has been repeatedly debated [1, 2]. The studies from the Zurich group [3, 5, 8] have shown that pain decreases with increasing duration of the disease. In one long-term study, 85% of 145 patients with chronic pancreatitis felt no more pain after a 4.5 years' (median) duration of the disease. Furthermore, an increasing incidence of patients with pancreatic calcifications was observed along with a steady decrease of exocrine pancreatic insufficiency [5].

These two reports are at variance with two other more recent studies. Miyake et al. [41] found that only 48.2% of the patients with chronic pancreatitis became free of pain within 5 years, and 66%–73% after more than 5 years. That meant that every third or fourth patient still suffered from relapsing pain attacks, even after a longer observation time. Lankisch et al. [32] reported that the incidence of relapsing pain attacks decreased during the observation period, but more than half of the patients (53%) still suffered from relapsing pain attacks even after a more than 10 years' observation (Table 20.1). Finally, Layer et al. [34] reported that in alcoholics pain decreased or disappeared in 77% of the patients after 14 years of observation, whereas the corresponding percentages were 67% and 64% for early and late idiopathic onset after 27 and 13 years, respectively.

20.2.4
Does Pain Decrease With Progressing Exocrine Pancreatic Insufficiency?

Ammann and coworkers in Zurich [1–3, 8] repeatedly observed a decrease in pain as exocrine and endocrine pancreatic function declined. Similarly, Girdwood et al. [24]

Table 20.1. Pain in relation to the duration of the disease in 311 patients with initially painful chronic pancreatitis. With increasing observation time, the number of patients still having attacks of pain or becoming free from pain changed significantly ($p < 0.0001$). Even after follow-up for more than 10 years, the majority of patients (81/152: 53%) still suffered from pain [32]

Follow-up (years)	n	Patients still having attacks of pain ($n = 202$)	Patients who became free from pain ($n = 109$)
<5	79	67 (33%)	12 (11%)
5–10	80	54 (27%)	26 (24%)
>10	152	81 (40%)	71 (65%)

Table 20.2. Influence of exocrine pancreatic insufficiency on pain in 311 patients with initially painful chronic pancreatitis. At the end of observation, exocrine pancreatic insufficiency differed significantly between patients with persisting pain and those having obtained pain relief ($p=0.03$). The majority of patients with severe exocrine pancreatic insufficiency (81/141: 57%) still suffered from pain [32]

Exocrine pancreatic insufficiency ($n=311$)	n	At end of observation period	
		Persisting pain ($n=202$)	Pain relief ($n=109$)
Mild	78 (25%)	53 (26%)	25 (23%)
Moderate	92 (30%)	68 (34%)	24 (22%)
Severe	141 (45%)	81 (40%)	60 (55%)

reported that pain decreased as exocrine pancreatic function deteriorated, independent of pancreatic duct changes and alcohol abuse.

Thorsgaard Pedersen et al. [45] in Copenhagen, however, found no correlation between pain and exocrine pancreatic function.

Similarly, in a more recent study, the influence of exocrine pancreatic insufficiency on pain was limited [32]. Instead of using chymotrypsin measurements, as was done in Zurich [5], Lankisch et al. [32] used in their study the secretin-pancreozymin test and fecal fat analysis to evaluate exocrine pancreatic insufficiency. Mild exocrine pancreatic insufficiency was defined as reduced enzyme output; moderate, as a decreased bicarbonate concentration along with reduced enzyme output but normal fecal fat excretion; and severe exocrine pancreatic insufficiency was equated with an abnormal secretin-pancreozymin test plus steatorrhea. At the end of observation period, the majority (57%) of patients with severe pancreatic insufficiency still had relapsing pain attacks (Table 20.2) [32].

20.2.5
Does Pain Decrease When Pancreatic Calcifications and/or Duct Abnormalities Occur?

Ammann et al. [5, 8] showed that the development of pancreatic calcifications was associated with decrease in pain.

This result is at variance with several other studies. Malfertheiner et al. [40] found that 89% of patients had pain despite pancreatic calcifications observed on computed tomography, and 39% very intense pain. In two further studies, the incidence of patients free of pain was higher in the group in which calcifications were seen [31,32]. Finally, Ammann et al. [9] found that pancreatic calcifications may decrease in the course of the disease. Therefore, the prognostic role of pancreatic calcifications and their influence on the course of pain in chronic pancreatitis is presently uncertain.

Ebbehøj et al. [19, 20] measured percutaneously or intraoperatively pancreatic tissue fluid pressure and found a significant correlation between pressure and pain, but not between pressure and pancreatic duct diameter as measured by endoscopic retrograde cholangiopancreatography (ERCP) in patients with chronic pancreatitis. In a variety of studies, the correlation between pain and pancreatic duct changes demonstrated by ERCP or measured duct pressure has been imprecise. Whereas Bradley [14] intraoperatively found increased pancreatic duct pressure in patients with painful chronic pancreatitis, Jensen et al. [29] found no correlation between pancreatic duct changes and pain. Warshaw et al. [50] found in 2 of 10 of his patients, 1 year after a lateral pancreaticojejunostomy, no pain relief in spite of a patent anastomosis detected by ERCP. Two recent investigations confirmed the nonparallelism between pancreatic duct changes and pain relief. Malfertheiner et al. [40] reported severe pain in only 62% of patients who had advanced pancreatic duct changes demonstrated by ERCP. Lankisch et al. [32] found no significant correlation between pancreatic duct abnormalities detected by ERCP, and pain in 88 patients with chronic pancreatitis. Severe pancreatic duct abnormalities – as defined by the Cambridge classification [11] – were present in 42 patients, but only 16 (31%) of these became free of pain. Despite a normal pancreatic duct in 14 patients, 10 (71%) of them suffered from persisting pain (Table 20.3) [32].

Thus, morphological changes, such as pancreatic calcifications or pancreatic duct abnormalities, are not necessarily helpful in establishing prognosis of chronic pancreatitis or predicting the course of pain.

20.2.6
Does Pain Decrease With Alcohol Abstinence?

In regard to alcoholism, the leading etiological factor in chronic pancreatitis, it is unclear whether alcohol abstinence influences pain or the progression of the disease. When alcohol was discontinued, 50% of the patients with chronic pancreatitis in one study [42] and 75% in another [48] experienced relief of pain.

Two recent investigations confirmed that abstinence can be helpful: Miyake et al. [41] demonstrated pain relief in 60% of their patients who discontinued or reduced alcohol intake, whereas in the group of patients who continued drinking, spontaneous pain relief was only 26%. In another study [32], pain relief occurred in 52% of patients who discontinued alcohol and only in 37% who continued to consume alcohol. Thus,

Table 20.3. Pancreatic duct abnormalities upon endoscopic retrograde cholangiopancreatography (ERCP) and pain in 88 patients with chronic pancreatitis. Pain was independent of duct abnormalities ($p = 0.45$, not significant) [32]

Pancreatic duct abnormalities ($n = 88$)	n	At end of observation period	
		Persisting pain ($n = 60$)	Pain relief ($n = 28$)
Absent	14 (16%)	10 (17%)	4 (14%)
Mild	3 (3%)	2 (3%)	1 (4%)
Moderate	29 (33%)	22 (37%)	7 (25%)
Severe	42 (48%)	26 (43%)	16 (57%)

alcohol abstinence may lead to improvement of pain, but why in some cases, but not in others, remains to be investigated.

20.2.7
Does Pain Decrease After Surgery?

Whether surgery or conservative treatment should be utilized in cases of severe pain in chronic pancreatitis is a controversial and much discussed point [5, 50].

It is clear, however, that surgical treatment is necessary in every second to fourth patient due to pain and/or to complications such as pancreatic pseudocysts [5, 32]. The influence of surgical treatment on pain is difficult to evaluate, as well as comparison between the different studies, because of the following reasons:
- The definition of freedom of pain is often vague. Pain is usually not measured, for example on an analogue scale.
- Not all patients received the same surgical treatment for the same indication. Several authors recommend not performing an indicated resection operation in alcoholics because of the postoperatively difficult treatment of diabetes mellitus in these patients [21, 51].
- Continued alcohol abuse distinctly worsens the effect of surgical treatment [15, 28, 35]. It is, therefore, difficult to decide whether a postoperative deterioration results from chronic pancreatitis, or from continued alcohol abuse, or from the surgical treatment.
- In the course of a longer follow-up, pain increases (see Table 19.7) [44]. Thus, an initial beneficial effect may be misleading.

The choice of the surgical procedure is definitely dependent on the special circumstances of each patient. Earlier reports on postoperative results show that independent of the surgical procedure freedom of pain will be obtained in up to 100% of the cases over several years of follow-up (see Table 19.8).

20.3
Exocrine Pancreatic Insufficiency

Compared to pain, exocrine pancreatic insufficiency does not play a major prognostic role. Occasionally, massive steatorrhea leading to cachexia and susceptibility to infection has prognostic significance.

There is controversy regarding the deterioration of exocrine pancreatic insufficiency in the course of the disease. Ammann et al. [5] found that severe exocrine pancreatic insufficiency (defined as fecal chymotrypsin < 40 µg/g) developed within 5.65 years (median) in 122 (84.1%) of·145 patients, whereas Thorsgaard Pedersen et al. [45] observed no significant changes in their patients. According to reports by Lankisch et al. [32] on secretin-pancreozymin tests in 143 patients, exocrine pancreatic insufficiency may not be progressive. In 66 (46.2%) patients the degree of severity of exocrine pancreatic insufficiency remained unchanged, whereas in 61 (42.6%) patients there was deterioration. Functional improvement was even seen in 16 (11.2%) of their patients, several of whom required no more pancreatic enzyme substitution.

Several other studies furnish evidence of functional improvement in exocrine pancreatic insufficiency in chronic pancreatitis [13, 22, 31, 41]. Improvement was observed in patients, who stopped drinking and/or in whom exocrine pancreatic insufficiency was moderate, not severe, prior to conservative and/or surgical treatment [32].

20.4
Endocrine Pancreatic Insufficiency

The course of endocrine pancreatic insufficiency differs from that of exocrine pancreatic insufficiency. Whereas the latter is present in all patients upon onset of the symptoms of chronic pancreatitis, endocrine pancreatic insufficiency may be absent. In a recent study, only 28 (8%) of 335 patients suffered at the start of the observation time from diabetes mellitus, of whom the majority needed insulin treatment. After a 9.8 years' (median) observation time, the incidence of diabetes had increased 10-fold: 260 (78%) patients suffered from diabetes and 51 of them needed insulin treatment. Remarkably, 75 (22%) patients still had no diabetes (Table 20.4). A comparison of the severity of exocrine and endocrine pancreatic insufficiency showed that the degree of insufficiency was not parallel. Only 46 (45%) of 102 patients with severe exocrine pancreatic insufficiency also had severe endocrine pancreatic failure. On the other hand, only 46 (67%) of 69 patients with severe endocrine pancreatic insufficiency also had severe exocrine pancreatic failure (Fig. 20.1) [32].

Endocrine complication of chronic pancreatitis may play a major prognostic role, especially after surgical treatment of chronic pancreatitis, because of hypoglycemia [37]. Hypoglycemia frequently occurs after subtotal left-sided pancreatic resection [21] and may contribute to an unfavorable prognosis.

The frequency of some complications of diabetes mellitus secondary to chronic pancreatitis has been studied. Earlier investigations suggested that diabetic retinopathy was a rare complication of pancreatogenic diabetes, occurring in 7.4%–18% [18, 43, 49]. More recently, Tiengo et al. [46] and Couet et al. [16] had found retinopathy in 31% and 41%, respectively, of patients with chronic pancreatitis. Finally, Gullo et al. [27] have shown that the risk of retinopathy in patients with diabetes caused by chronic pancreatitis is the same as in patients with type I diabetes. About half of the patients studied in both groups had retinopathy, that occurred particularly in longstanding diabetes.

Table 20.4. Endocrine pancreatic insufficiency in 335 patients with chronic pancreatitis [32]

Endocrine pancreatic insufficiency	At onset of disease	At end of observation
Absent	307 (92%)	75 (22%)
Present	28 (8%)	260 (78%)
– Moderate	13 (4%)	127 (38%)
– Severe	15 (4%)	133 (40%)

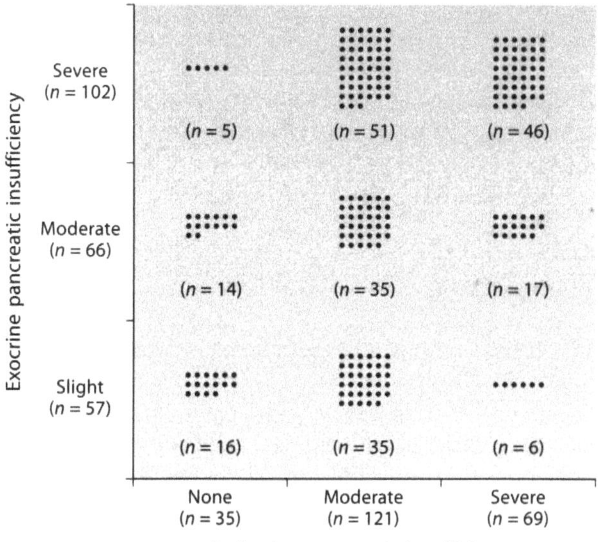

Fig. 20.1. Comparison of the severity of exocrine and endocrine pancreatic insufficiency in 214 patients with chronic pancreatitis. The degree of insufficiency was not parallel ($p = 0.001$). Double investigations were also considered so that 225 cases were evaluated. (From [32] with permission)

Similarly, in 1995, Levitt et al. [36] have shown that microvascular complications (retinopathy, nephropathy) in pancreatic diabetes and insulin-dependent diabetes mellitus are equally common and severe.

Nondiabetic retinal lesions and retinal function abnormalities are also common in patients with chronic pancreatitis, even in the absence of steatorrhea [47].

Electrocardiographic evidence of ischemic heart disease has been reported in 18% [30] and diabetic neuropathy in about 30% [12] of patients with chronic pancreatitis. Finally, arteriopathy has the same prevalence and distribution in chronic pancreatitis and idiopathic diabetes [53].

Whether these complications have major prognostic significance has not yet been investigated.

20.5
Complications

The list of complications in chronic pancreatitis includes pancreatic pseudocysts and abscesses, stenosis of the common bile duct, the duodenum, and the colon, development of pleural or pericardial effusions, ascites, and gastrointestinal bleeding. All of these complications surely have severe implications for the prognosis of the disease. However, since these have not been dealt with in larger studies, the exact influence on the outcome of the disease is even less certain.

20.6
Pancreatic and Extrapancreatic Carcinomas

Pancreatic carcinoma (see Sect. 18.2.5) and extrapancreatic carcinomas (see Sect. 18.3.11) are not rare events and limit the prognosis of a patient with chronic pancreatitis.

20.7
Quality of Life

In comparison with the three dominant symptoms of chronic pancreatitis, other symptoms have received little attention. The frequency of problems such as diarrhea and weight loss is hardly mentioned in the literature. It seems, however, that more than half of the patients, even during a lengthy observation period, were of normal body weight or even overweight [52]. About half of the patients had at no point suffered from any mentionable diarrhea [32, 39]. This is in agreement with figures by Creutzfeldt et al. [17] and Andersen et al. [10]. Both observed diarrhea in 42%, and 27%, respectively, mainly caused by exocrine pancreatic insufficiency with steatorrhea.

Some general attention has been paid to the socioeconomic situation of the patients. Gastard et al. [23] found that 1 out of 2 male patients continued to work normally, in spite of pain or diabetes; 1 out of 3 was regarded as unfit for regular work, being totally incapacitated or absent from work for more than 3 months a year. The figures improved after the 15th year due to the death of patients with severe forms of the disease; at this stage, 68% of the patients were working regularly, and 6% were totally incapacitated. Thorsgaard Pedersen et al. [45] found a decline during an observation period of 5 years (median). Only 15 (40%) of their 38 surviving patients still worked, whereas the remaining were either on prolonged sickleave or retired. Miyake et al. [41] reported that while 63 (71%) of their 89 patients continued to work, almost all other patients, who were either retired or who suffered socioeconomically, continued their alcohol abuse. In a recent study [32], the incidence of unemployed patients increased from 3% to 15%, and that of the retired, from 3% to 25% during an observation time of about 11 years. Almost half of the retirements were due to pancreatitis.

20.8
Mortality

Data on the mortality rate in chronic pancreatitis are difficult to interpret since etiology and mean observation times vary from study to study. Three studies with a comparatively similar observation time (median 6.3–9.8 years) reveal a general mortality rate of 20.8%–35%, but the mortality rate when related to chronic pancreatitis was of only 12.8%–19.8% [5, 32, 41]. Continued alcohol abuse after conservative and/or surgical treatment has been associated with significantly lower survival rates (Figs. 20.2, 20.3) [5, 21, 32, 41, 51].

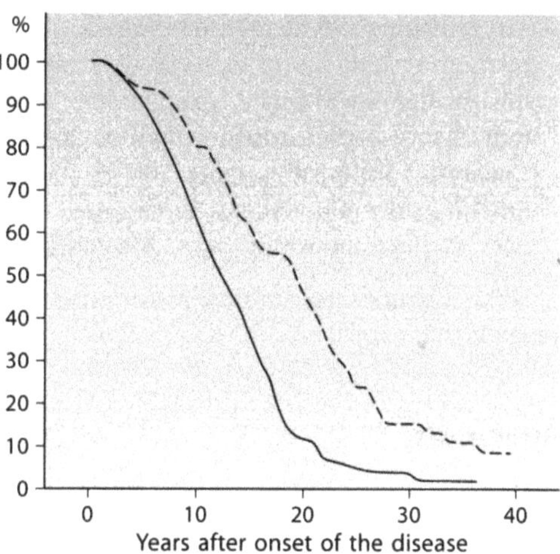

Fig. 20.2. Cumulative survival curve for 230 patients with alcoholic (*continuous line*) and 105 patients with nonalcoholic (*broken line*) chronic pancreatitis ($p=0.0001$). The mean age of onset of the disease (i.e., first pancreatitis-related symptoms) was 37 ± 9 (mean$\pm$SD) years in patients with alcoholic and 39 ± 17 in patients with nonalcoholic chronic pancreatitis. (From [32] with permission)

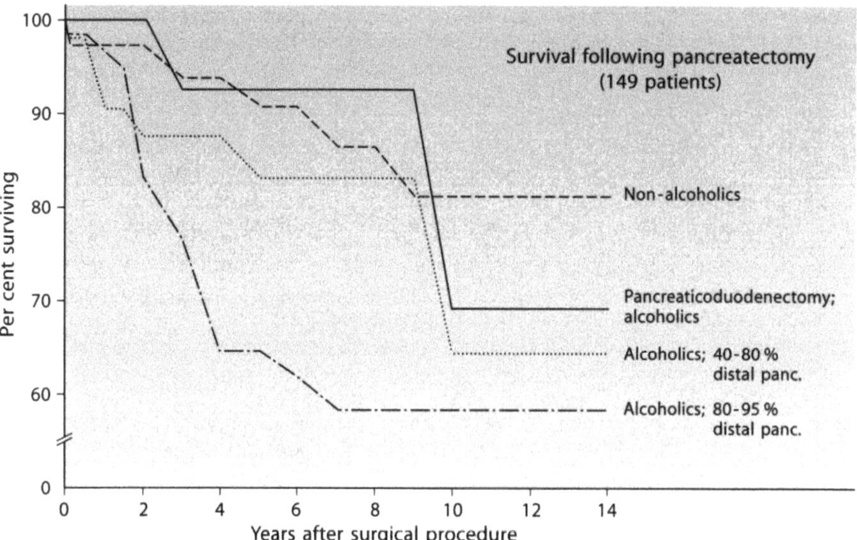

Fig. 20.3. Survival rate of 149 alcoholics and nonalcoholics with chronic pancreatitis following surgical therapy. In the majority of nonalcoholics, an 80%–95% distal pancreatectomy (panc.) was performed. (From [21] with permission)

20.9
Factors of Prognosis

The prognosis of chronic pancreatitis is independent of conservative or surgical treatment. A multicenter investigation in 7 hospitals of 6 countries including 2015 patients with chronic pancreatitis shows that mortality rate was 3.6-fold higher than in patients without pancreatitis. The 10-years' survival rate was 70%, the 20-years' survival rate 45%, as compared to 93%, and 65%, respectively, in patients without pancreatitis.

The following risk factors were found:
- Medium or high age at the time of diagnosis. The mortality rate in patients medium- or high-aged was 2.3-fold, and 6.3-fold, respectively, higher than in patients with chronic pancreatitis in whom the disease was diagnosed before the age 40
- Consistent alcohol abuse: mortality risk 1.6-fold higher
- Smoking: mortality risk 1.4-fold higher
- Liver cirrhosis: mortality rate 2.5-fold higher

Neither gender nor surgical history had any influence on the prognosis of the disease [38].

References

1. Ammann R (1970) Die Behandlung der chronischen Pankreatitis. Dtsch Med Wochenschr 95: 1234–1235
2. Ammann R (1970) Die chronische Pankreatitis. Zur Frage der Operationsindikation und Beitrag zum Spontanverlauf der chronisch-rezidivierenden Pankreatitis. Dtsch Med Wochenschr 95:1–7
3. Ammann R (1989) Klinik, Spontanverlauf und Therapie der chronischen Pankreatitis. Unter spezieller Berücksichtigung der Nomenklaturprobleme. Schweiz Med Wochenschr 119:696–706
4. Ammann RW (1992) Alcohol- and non-alcohol-induced pancreatitis: clinical aspects. In: Burns GP, Bank S (eds) Disorders of the Pancreas. Current Issues in Diagnosis and Management. McGraw-Hill, New York, pp 253–272
5. Ammann RW, Akovbiantz A, Largiadèr F, Schueler G (1984) Course and outcome of chronic pancreatitis. Longitudinal study of a mixed medical-surgical series of 245 patients. Gastroenterology 86:820–828
6. Ammann RW, Buehler H, Muench R, Freiburghaus AW, Siegenthaler W (1987) Differences in the natural history of idiopathic (nonalcoholic) and alcoholic chronic pancreatitis. A comparative long-term study of 287 patients. Pancreas 2:368–377
7. Ammann RW, Hammer B, Fumagalli I (1973) Chronic pancreatitis in Zurich, 1963–1972. Clinical findings and follow-up studies of 102 cases. Digestion 9:404–415
8. Ammann RW, Largiadèr F, Akovbiantz A (1979) Pain relief by surgery in chronic pancreatitis? Relationship between pain relief, pancreatic dysfunction, and alcohol withdrawal. Scand J Gastroenterol 14:209–215
9. Ammann RW, Muench R, Otto R, Buehler H, Freiburghaus AU, Siegenthaler W (1988) Evolution and regression of pancreatic calcification in chronic pancreatitis. A prospective long-term study of 107 patients. Gastroenterology 95:1018–1028
10. Andersen BN, Scheel J, Rune SJ, Worning H (1982) Exocrine pancreatic function in patients with dyspepsia. Hepatogastroenterology 29:35–37
11. Axon ATR, Classen M, Cotton PB, Cremer M, Freeny PC, Lees WR (1984) Pancreatography in chronic pancreatitis: international definitions. Gut 25:1107–1112
12. Bank S, Marks IN, Vinik AI (1975) Clinical and hormonal aspects of pancreatic diabetes. Am J Gastroenterol 64:13–22
13. Begley CG, Roberts-Thomson IC (1985) Spontaneous improvement in pancreatic function in chronic pancreatitis. Dig Dis Sci 30:1117–1120
14. Bradley III EL (1982) Pancreatic duct pressure in chronic pancreatitis. Am J Surg 144:313–316
15. Capitaine Y, Roche B, Wiesner L, Hahnloser P (1988) Pancréatite chronique: histoire naturelle et évolution en relation avec l'alcoolisme. Schweiz Med Wochenschr 118:817–820
16. Couet C, Genton P, Pointel JP, Louis J, Gross P, Saudax E, Debry G, Drouin P (1985) The prevalence of retinopathy is similar in diabetes mellitus secondary to chronic pancreatitis with or without pancreatectomy and in idiopathic diabetes mellitus. Diabetes Care 8:323–328
17. Creutzfeldt W, Fehr H, Schmidt H (1970) Verlaufsbeobachtungen und diagnostische Verfahren bei der chronisch-rezidivierenden und chronischen Pankreatitis. Schweiz Med Wochenschr 100: 1180–1189

18. Creutzfeldt W, Perings E (1972) Is the infrequency of vascular complications in human secondary diabetes related to nutritional factors? Acta Diabetol Lat 9, Suppl. 1:432–445
19. Ebbehøj N, Borly L, Bülow J, Rasmussen SG, Madsen P (1990) Evaluation of pancreatic tissue fluid pressure and pain in chronic pancreatitis. A longitudinal study. Scand J Gastroenterol 25:462–466
20. Ebbehøj N, Borly L, Madsen P, Matzen P (1990) Comparison of regional pancreatic tissue fluid pressure and endoscopic retrograde pancreatographic morphology in chronic pancreatitis. Scand J Gastroenterol 25:756–760
21. Frey CF, Child III CG, Fry W (1976) Pancreatectomy for chronic pancreatitis. Ann Surg 184: 403–414
22. García-Pugés AM, Navarro S, Ros E, Elena M, Ballesta A, Aused R, Vilar-Bonet J (1986) Reversibility of exocrine pancreatic failure in chronic pancreatitis. Gastroenterology 91:17–24
23. Gastard J, Joubaud F, Farbos T, Loussouarn J, Marion J, Pannier M, Renaudet F, Valdazo R, Gosselin M (1973) Etiology and course of primary chronic pancreatitis in Western France. Digestion 9:416–428
24. Girdwood AH, Marks IN, Bornman PC, Kottler RE, Cohen M (1981) Does progressive pancreatic insufficiency limit pain in calcific pancreatitis with duct stricture or continued alcohol insult? J Clin Gastroenterol 3:241–245
25. Goebell H (1986) Beginn und Entwicklung der chronischen Pankreatitis. Internist 27:172–174
26. Gullo L, Costa PL, Labò G (1977) Chronic pancreatitis in Italy. Aetiological, clinical and histological observations based on 253 cases. Rendic Gastroenterol 9:97–104
27. Gullo L, Parenti M, Monti L, Pezzilli R, Barbara L (1990) Diabetic retinopathy in chronic pancreatitis. Gastroenterology 98:1577–1581
28. Holmberg JT, Isaksson G, Ihse I (1985) Long term results of pancreticojejunostomy in chronic pancreatitis. Surg Gynecol Obstet 160:339–346
29. Jensen AR, Matzen P, Malchow-Møller A, Christoffersen I, The Copenhagen Pancreatitis Study Group (1984) Pattern of pain, duct morphology, and pancreatic function in chronic pancreatitis. A comparative study. Scand J Gastroenterol 19:334–338
30. Joffe BI, Novis B, Seftel HC, Krut L, Bank S (1971) Ischaemic heart-disease and pancreatic diabetes. Lancet 2:269
31. Kondo T, Hayakawa T, Noda A, Ito K, Yamazaki Y, Iinuma Y, Okumura N, Sakakibara A, Mizuno R, Naruse S (1981) Follow-up study of chronic pancreatitis. Gastroenterol Jpn 16:46–53
32. Lankisch PG, Löhr-Happe A, Otto J, Creutzfeldt W (1993) Natural course in chronic pancreatitis. Pain, exocrine and endocrine pancreatic insufficiency and prognosis of the disease. Digestion 54: 148–155
33. Lankisch PG, Seidensticker F, Löhr-Happe A, Otto J, Creutzfeldt W (1995) The course of pain is the same in alcohol- and nonalcohol-induced chronic pancreatitis. Pancreas 10:338–341
34. Layer P, Yamamoto H, Kalthoff L, Clain JE, Bakken LJ, DiMagno EP (1994) The different courses of early- and late-onset idiopathic and alcoholic chronic pancreatitis. Gastroenterology 107: 1481–1487
35. Leger L, Lenriot JP, Lemaigre G (1974) Five to twenty year followup after surgery for chronic pancreatitis in 148 patients. Ann Surg 180:185–191
36. Levitt NS, Adams G, Salmon J, Marks INS, Musson G, Swanepoel C, Levy M, Byrne MJ (1995) The prevalence and severity of microvascular complications in pancreatic diabetes and IDDM. Diabetes Care 18:971–974
37. Linde J, Nilsson LH, Bárány FR (1977) Diabetes and hypoglycemia in chronic pancreatitis. Scand J Gastroenterol 12:369–373
38. Lowenfels AB, Maisonneuve P, Cavallini G, Ammann RW, Lankisch PG, Andersen JR, DiMagno EP, Andrén-Sandberg Å, Domellöf L, International Pancreatitis Study Group (1994) Prognosis of chronic pancreatitis: an international multicenter study. Am J Gastroenterol 89:1467–1471
39. Löhr A (1990) Der natürliche Verlauf der chronischen Pankreatitis. Die Entwicklung der Leitsymptome Schmerzen, exokrine und endokrine Pankreasinsuffizienz und die Prognose der Erkrankung. Med Diss Göttingen
40. Malfertheiner P, Büchler M, Stanescu A, Ditschuneit H (1987) Pancreatic morphology and function in relationship to pain in chronic pancreatitis. Int J Pancreatol 2:59–66
41. Miyake H, Harada H, Kunichika K, Ochi K, Kimura I (1987) Clinical course and prognosis of chronic pancreatitis. Pancreas 2:378–385

42. Sarles H, Sahel J (1976) Die chronische Pankreatitis. In: Forell M (ed) Handbuch der Inneren Medizin, Vol. 3/6, Pankreas, 5th edn. Springer, Berlin–Heidelberg–New York, pp 737–844
43. Sevel D, Bristow JH, Bank S, Marks I, Jackson P (1971) Diabetic retinopathy in chronic pancreatitis. Arch Ophthalmol 86:245–250
44. Taylor RH, Bagley FH, Braasch JW, Warren KW (1981) Ductal drainage or resection for chronic pancreatitis. Am J Surg 141:28–33
45. Thorsgaard Pedersen N, Andersen BN, Pedersen G, Worning H (1982) Chronic pancreatitis in Copenhagen. A retrospective study of 64 consecutive patients. Scand J Gastroenterol 17:925–931
46. Tiengo A, Segato T, Briani G, Setti A, del Prato S, Devidé A, Padovan D, Virgili F, Crepaldi G (1983) The presence of retinopathy in patients with secondary diabetes following pancreatectomy or chronic pancreatitis. Diabetes Care 6:570–574
47. Toskes PP, Dawson W, Curington C, Levy NS, Fitzgerald C (1979) Non-diabetic retinal abnormalities in chronic pancreatitis. N Engl J Med 300:942–946
48. Trapnell JE (1979) Chronic relapsing pancreatitis: a review of 64 cases. Br J Surg 66:471–475
49. Verdonk CA, Palumbo PJ, Gharib H, Bartholomew LG (1975) Diabetic microangiopathy in patients with pancreatic diabetes mellitus. Diabetologia 11:395–400
50. Warshaw AL, Popp JW Jr, Schapiro RH (1980) Long-term patency, pancreatic function, and pain relief after lateral pancreaticojejunostomy for chronic pancreatitis. Gastroenterology 79:289–293
51. White TT, Keith RG (1973) Long term follow-up study of fifty patients with pancreaticojejunostomy. Surg Gynecol Obstet 136:353–358
52. Worning H (1984) Chronic pancreatitis: pathogenesis, natural history and conservative treatment. Clin Gastroenterol 13:871–894
53. Ziegler O, Candiloros H, Guerci B, Got I, Crea T, Drouin P (1994) Lower-extremity arterial disease in diabetes mellitus due to chronic pancreatitis. Diabete Metab 20:540–545

21 Addendum: Hereditary Pancreatic Diseases

Hereditary diseases of the pancreas may be divided in those presenting with exocrine pancreatic insufficiency and those with acute or chronic pancreatitis as the first manifestation. In some inherited diseases, a combination of both manifestations is possible (Table 21.1).

21.1
Hereditary Pancreatic Diseases Associated With Exocrine Pancreatic Insufficiency

21.1.1
Cystic Fibrosis

21.1.1.1
General

Cystic fibrosis, inherited in an autosomal-recessive process, is by far the most common inherited disease of the exocrine pancreas. It involves all exocrine glands and has been diagnosed in all ethnic groups. Its incidence varies greatly from 1 in 2000 live births in the Caucasian population to 1 in 17000 in the Black population of the United States. The pathogenetic mechanisms are not fully understood at present [31]. It is believed that the underlying pathogenetic mechanism involves a defect in the regulation of apical membrane-chloride channels of epithelial cells, resulting in highly viscous

Table 21.1. Hereditary pancreatic diseases

- Associated with exocrine pancreatic insufficiency
  Cystic fibrosis
  Shwachman syndrome
  Johanson-Blizzard syndrome
  Sideroblastic anemia
  Isolated enzyme defects
- Associated with pancreatitis
  Cystic fibrosis
  Hereditary pancreatitis
  Antitrypsin deficiency
  Inborn errors of metabolism

secretions [39]. A protein named *cystic fibrosis transmembrane conductance regulator* either acts as a chloride channel itself or is involved in its regulation, since its expression in epithelial cells of cystic fibrosis patients is able to overcome the specific Cl^--transport defect [47]. In the corresponding gene, a deletion of 3 base pairs that results in the loss of a phenylalanine residue at amino acid position 508, has been shown to be responsible for the disease in approximately 70% of the patients [24].

There are a number of extensive reviews on cystic fibrosis. Therefore, within the limits of this chapter, only features of hereditary diseases relevant to an association with acute or chronic pancreatitis, or exocrine pancreatic insufficiency, are discussed.

21.1.1.2
Pathology

Upon general examination, the pancreas may be normal, but usually appears small with evidence of fibrosis, fatty change, and cysts. Histologically, the pancreatic lesion is initiated by the obstruction of small ducts with eosinophilic concretions. Newborns may show only minimal and nonspecific changes, although the characteristic lesions of cystic fibrosis may be present even then with luminal concretions, distension of ducts and acini, mild inflammation and fibrosis, and cysts lined by a single layer of epithelial cells. Older children with established disease usually demonstrate these lesions. The cysts may occasionally be as large as 2–3 mm in diameter. Calcification is seen, but the main pancreatic ducts and islet cells are usually normal.

Late in the course of the disease, these characteristic lesions may not be visible. Glands may be replaced by fat with interspersed fibrous strands and residual islets. At this stage, it may be very difficult to differentiate histologically between cystic fibrosis and chronic pancreatitis [57].

21.1.1.3
Clinical Presentation

Exocrine pancreatic insufficiency occurs in approximately 85% of patients with cystic fibrosis [51]. Pancreatic secretions are scant, viscous, and deficient in both enzymes and bicarbonate [16]. For these patients, malabsorption, azotorrhea, and steatorrhea are the most frequent gastrointestinal manifestations. The remaining 15%–20% of patients with cystic fibrosis do not manifest clinical exocrine pancreatic insufficiency.

Shwachman et al. [54] reported acute pancreatitis in 0.5% of all cystic fibrosis patients and about 2%–3% of those without steatorrhea. Several other reports have also shown that acute pancreatitis may be a complication of cystic fibrosis and even be the initial presentation of the disease in the adult [5, 15, 37].

Since cystic fibrosis patients without clinical exocrine pancreatic insufficiency may have elevated serum levels of pancreatic isoamylase in the absence of gastrointestinal symptoms [61, 64], clinical correlation is essential.

21.1.1.4
Diagnosis

The diagnosis of pancreatic involvement in cystic fibrosis is the same in regard to estimation of exocrine pancreatic insufficiency (see Sect. 17.2.2).

Endoscopic retrograde cholangiopancreatography (ERCP) examination should be performed only if absolutely necessary. It is the authors' and others' experience [54] that due to the high viscosity of pancreatic secretion, drainage of contrast medium is delayed, which may lead to post-ERCP pancreatitis. Interestingly, even the exocrine pancreatic function test, such as the secretin-pancreozymin test (SPT), has led to abdominal pain and an increase in serum amylase [54].

21.1.1.5
Treatment

Management of exocrine pancreatic insufficiency with pancreatic enzymes is the same as in chronic pancreatitis. However, several reports have been published on the occurrence of large-bowel strictures in patients with cystic fibrosis caused by high-strength pancreatic enzyme supplements [8, 43, 55, 56]. The use of high-strength pancreatin preparations in conjunction with a high protease intake probably causes thickening of the wall of the colon [35]. Ultrasound examination detects characteristic ileocecal wall lesions which may lead to wall thickness, which is correlated but not restricted to high-strength enzyme preparations [32].

21.1.2
Shwachman Syndrome

21.1.2.1
General

Shwachman syndrome is the second most common cause of exocrine pancreatic insufficiency in childhood. It is characterized by exocrine pancreatic insufficiency, cyclic neutropenia, metaphyseal dysostosis, and growth retardation. Sweat electrolytes are normal. This syndrome has been expanded greatly in the last decades to include abnormalities in most organ systems (Table 21.2). Its estimated incidence is 1 in 20 000 live births. Both sexes are equally affected. The suggested mode of inheritance is autosomal-recessive. The pathogenetic mechanism is unknown.

21.1.2.2
Pathology

At an early stage, the pancreas may be nearly normal [6]. Later on, the gland varies in size from normal to small, and usually has a fatty degeneration. The main pancreatic

Table 21.2. Clinical features of Shwachman syndrome [33]

Major features
- Pancreatic insufficiency
- Cyclic selective bone marrow depression
- Metaphyseal dysostosis
- Short stature
- Normal sweat electrolytes

Associated features
- Subtle disturbances in lung function
- Hepatomegaly
- Dental abnormalities
- Renal dysfunction
- Delayed puberty
- Ichthyosis

Infrequent features
- Cardiac lesions
- Testicular fibrosis
- Diabetes mellitus
- Hirschsprung's disease

ducts are normal. Histologically, a predominance of fatty cells is seen, with scattered normal islets and minimal remaining acinar tissue [57].

21.1.2.3
Clinical Presentation

Children almost always become ill with symptoms of malabsorption at 4–6 months of age [4, 50, 52]. Other problems are generally poor health and growth retardation. Infections are very frequent, occasionally leading to death [57].

During the course of the disease, malabsorption may disappear. We saw a patient with Shwachman syndrome, who had severe exocrine pancreatic insufficiency documented by SPT, and significant steatorrhea at the age of 14 years. Eighteen years later, steatorrhea had disappeared, and she had overweight [28]. The increased weight was probably due to a nonpancreatic lipolytic activity [1–3].

Endocrine pancreatic insufficiency is rare in Shwachman syndrome [53, 57]; histologically, the islets of Langerhans are almost normal [18].

The hematologic picture is variable and dominated by neutropenia in 95%, thrombocytopenia in 70%, and anemia in 50% of the patients [4]. The most common bone lesion, metaphyseal dysostosis, has been reported in 10%–15% of the patients. The skeletal parts affected are the femur, tibia, and ribs. The femoral neck is most often affected, and the lesion is generally symmetric and progressive and may result in disturbance of gait and coxa vara deformity [6, 14, 33, 38, 50]. Besides exocrine pancreatic insufficiency, cyclic selective bone marrow depression, metaphyseal dysostosis, short stature, and a variety of other features have been described (Table 21.2)

21.1.2.4
Diagnosis

The diagnosis of exocrine pancreatic insufficiency in Shwachman syndrome is the same as for other causes of this symptom (see Sect. 17.2.2).

In the later course of the disease, complete fatty degeneration of the pancreas is seen on computed tomography [13, 17, 27].

21.1.2.5
Treatment

Treatment is symptomatic. Pancreatic enzyme replacement is aimed at decreasing steatorrhea and improving the child's nutrition. Growth is rarely improved. Since spontaneous or nonpancreatic lipolytic activity-induced improvement is possible [19, 28], the need for enzyme replacement should be checked periodically during the course of the disease.

21.1.3
Johanson-Blizzard Syndrome

21.1.3.1
General

The Johanson-Blizzard syndrome was first described in 1971; since then 35 cases have been published. Still, the syndrome is not well defined. Main features are congenital aplasia of the alae nasi, deafness, hypothyroidism, dwarfism, microcephaly, absence of permanent teeth, and malabsorption. More recently, hypopituitarism and growth hormone insufficiency have been added.

An association with cystic fibrosis in the same family has been described.

The pathogenetic mechanism and the genetic abnormality are unknown [33].

21.1.3.2
Pathology

At autopsy the pancreas may be absent or replaced by fat.

21.1.3.3
Clinical Presentation

Of all above described features of the syndrome, exocrine pancreatic insufficiency is the most consistent (for diagnosis see Sect. 17.2.2). Patients with Johanson-Blizzard syndrome show preservation of ductular output of fluid and electrolytes, as in patients with Shwachman syndrome, but differing from those with cystic fibrosis, who have a primary ductular defect. They have been reported to have a decreased acinar secretion of trypsin, colipase, and total lipase, and low serum immunoreactive trypsin levels, consistent with a primary acinar cell defect [20].

21.1.3.4
Treatment

Early treatment of malabsorption (see Sect. 19.2.3) is critical for prevention of growth retardation and failure to thrive. The most common causes of death in reported cases have been related to malabsorption and its consequences [60].

21.1.4
Sideroblastic Anemia

Pearson et al. [44] described four patients with sideroblastic anemia and generalized pancreatic insufficiency. Two had splenic atrophy. This is another syndrome suggesting an interaction between the bone marrow and the exocrine pancreas. Although a few more patients with this syndrome have been described [33], it seems too early for a final clinical description of this syndrome.

21.1.5
Isolated Defects

Isolated enzyme defects as well as enterokinase deficiency have been reported (Table 21.3), but the frequency of such occurrences is rare. All patients described have malabsorption as a clinical manifestation requiring pancreatic enzyme replacement therapy [33, 57].

Table 21.3. Isolated pancreatic enzyme deficiency

- Lipase
- Lipase-colipase
- Colipase
- Amylase
- Trypsinogen
- Enterokinase

21.2
Hereditary Diseases of the Exocrine Pancreas Associated With Pancreatitis

21.2.1
Hereditary Pancreatitis

21.2.1.1.
Definition

Hereditary pancreatitis is defined as recurrent pancreatitis which occurs in blood-related persons over two and more generations. It is inherited as an autosomal-dominant trait with apparently complete penetrance but variable expressivity [36].

Since the first report by Comfort and Steinberg [10] in 1952, more than 400 patients and 95 kindreds have been described in over 20 countries around the world [36].

The exact incidence is unknown, but in three separate reports, an incidence of 0.6, 0.9, and 1.5, respectively, was reported [11, 34, 59].

21.2.1.2
Pathology

Recently, two forms of hereditary pancreatitis have been described, one classified as calcific and one as protein lithiasis [49]. The consequence of these findings needs clarification.

Furthermore, a linkage between the hereditary pancreatitis phenotype and chromosome 7q has been established [30, 62].

21.2.1.3
Clinical Presentation

Symptoms may start at any age, but most cases first present in childhood. With this exception, signs and symptoms as well as complications of hereditary pancreatitis do not differ from that of nonhereditary chronic pancreatitis. However, a comparison of patients having hereditary pancreatitis with young patients having idiopathic chronic pancreatitis showed that the hereditary form seems to be a more severe variant of chronic pancreatitis, inasmuch as it is associated with more frequent complications and need for surgical intervention [26, 45].

21.2.1.4
Diagnosis

The diagnosis of hereditary pancreatitis does not differ from that of chronic pancreatitis (see Chap. 17).

It has been earlier believed that aminoaciduria (cystine, arginine, and lysine) is specific for hereditary pancreatitis, but this has not been confirmed [46].

21.2.1.5
Treatment

Management of acute attacks and of the chronic state of hereditary pancreatitis does not differ from that of acute pancreatitis due to other causes and of chronic pancreatitis.

21.2.1.6
Prognosis

Earlier, a serious complication, the development of intraabdominal tumors, has been described. Kattwinkel et al. [23] reported 8 (15%) cases of pancreatic carcinoma and 5 (9%) cases with other abdominal tumors among 54 deceased patients with definite or suspected hereditary pancreatitis in 21 kindreds.

21.2.2
Antitrypsin Deficiency

α_1-antitrypsin is a serum protease inhibitor inherited through 2 codominant alleles.
    Several studies suggested that a1-deficiency renders the pancreas more vulnerable to etiological agents such as alcohol [12, 41, 42], but a large-scale study failed to confirm this hypothesis [29].

21.2.3
Inborn Errors of Metabolism

Acute and chronic pancreatitis have been reported in some patients with inborn errors of metabolism, such as maple-syrup urine disease, isovaleric and methylmalonic acidemia [21], 3-hydroxy-3-methylglutaric aciduria [63], homocystinuria [9], respiratory-chain defects [22, 48], glycogen storage disease type I [25], carnitine palmitoyl-transferase-II deficiency [40, 58], and propionic acidemia [7].

References

1. Abrams CK, Hamosh M, Dutta SK, Hubbard VS, Hamosh P (1987) Role of nonpancreatic lipolytic activity in exocrine pancreatic insufficiency. Gastroenterology 92:125–129
2. Abrams CK, Hamosh M, Hubbard VS, Dutta SK, Hamosh P (1984) Lingual lipase in cystic fibrosis. Quantitation of enzyme activity in the upper small intestine of patients with exocrine pancreatic insufficiency. J Clin Invest 73:374–382

3. Abrams CK, Hamosh M, Lee TC, Ansher AF, Collen MJ, Lewis JH, Benjamin SB, Hamosh P (1988) Gastric lipase: localization in the human stomach. Gastroenterology 95:1460–1464

4. Aggett PJ, Cavanagh NPC, Matthew DJ, Pincott JR, Sutcliffe J, Harries JT (1980) Shwachman's syndrome. A review of 21 cases. Arch Dis Child 55:331–347

5. Atlas AB, Orenstein SR, Orenstein DM (1992) Pancreatitis in young children with cystic fibrosis. J Pediatr 120:756–759

6. Burke V, Colebatch JH, Anderson CM, Simons MJ (1967) Association of pancreatic insufficiency and chronic neutropenia in childhood. Arch Dis Child 42:147–157

7. Burlina AB, Dionisi-Vici C, Piovan S, Saponara I, Bartuli A, Sabetta G, Zacchello F (1995) Acute pancreatitis in propionic acidaemia. J Inher Metab Dis 18:169–172

8. Campbell CA, Forrest J, Musgrove C (1994) High-strength pancreatic enzyme supplements and large-bowel stricture in cystic fibrosis. Lancet 343:109–110

9. Collins JE, Brenton DP (1990) Pancreatitis and homocystinuria. J Inher Metab Dis 13:232–233

10. Comfort MW, Steinberg AG (1952) Pedigree of a family with hereditary chronic relapsing pancreatitis. Gastroenterology 21:54–63

11. DiMagno EP, Layer P, Clain JE (1993) Chronic pancreatitis. In: Go VLW, DiMagno EP, Gardner JD, Lebenthal E, Reber HA, Scheele GA (eds) The Pancreas: Biology, Pathobiology, and Disease, 2nd edn. Raven Press, New York, pp 665–706

12. Freeman HJ, Weinstein WM, Shnitka TK, Crockford PM, Herbert FA (1976) Alpha$_1$-antitrypsin deficiency and pancreatic fibrosis. Ann Intern Med 85:73–76

13. Genieser NB, Halac ER, Greco MA, Richards HMS (1982) Shwachman-Bodian syndrome. J Comput Assist Tomogr 6:1191–1192

14. Giedion A, Prader A, Hadorn B, Shmerling DH, Auricchio S (1968) Metaphysäre Dysostose und angeborene Pankreasinsuffizienz. Fortschr Röntgenstr 108:51–57

15. Gross V, Schoelmerich J, Denzel K, Gerok W (1989) Relapsing pancreatitis as initial manifestation of cystic fibrosis in a young man without pulmonary disease. Int J Pancreatol 4:221–228

16. Hadorn B, Johansen PG, Anderson CM (1968) Pancreozymin secretin test of exocrine pancreatic function in cystic fibrosis and the significance of the result for the pathogenesis of the disease. Can Med Assoc J 98:377–385

17. Henze E, Hitzemann T (1990) Die Kriterien eines Shwachman-Diamond-Syndroms bei zwei Brüdern. Fortschr Röntgenstr 152:100–102

18. Higashi O, Hayashi T, Ohara K, Honda Y, Konno T, Sato Y, Yoshida T (1967) Pancreatic insufficiency with bone marrow dysfunction (Shwachman-Diamond-Oski-Khaw's syndrome). Report of a case. Tohoku J Exp Med 92:1–12

19. Hill RE, Durie PR, Gaskin KJ, Davidson GP, Forstner GG (1982) Steatorrhea and pancreatic insufficiency in Shwachman syndrome. Gastroenterology 83:22–27

20. Jones NL, Hofley PM, Durie PR (1994) Pathophysiology of the pancreatic defect in Johanson-Blizzard syndrome: a disorder of acinar development. J Pediatr 125:406–408

21. Kahler SG, Sherwood WG, Woolf D, Lawless ST, Zaritsky A, Bonham J, Taylor CJ, Clarke JTR, Durie P, Leonard JV (1994) Pancreatitis in patients with organic acidemias. J Pediatr 124:239–243

22. Kato S, Miyabayashi S, Ohi R, Nakagawa H, Abe J, Yamamoto K, Watanabe S, Tada K (1990) Chronic pancreatitis in muscular cytochrome c oxidase deficiency. J Pediatr Gastroenterol Nutr 11:549–552

23. Kattwinkel J, Lapey A, di Sant'Agnese PA, Edwards WA (1973) Hereditary pancreatitis: three new kindreds and a critical review of the literature. Pediatrics 51:55–69

24. Kerem B-S, Rommens JM, Buchanan JA, Markiewicz D, Cox TK, Chakravarti A, Buchwald M, Tsui L-C (1989) Identification of the cystic fibrosis gene: genetic analysis. Science 245:1073–1080

25. Kikuchi M, Hasegawa K, Handa I, Watabe M, Narisawa K, Tada K (1991) Chronic pancreatitis in a child with glycogen storage disease type 1. Eur J Pediatr 150:852–853

26. Konzen KM, Perrault J, Moir C, Zinsmeister AR (1993) Long-term follow-up of young patients with chronic hereditary or idiopathic pancreatitis. Mayo Clin Proc 68:449–453

27. Kurdziel JC, Dondelinger R (1984) Fatty infiltration of the pancreas in Shwachman's syndrome: computed tomography demonstration. Eur J Radiol 4:202–204

28. Lankisch PG (1991) Shwachman-Syndrom. Exokrine Pankreasinsuffizienz, Minderwuchs, periphere Dysostosen, Neutropenie. Dtsch Med Wochenschr 116:812–815

29. Lankisch PG, Koop H, Winckler K, Kaboth U (1978) α_1-Antitrypsin in pancreatic diseases. Digestion 18:138–140

30. Le Bodic L, Bignon J-D, Raguénès O, Mercier B, Georgelin T, Schnee M, Soulard F, Gagne K, Bonneville F, Muller J-Y, Bachner L, Férec C (1996) The hereditary pancreatitis gene maps to long arm of chromosome 7. Hum Molec Genet 5:549–554

31. Lebenthal E, Lerner A, Rolston DDK (1993) The pancreas in cystic fibrosis. In: Go VLW, DiMagno EP, Gardner JD, Lebenthal E, Reber HA, Scheele GA (eds) The Pancreas: Biology, Pathobiology, and Disease, 2nd edn. Raven Press, New York, pp 1041–1081

32. Lembcke B, Pohl M, Krackhardt B, Posselt HG (1995) A unique pattern of ileocaecal gut wall morphology related to pancreatic enzyme replacement therapy: an ultrasonography study in 200 cystic fibrosis patients. Gastroenterology 108:A369 (abstr)

33. Lerner A, Lebenthal E (1993) Hereditary diseases of the pancreas. In: Go VLW, DiMagno EP, Gardner JD, Lebenthal E, Reber HA, Scheele GA (eds) The Pancreas: Biology, Pathobiology, and Disease, 2nd edn. Raven Press, New York, pp 1083–1094

34. Löhr A (1990) Der natürliche Verlauf der chronischen Pankreatitis. Die Entwicklung der Leitsymptome Schmerzen, exokrine und endokrine Pankreasinsuffizienz und die Prognose der Erkrankung. Med Diss Göttingen

35. Mac Sweeney EJ, Oades PJ, Buchdahl R, Rosenthal M, Bush A (1995) Relation of thickening of colon wall to pancreatic-enzyme treatment in cystic fibrosis. Lancet 345:752–756

36. Madrazo-de la Garza JA, Hill ID, Lebenthal E (1993) Hereditary pancreatitis. In: Go VLW, DiMagno EP, Gardner JD, Lebenthal E, Reber HA, Scheele GA (eds) The Pancreas: Biology, Pathobiology, and Disease, 2nd edn. Raven Press, New York, pp 1095–1101

37. Masaryk TJ, Achkar E (1983) Pancreatitis as initial presentation of cystic fibrosis in young adults. A report of two cases. Dig Dis Sci 28:874–878

38. McLennan TW, Steinbach HL (1974) Shwachman's syndrome: the broad spectrum of bony abnormalities. Radiology 112:167–173

39. McPherson MA, Dormer RL (1991) Molecular and cellular biology of cystic fibrosis. Molec Aspects Med 12:1–81

40. Michels VV, Beaudet AL (1980) Hemorrhagic pancreatitis in a patient with glycogen storage disease type I. Clin Genet 17:220–222

41. Mihas AA, Hirschowitz BI (1976) Alpha$_1$-antitrypsin and chronic pancreatitis. Lancet 2:1032–1033

42. Novis BH, Young GO, Bank S, Marks IN (1975) Chronic pancreatitis and α_1-antitrypsin. Lancet 2:748–749

43. Oades PJ, Bush A, Ong PS, Brereton RJ (1994) High-strength pancreatic enzyme supplements and large-bowel stricture in cystic fibrosis. Lancet 343:109

44. Pearson HA, Lebel JS, Kocoshis SA, Naiman JL, Windmiller J, Lammi AT, Hoffman R, Marsh JC (1979) A new syndrome of refractory sideroblastic anemia with vacuolization of marrow precursors and exocrine pancreatic dysfunction. J Pediatr 95:976–984

45. Perrault J (1994) Hereditary pancreatitis. Gastroenterol Clin North Am 23:743–752

46. Riccardi VM, Shih VE, Holmes LB, Nardi GL (1975) Hereditary pancreatitis. Nonspecificity of aminoaciduria and diagnosis of occult disease. Arch Intern Med 135:822–825

47. Rich DP, Anderson MP, Gregory RJ, Cheng SH, Paul S, Jefferson DM, McCann JD, Klinger KW, Smith AE, Welsh MJ (1990) Expression of cystic fibrosis transmembrane conductance regulator corrects defective chloride channel regulation in cystic fibrosis airway epithelial cells. Nature 347:358–363

48. Rötig A, Cormier V, Blanche S, Bonnefont J-P, Ledeist F, Romero N, Schmitz J, Rustin P, Fischer A, Saudubray J-M, Munnich A (1990) Pearson's marrow-pancreas syndrome. A multisystem mitochondrial disorder in infancy. J Clin Invest 86:1601–1608

49. Sarles H, Camarena J, Bernard JP, Sahel J, Laugier R (1996) Two forms of hereditary chronic pancreatitis. Pancreas 12:138–141

50. Shmerling DH, Prader A, Hitzig WH, Giedion A, Hadorn B, Kühni M (1969) The syndrome of exocrine pancreatic insufficiency, neutropenia, metaphyseal dysostosis and dwarfism. Helv Paediatr Acta 24:547–575

51. Shwachman H (1975) Gastrointestinal manifestations of cystic fibrosis. Pediatr Clin North Am 22:787–805

52. Shwachman H, Diamond LK, Oski FA, Khaw K-T (1964) The syndrome of pancreatic insufficiency and bone marrow dysfunction. J Pediatr 65:645–663

53. Shwachman H, Holsclaw D (1972) Some clinical observations on the Shwachman syndrome (pancreatic insufficiency and bone marrow hypoplasia). Birth Defects: Original Article Series 8, No. 3: 46–49
54. Shwachman H, Lebenthal E, Khaw K-T (1975) Recurrent acute pancreatitis in patients with cystic fibrosis with normal pancreatic enzymes. Pediatrics 55:86–95
55. Smyth RL, Ashby D, O'Hea U, Burrows E, Lewis P, van Velzen D, Dodge JA (1995) Fibrosing colonopathy in cystic fibrosis: results of a case-control study. Lancet 346:1247–1251
56. Smyth RL, van Velzen D, Smyth AR, Lloyd DA, Heaf DP (1994) Strictures of ascending colon in cystic fibrosis and high-strength pancreatic enzymes. Lancet 343:85–86
57. Stafford RJ, Grand RJ (1982) Hereditary disease of the exocrine pancreas. Clin Gastroenterol 11: 141–170
58. Tein I, Christodoulou J, Donner E, McInnes RR (1994) Carnitine palmitoyltransferase II deficiency: a new cause of recurrent pancreatitis. J Pediatr 124:938–940
59. The Copenhagen Pancreatitis Study Group (1981) Copenhagen Pancreatitis Study. An interim report from a prospective epidemiological multicentre study. Scand J Gastroenterol 16:305–312
60. Trellis DR, Clouse RE (1991) Johanson-Blizzard syndrome. Progression of pancreatic involvement in adulthood. Dig Dis Sci 36:365–369
61. Van Hubbard S, Wolf RO (1978) Pancreatitis in children. J Pediatr 92:685–686
62. Whitcomb DC, Preston RA, Aston CE, Sossenheimer MJ, Barua PS, Zhang Y, Wong-Chong A, White GJ, Wood PG, Gates LK Jr, Ulrich C, Martin SP, Post C, Ehrlich GD (1996) A gene for hereditary pancreatitis maps to chromosome 7q35. Gastroenterology 110:1975–1980
63. Wilson WG, Cass MB, Søvik O, Gibson KM, Sweetman L (1984) A child with acute pancreatitis and recurrent hypoglycemia due to 3-hydroxy-3-methylglutaryl-CoA lyase deficiency. Eur J Pediatr 142:289–291
64. Wolf RO, Taussig LM, Ross ME, Wood RE (1976) Quantitative evaluation of serum pancreatic isoamylases in cystic fibrosis. J Lab Clin Med 87:164–168

Subject Index

MIX
Papier aus verantwortungsvollen Quellen
Paper from responsible sources
FSC® C105338

If you have any concerns about our products,
you can contact us on
ProductSafety@springernature.com

In case Publisher is established outside the EU,
the EU authorized representative is:
Springer Nature Customer Service Center GmbH
Europaplatz 3, 69115 Heidelberg, Germany

Printed by Libri Plureos GmbH
in Hamburg, Germany